Sexual Medicine

AF665687

Karthik Gunasekaran • Shah Dupesh Khan
Editors

Sexual Medicine

Principles and Practice

Springer

Editors
Karthik Gunasekaran
The Metromale Clinic and Fertility Center
Chennai
India

Shah Dupesh Khan
The Metromale Clinic and Fertility Center
Chennai
India

ISBN 978-981-13-4587-6 ISBN 978-981-13-1226-7 (eBook)
https://doi.org/10.1007/978-981-13-1226-7

© Springer Nature Singapore Pte Ltd. 2019
Softcover re-print of the Hardcover 1st edition 2019
This work is subject to copyright. All rights are reserved by the Publisher, whether the whole or part of the material is concerned, specifically the rights of translation, reprinting, reuse of illustrations, recitation, broadcasting, reproduction on microfilms or in any other physical way, and transmission or information storage and retrieval, electronic adaptation, computer software, or by similar or dissimilar methodology now known or hereafter developed.
The use of general descriptive names, registered names, trademarks, service marks, etc. in this publication does not imply, even in the absence of a specific statement, that such names are exempt from the relevant protective laws and regulations and therefore free for general use.
The publisher, the authors, and the editors are safe to assume that the advice and information in this book are believed to be true and accurate at the date of publication. Neither the publisher nor the authors or the editors give a warranty, express or implied, with respect to the material contained herein or for any errors or omissions that may have been made. The publisher remains neutral with regard to jurisdictional claims in published maps and institutional affiliations.

This Springer imprint is published by the registered company Springer Nature Singapore Pte Ltd.
The registered company address is: 152 Beach Road, #21-01/04 Gateway East, Singapore 189721, Singapore

Foreword

Reproduction is the law of life. We all live to reproduce and continue to live through our offspring. Species that are able to reproduce successfully grow and thrive. Others decline and disappear.

Sex is the driving force that keeps reproduction going. Sex seems to be the only way for the large majority of people to reproduce. The advent of assisted reproduction and the newer reproductive technologies would hardly make any change in the reproductive lives of most of the people. They may have to and will continue to reproduce in the old fashion way—sexual intercourse-related reproduction.

Sexual problems are rampant and are almost universal. They occur with equal frequencies in both men and women. As men are expected to perform, it is often felt that sexual problems are more prevalent in men. However, sexual problems in women occur with equal frequency but are often untold and often go unnoticed. Bedroom tragedies are often worse than boardroom tragedies and often lead to problems in both the fronts.

Sexual medicine is an uncharted territory. There are very few qualified, trained, or self-trained practitioners of sexual medicine. The field is often dominated by sexual medicine charlatans and mavericks who continue to sell wrong ideas to people, such as "masturbation is harmful" and many other sexual myths.

Medical education in India and in many other countries is bereft of formal or informal training in sexual medicine at all levels. This has not helped the situation improve any further. Neither the gynecologist who is often the primary physician for the woman, nor the urologist who may be the primary physician for men, nor the general practitioner or the family physician enquires about the sexual health of their clients.

Men and women are sexual beings with varying sexual needs from puberty to, often, the grave. This need varies in different phases of life in both sexes. A proper history taking in all adolescents, adults, and elderly patients requires proper knowledge.

This book edited by two eminent andrologists with contributions from experts in sexual medicine from India and abroad attempts to fulfill the lacunae in sexual medicine education. The chapters cover a wide range of topics written by practitioners of sexual medicine, intended for general practitioners and early career gynecologists, urologists, andrologists, and sexual medicine specialists. The chapters include physiology of sexual response, importance of history taking, and sexual dysfunction in men and women and in the young and not so young.

The book, however, does not address sex during pregnancy, sex in the postpartum period, and sex in special situations. I am sure the next edition of the book will address these issues. This concise book I hope would find a place in the library of all practitioners of gynecology, urology, andrology, and family medicine.

Chennai, India Pandiyan Natarajan

Contents

About the Editors

Karthik Gunasekaran, MS, FRCS (Glasgow), FECSM is an andrologist, embryologist, and sexual medicine specialist. Dr. Karthik graduated from Madras Medical College and completed his master's in surgery there. During this time, he was awarded the Prof. Venugopal gold medal in urology. He completed his fellowship in pelvic surgery at the Cleveland Clinic Foundation, USA. His andrology and embryology training were from Chettinad University, Chennai. He completed the ESSM course in Hungary and secured the FECSM in 2014, prior to obtaining his FRCS from the Royal College of Physicians and Surgeons of Glasgow. He has been serving as Lead Andrologist and Reproductive Microsurgeon at Metromale Clinic and Fertility Center since 2013.

Shah Dupesh Khan, MBBS, DCE, FASM, (PhD) is the Lead Consultant for Andrology and Sexual Medicine at the Metromale Clinic and Fertility Center. He graduated from Chengalpattu Government Medical College and finished his post-graduation in embryology, which he passed with honors. He then pursued his fellowship in andrology and sexual medicine at the Department of Reproductive Medicine, Chettinad Health City, completing it with double honors. He also received the Rajah Muthiah award for his academic achievements. He has filed for a patent on human sperm lyophilization and was shortlisted for the 2014 Medical Healthcare Innovation award in recognition of his contributions. Dr. Shah has presented four prize-winning papers at the ISAR (Indian Society of Assisted Reproduction) and Chettinad International Fertility colloquiums. He has eight publications and one textbook on Male Infertility to his credit and is currently investigating stem cells and cryobiology.

The Human Sexual Response

1

Shah Dupesh Khan and Karthik Gunasekaran

Introduction

Sex remains highly controversial and is a major driving force for the human brain [1]. The brain is the master seat control for all sexual behaviour. Human beings are sexual through a better part of their entire lives [1]. Sexuality of humans manifests in different ways with increasing age. Despite the controversies that surround human sex, for a majority of us, sex is a highly pleasurable process [2]. In the boarder context things, good sexual health definitely goes hand in hand with general wellness and good health [2]. But why engage in sex in the first place? Sex is definitely more wasteful compared to asexual modalities of reproduction [3]. Moreover sex and sexual reproduction are far less efficient in propagating a species as compared to asexual reproduction [3]. The exact answer however has eluded researchers for years despite excellent studies on animal sexual behaviour.

Human beings seem to engage in sex for a variety of reasons. In a study by Meston and Buss, that involved over 1500 young men and women, a total of 237 unique reasons were found that motivated participants to engage in sexual activity [4, 5]. The reasons could be broadly categorized as physical needs, emotional, attainment of a goal and lastly insecurity. Emotional reasons were love and/or commitment along with the need to express it. Physical reasons included pleasure seeking and fulfilment [4, 5]. Goals included resources, status and even revenge. Insecurity included 'guarding the mate' and fulfilling a sense of duty. Emotional reasons predominated over all other reasons for partnered sex, closely followed by physical needs [4, 5].

S. D. Khan · K. Gunasekaran, MS, FRCS (Glasgow), FECSM (✉)
The Metromale Clinic and Fertility Center,
No 1, Crescent Park Street, T-Nagar, Chennai, India

© Springer Nature Singapore Pte Ltd. 2019

K. Gunasekaran, S. D. Khan (eds.), *Sexual Medicine*,
https://doi.org/10.1007/978-981-13-1226-7_1

Human Sexual Behaviour and Culture

Sexual behaviour definitely plays an important role in species survival, yet it is highly influenced by an individual's society and cultural context of the individual's upbringing. Unlike other species where sexual behaviour is adaptive, higher brain functions like 'morality' constantly affect sexual behaviour [6]. Across cultures and societies in different parts of the world, human sex is not always tailored towards reproduction as compared to other animals [7]. Human sex and biological reproduction share a complex yet intricate relationship that is non-linear [6, 7]. Sexual behaviour is intensely social and is influenced by culture, biology and/or one's own fantasies and/or beliefs. Sexual behaviour also changes through the years depending on the individual's health, social interaction and choice of partners. Sex is influenced by an individual's social boundaries along the frameworks of his or her past sexual experience. A good example would be the shame felt by a woman when she is sexually abused [8]. This shame and guilt are strongly linked to the individual's sexuality and can affect the person's current and/or future sexual relationship throughout her sex life. Clearly, there are multiple routes to human sexual response and multiple cues to which human beings can sexually respond. Sex and social behaviour share a tangible link [9]. Understanding and responding to both sexual and non-sexual cues in day-to-day species interaction and watching porn and getting aroused suggest the presence of 'sexual mirror neurons' in the human brain. Although not directly proven, same regions of the brain are shown to fire while 'doing' as well as 'observing' the act [10–13]. The functionality of this neural network definitely varies among individuals and this variance also decides the individual's sexual susceptibility to sexual stimuli, for example watching pornography [12, 13].

The development of sexual response in the context of social interaction starts as early as the infant–parent relationship [14]. Male infants get erections and female infants lubricate as early as 24 h after birth. Infants are frequently found fondling their genitals and also showing curiosity in the genitals of adults and other infants [14]. With increasing age and brain development, the child learns to recognize the erotic nature of sexual interactions. Puberty and release of gonadal hormones play a cardinal role in this aspect. The complexity of sex is best viewed in terms of brain development both functionally and morphologically in terms of size with respect to human development and/or evolution [15].

Pitfalls of the Masters and Johnson's Model of Human Sexual Response

Masters and Johnson introduced the four-stage cycle of the human sexual response (HSRC) to describe the physiological sequence of changes that they observed during lab-performed sexual activities of coitus and masturbation [16]. One of the biggest pitfalls of the model was that it omitted the concept of sexual drive which was well emphasized in the much simpler two-phase model of sexual response proposed by Havelock Ellis in 1906 [17]. The concepts of sexual drive, passion and desire were all omitted in Masters and Johnson's model of sexual response. The HSRC seemed to be the trend in the twentieth century for sexologists who were more interested in operational definitions. Sex drive was highly subjective and vague and sexologists were happy to avoid any discussion on the topic. Frank Beach in 1956 argued at that time that sex drive was unproductive and had nothing to do with genuine biological need [18]. However, the recent discovery of 'desire' clearly indicated that ignoring the issue of sex drive or factors that initiate sex does not solve problems. Ignoring sex drive from the HSRC cycle removed a variable that was notoriously different within populations allowing Masters and Johnson to conveniently propose a universal model [16].

An important selection bias was made in the study, when only participants with a past history of positive coital experience and masturbation were included in the study. Any participant who could not respond to sexual stimulation and reach orgasm was excluded from the study. This itself introduced a significant bias, since the study was made with an aim to compress biological diversity by excluding such participants [16]. As early as 1953 Kinsey had reported that only about 58% of women ever reached orgasm, by masturbation at some time in their life [19]. Essential intraclass differences were also not accounted for, since only participants with a higher than average intelligence levels and socio-economic backgrounds were included in the study.

The HSRC also played an important role in contributing to understanding sexual function as a sequence of bodily functions that work in a preset and defined manner one stage after the other. This compartmentalization of sexual function and the fact that the very concept of sexual satisfaction was ruled out are among the major pitfalls of the HSRC model. Even today we do not have the right answer to subjective questions of sexual function, like how rigid is normal, how early is premature or how delayed is actually delayed. The right answers to all these questions depend on the couple's expectations and/or cultural background. Despite the strong emphasis that has been placed on individualizing treatments, the use of rigid scales and tests still dominates the field [20].

This is clear indication of the medical trend towards increased dependency on scales/technology with an aim to obtain objective information versus subjective individualized information for clinical management. The HSRC set the stage for proper clinical occupation with measuring individual parts of human sexual function rather than looking at sexuality as a whole. The vast focus of Masters and Johnson's research was narrowed down to performance of the genitals.

Current Concepts in Human Sexual Response

Sexual behaviour is a very broad term and includes a variety of parameters related to sexual function [21]. Sexual behaviour is highly cyclical in nature and can wax and wane over an individual's lifespan depending on goals, desires and circumstances [22]. The human sexual response cycle can thus be described as a cycle of repeating events and behaviours that ultimately culminate in human reproduction [6]. The human sexual response can be best viewed as a motivation/incentive-based cycle that includes different phases of physiological response and subjective experiences [21–23]. Sexual urge may not be usually felt initially but can be triggered by sexual stimuli that cause sexual excitement [24]. Some researchers also state that all arousal and desire are responses to sexual stimuli [25]. Neuroimaging studies also confirm a significant overlap of phases [26]. Studies have shown that men and women at the outset of sexual activity are not aware of desire [25]. Frequently, men and women both find it difficult to distinguish arousal from desire and report that sexual stimuli usually stimulate both simultaneously [25, 26]. This fact is well represented in the DSM 5 manual (Diagnostic and Statistical Manual of Mental Disorders), where women with sexual dysfunction receive a separate category of sexual interest arousal disorder [27].

Numerous factors, both biological and psychological, influence the cycle, and both sexual/non-sexual outcomes decide sexual motivation [28]. During a given encounter the cycle may or may not be complete and this varies both within individuals and between individuals and is influenced by the individual's age, health status, relationship and mental health [29]. Human sexual response can be better understood in the context of rewards associated with sex in general.

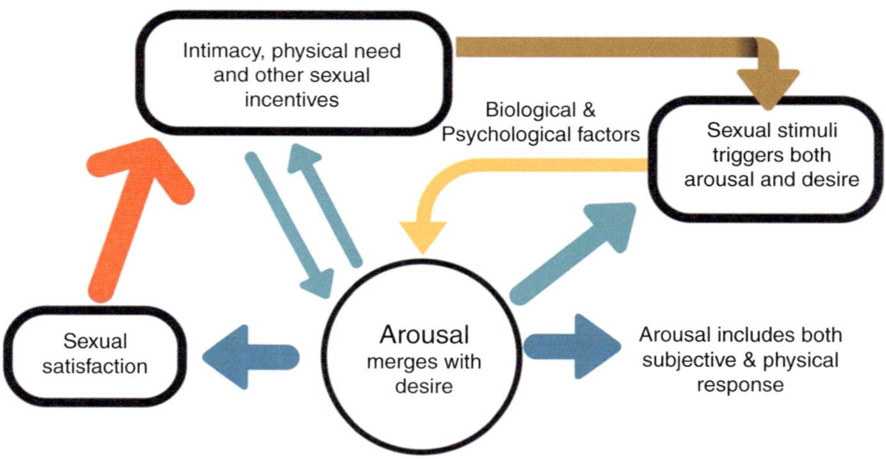

Factors that Influence Sexual Arousal

Liking sex is different from wanting sex: Sexual activity is associated with an extraordinary degree of pleasure; this is probably why it has nearly been impossible to control sexual abuse and other sex-related crimes. Higher order brain functions definitely play a role in the physiology of sex. 'Liking sex' and 'wanting sex' are probably two different behaviours, although studies have found it difficult to prove it, strictly from a behavioural perspective [30].

The first crucial step of the sexual response cycle involves the inculcating of a need or want or desire of sex that can lead to or culminate in suitable rewards. This 'wanting' is thus dependant on sensory inputs, at least partly. Dopamine release is closely associated with 'wanting' and is different compared to liking from a neuro-anatomical perspective [31]. Both primary and secondary cortices along with higher order regions of the human brain are involved in processing the complex sensory inputs. There is a dispute over how to differentiate and dissociate the two conditions. In our clinic, in over 63 female patients who presented to us over a 2-year period, we found over 40% of women wanting sex and still attempting at coitus twice/week despite a disliking stimulus, i.e. pain (unpublished data).

Sensory gateways to arousal: The olfactory inputs and its exact role in human sexual response have eluded researchers. It is yet unclear on as to how pheromones influence the human brain [32]. PET studies have found that artificial pheromones can effect a significant change in the activity of the hypothalamus, amygdala, occipitotemporal cortex and orbitofrontal cortex [6, 32]. This network of brain areas is also strongly involved in processing visual sexual stimuli. Thus, this suggests that both olfactory and visual routes of sensory stimuli can together play a cardinal role in making an individual ready and primed for sexual arousal and/or consummation. Touch is another intriguing aspect of sensory input. Pleasant touch in human species is taken care by low-threshold mechanoreceptor C-afferents [33]. For example, stimulation of the nipple and/or genital areas both in an erotic and a non-erotic context does lead to sexual arousal [33–35]. Miyagawa's study looked at unimodal auditory stimulus with erotic content, and found that erotic auditory inputs instigated sexual arousal [36].

Visual stimulus is the most robust of all cues; proof is in the overwhelming growth and profits made by the porn industry. Primate studies have found that visual cues and coloration drive specific mate selection in few monkey species [37]. Visual erotica directly taps into the brain's motivational circuits, and this is exactly why an overwhelming number of studies have adopted the visual sexual stimulation (VSS) route to assess brain activity in relation to an erotic visual stimulus [38]. These studies however can be puzzling since a majority of these studies have used different types of images/erotic material with different durations of exposure time. The brain activity recorded would be expected to be different largely due to these uncontrolled factors in different studies. Eye tracking studies on heterosexual men, when shown erotica, frequently show that the focus is on the women's genitals, face and body parts. When the VSS consisted specifically movies showing sexually explicit interactions, changes in the occipitotemporal areas of the brain were observed [39]. Subcortical areas of the brain, specifically the ventral striatum (VS) and nucleus accumbens (NAC), show activity when heterosexual men are shown series of image of single nude women, though the same brain areas are not active during watching of a movie clip where couples engage in sex [40]. This suggests that both the VS and NAC are involved in the early part of the human sexual response cycle [40]. Studies have also suggested that both the VS and NAC may be involved in 'sexual learning'. Other areas of the brain that have been implicated in sexual arousal include the amygdale, hypothalamus, anterior cingulate cortex and insular cortex [41]. Studies have also shown that these brain areas have strong anatomical connections between them. Interestingly, these areas were not found to be associated with genital responses suggesting that their fundamental role is in identifying a sexual opportunity and/or directing motivational behaviour towards achieving the activity [42].

On the other hand, the ventral and lateral occipitotemporal cortices, ventral aspect of the premotor cortex, anterior part of the middle cingulate cortex and posterior insula were involved during VSS that included video of couples interacting along with genital arousal [41, 42]. This clearly shows that different areas of the brain are involved in both interest and arousal at least from a neuroanatomical perspective. Hypothalamic activity though was recorded during both photos and videos. Interestingly, some brain areas seem to have a duality in the sexual response cycle [43]. The amygdale, for instance, responds during direct stimulation with visual erotica, but its activity definitely decreases, when direct sexual stimulation occurs [43]. This finding suggests that both sexual anticipation and sexual consummation are entirely different and are coordinated through complex neural networks.

Studies suggest that there seem to be significant differences between males and females in VSS-related brain activity. Yet, women's sexual response can be stimulated by a much wider range of stimulus compared to men and is not sex specific, especially for self-identified heterosexual women. Furthermore, the menstrual cycle and the variable hormonal milieu during the follicular and luteal phase further complicate research [44]. There is adequate consensus in the fact that sexual receptivity usually peaks during the follicular phase and VSS data also indicate that women show more interest in pictures of nude men closer to ovulation [45]. In general, there is much more noise to be filtered out in female sexual response.

Women seem to show less sensitivity and show higher non-specific responses to visual sexual stimuli. Their sexual arousal and physiological arousal also seem to be discordant and highly variable. Studies have shown that there is variable correlation between objective measures of genital congestion, subjective arousal and functional magnetic imaging (fMRI) in women [46]. Women cannot accurately perceive clitoral congestion and vaginal congestion, and an accurate estimate of their arousal, both physical and subjective, hence cannot be made. Paradoxically, the objective measurement of genital arousal in women complaining of interest/arousal disorder equals that of sexually healthy normal women when exposed to audiovisual stimuli [47]. For women, the context of the act is more important; a longitudinal study for 8 years on women transitioning through menopause found that their feelings for their partner along with their mood was the important deciding factor for their sexual motivation [48].

Orgasm and Post-orgasm in Sexual Response

Orgasm is a unique and/or eccentric phase of the sexual response cycle. Orgasm as a process is highly distinct and phenomenal in the sense that it includes a series of overlapping events like involuntary muscular contractions, a sense of loss of control, altered perception of space-time, cardiovascular arousal and a feeling of release [49]. How the brain produces these effects? The answer is not yet clear. Orgasms however can occur independently of genital stimulation; a good example of the same would be the sexual ictal manifestations of arousal and/or orgasm perceived by patients with temporal lobe epilepsy [50].

Neuroimaging studies have suggested that much of the brain activity during an orgasm seems to involve the prefrontal cortex, specifically the left orbitofrontal cortex and medial orbitofrontal cortex [35, 51, 52]. Emerging studies also suggest that these areas of brain are involved in reward processing to a variety of stimuli, like food, music, chocolate consumption and drugs [6]. Interestingly, recent studies have also suggested the role of cerebellum in processing orgasm; incremental blood flow increase was seen in the left vermis and deep cerebellar nuclei in both men and women [6].

The post-ejaculatory phase of refraction is usually the final stage/phase of the human sexual response cycle [53]. Very little is actually known about the exact neural correlates of this phase. Invariably, in all men orgasm is followed by a refractory period, a period of decreased and/or unresponsiveness to sexual stimuli. However, women retain the ability to respond to sexual stimuli multiple times in a given sexual cycle [53]. The period of the refractory phase can vary both within and between individuals.

Conclusion

The human sexual response cycle is not a simple set of stages that an individual will automatically progress through one after the other. The human sexual response should be best viewed in an incentive/motivation-based model, where the individual actively searches for sex, driven by both his or her urge and his or her need for a prospective reward after sex. Complex neural networks regulate the different phases of the sexual response cycle. While sexual interest and arousal seem to be well researched in the context of neuroanatomy, limited information is actually available about the neural correlates of orgasm and/or refractory phase. From a clinical viewpoint, the clinician should bear in mind the vast complexity of the sexual response and the various biological, social and psychological factors that can influence and confound apparently accurate clinical findings.

References

1. DeLamater J, Friedrich WN. Human sexual development. J Sex Res. 2002;39(1):10–4.
2. Jannini EA, Fisher WA, Bitzer J, McMahon CG. Is sex just fun? How sexual activity improves health. J Sex Med. 2009;6:2640–8.
3. Morran LT, Schmidt OG, Gelarden IA, Parris RC II, Lively CM. Running with the red queen: host–parasite coevolution selects for biparental sex. Science. 2011:333:216–8.
4. Meston CM, Buss DM. Why humans have sex. Arch Sex Behav. 2007;36:477–507.
5. Meston CM, Hamilton LD, Harte CB. Sexual motivation in women as a function of age. J Sex Med. 2009;6:3305–19.

6. Georgiadis JR, Kringelbach ML. The human sexual response cycle: brain imaging evidence linking sex to other pleasures. Prog Neurobiol. 2012;98(1):49–81.
7. Pfaus JG, Kippin TE, Coria-Avila G. What can animal models tell us about human sexual response? Ann Rev Sex Res. 2003;14(1):1–63.
8. Feiring C, Cleland CM, Simon VA. Abuse-specific self-schemas and self functioning: a prospective study of sexually abused youth. J Clin Child Adolesc Psychol. 2010;39:35–50.
9. Ferretti A, Caulo M, Del Gratta C, Di Matteo R, Merla A, Montorsi F, Pizzella V, Pompa P, Rigatti P, Rossini PM, Salonia A, Tartaro A, Romani GL. Dynamics of male sexual arousal: distinct components of brain activation revealed by fMRI. NeuroImage. 2005;26:1086–96.
10. Rizzolatti G, Craighero L. The mirror-neuron system. Annu Rev Neurosci. 2004;27:169–92.
11. Moulier V, Mouras H, Pelegrini-Issac M, Glutron D, Rouxel R, Grandjean B, Bittoun J, Stoleru S. Neuroanatomical correlates of penile erection evoked by photographic stimuli in human males. NeuroImage. 2006;33:689–99.
12. Mouras H, Stoleru S, Moulier V, Pelegrini-Issac M, Rouxel R, Grandjean B, Glutron D, Bittoun J. Activation of mirror-neuron system by erotic video clips predicts degree of induced erection: an fMRI study. NeuroImage. 2008;42:1142–50.
13. Ponseti J, Bosinski HA, Wolff S, Peller M, Jansen O, Mehdorn HM, Buchel C, Siebner HR. A functional endophenotype for sexual orientation in humans. NeuroImage. 2006;33:825–33.
14. Martinson FM. The sexual life of children. Westport, CT: Bergin and Garvey; 1994.
15. Bull JJ. Evolution of sex determining mechanisms. Menlo Park: The Benjamin/Cummings Publishing Company; 1983.
16. Masters WH, Johnson VE. Human sexual response. Boston, MA: Little, Brown & Company; 1966.
17. Robinson P. The modernization of sex. New York: Harper and Row; 1976.
18. Beach FA. Characteristics of masculine "sex drive". In: Jones MR, editor. Nebraska symposium on motivation. Lincoln: University of Nebraska Press; 1956. p. 1–32.
19. Kinsey AC, Pomeroy WB, Martln CE, Gebhard PH. Sexual behavior in the human female. Philadelphia: W. B. Saunders Co; 1953.
20. Hackett G. The use of questionnaires to assess sexual function. Trends Urol Mens Health. 2017;8(1):17–20.
21. Basson R. Human sex-response cycles. J Sex Marital Ther. 2001;27:33–43.
22. Janssen E, Everaerd W, Spiering M, et al. Automatic processes and the appraisal of sexual stimuli: toward an information processing model of sexual arousal. J Sex Res. 2000;37:8–23.
23. Laan E, van Driel EM, van Lunsen RHW. Genital responsiveness in healthy women with and without sexual arousal disorder. J Sex Med. 2008;5:1424–35.
24. Goldhammer DL, McCabe MP. A qualitative exploration of the meaning and experience of sexual desire among partnered women. Can J Hum Sex. 2011;20(1–2):19–34.
25. Vannier SA, O'Sullivan LF. Sex without desire: characteristics of occasions of sexual compliance in young adults' committed relationships. J Sex Res. 2010;47:429–39.
26. Stole'ru S, Fonteille V, Corne'lis C, et al. Functional neuroimaging studies of sexual arousal and orgasm in healthy men and women: a review and meta-analysis. Neurosci Biobehav Rev. 2012;36:1481–509.
27. American Psychiatric Association. Diagnostic and statistical manual of mental disorders (DSM-5®). San Francisco: American Psychiatric Publishing; 2013. p. 22.
28. King M, Holt V, Nazareth I. Women's view of their sexual difficulties: agreement and disagreement for the clinical diagnoses. Arch Sex Behav. 2007;36:281–8.
29. Levin RJ. The human sexual response cycle. In: The textbook of clinical sexual medicine. Cham: Springer; 2017. p. 39–51.
30. Havermans RC. How to tell where 'liking' ends and 'wanting' begins. Appetite. 2012;58:252–5.
31. Smith KS, Berridge KC, Aldridge JW. Disentangling pleasure from incentive salience and learning signals in brain reward circuitry. Proc Natl Acad Sci U S A. 2011;108:E255–64.
32. Mostafa T, El Khouly G, Hassan A. Pheromones in sex and reproduction: do they have a role in humans? J Adv Res. 2012;3:1–9.

33. Loken LS, Wessberg J, Morrison I, McGlone F, Olausson H. Coding of pleasant touch by unmyelinated afferents in humans. Nat Neurosci. 2009;12:547–8.
34. Michels L, Mehnert U, Boy S, Schurch B, Kollias S. The somatosensory representation of the human clitoris: an fMRI study. NeuroImage. 2010;49:177–84.
35. Georgiadis JR, Reinders AA, Paans AM, Renken R, Kortekaas R. Men versus women on sexual brain function: prominent differences during tactile genital stimulation but not during orgasm. Hum Brain Mapp. 2009;30:3089–101.
36. Miyagawa Y, Tsujimura A, Fujita K, Matsuoka Y, Takahashi T, Takao T, Takada S, Matsumiya K, Osaki Y, Takasawa M, Oku N, Hatazawa J, Kaneko S, Okuyama A. Differential brain processing of audiovisual sexual stimuli in men: comparative positron emission tomography study of the initiation and maintenance of penile erection during sexual arousal. NeuroImage. 2007;36:830–42.
37. Ghazanfar AA, Santos LR. Primate brains in the wild: the sensory bases for social interactions. Nat Rev Neurosci. 2004;5:603–16.
38. Childress AR, Ehrman RN, Wang Z, Li Y, Sciortino N, Hakun J, Jens W, Suh J, Listerud J, Marquez K, Franklin T, Langleben D, Detre J, O'Brien CP. Prelude to passion: limbic activation by unseen drug and sexual cues. PLoS One. 2008;3:e1506.
39. Rupp HA, Wallen K. Sex differences in response to visual sexual stimuli: a review. Arch Sex Behav. 2008;37:206–18.
40. Caspers S, Zilles K, Laird AR, Eickhoff SB. ALE meta-analysis of action observation and imitation in the human brain. NeuroImage. 2010;50:1148–67.
41. Buhler M, Vollstadt-Klein S, Klemen J, Smolka MN. Does erotic stimulus presentation design affect brain activation patterns? Event-related vs blocked fMRI designs. Behav Brain Funct. 2008;4:30.
42. Klucken T, Schweckendiek J, Merz CJ, Tabbert K, Walter B, Kagerer S, Vaitl D, Stark R. Neural activations of the acquisition of conditioned sexual arousal: effects of contingency awareness and sex. J Sex Med. 2009;6:3071–85.
43. Savic I, Lindstrom P. PET and MRI show differences in cerebral asymmetry and functional connectivity between homo- and heterosexual subjects. Proc Natl Acad Sci U S A. 2008;105:9403–8.
44. Clayton AH, Clavet GJ, McGarvey EL, Warnock JK, Weiss K. Assessment of sexual functioning during the menstrual cycle. J Sex Marital Ther. 1999;25:281–91.
45. Mass R, Holldorfer M, Moll B, Bauer R, Wolf K. Why we haven't died out yet: changes in women's mimic reactions to visual erotic stimuli during their menstrual cycles. Horm Behav. 2009;55:267–71.
46. Chivers ML, Seto MC, Blanchard R. Gender and sexual orientation differences in sexual response to sexual activities versus gender of actors in sexual films. J Pers Soc Psychol. 2007;93:1108–21.
47. Graham CA. The DSM diagnostic criteria for female sexual arousal disorder. Arch Sex Behav. 2010;39(2):240–55.
48. Dennerstein L, Lehert P, Guthrie J. The effects of the menopausal transition and biopsychosocial factors on well-being. Arch Womens Ment Health. 2002;5:15–22.
49. Mah K, Binik YM. The nature of human orgasm: a critical review of major trends. Clin Psychol Rev. 2001;21:823–56.
50. Warneke LB. A case of temporal lobe epilepsy with an orgasmic component. Can Psychiatr Assoc J. 1976;21(5):319–24.
51. Georgiadis JR, Kortekaas R, Kuipers R, Nieuwenburg A, Pruim J, Reinders AATS, Holstege G. Regional cerebral blood flow changes associated with clitorally induced orgasm in healthy women. Eur J Neurosci. 2006;24:3305–16.
52. Georgiadis JR, Reinders AA, van der Graaf FH, Paans AM, Kortekaas R. Brain activation during human male ejaculation revisited. Neuroreport. 2007;18:553–7.
53. Levin RJ. Revisiting post-ejaculation refractory time-what we know and what we do not know in males and in females. J Sex Med. 2009;6:2376–89.

How to Take a Sexual History

2

Narayana Reddy and Shah Dupesh Khan

Introduction

Sexual disorders and/or problems are exceedingly common and they significantly affect a patient's quality of life. Sexual health problems can be caused by an ongoing illness, medication use, past surgery and/or relationship issues. The WHO has defined 'sexual health as a state of physical, emotional, mental and social well being in relation to sexuality and it is not merely the absence of disease, dysfunction or infirmity' [1]. Good sexual health comprises an absence of sexually transmitted disease (STD), fertility problems and unwanted pregnancies and also the ability to enjoy one's sexuality without abuse and/or oppression [1]. The topic of sex and sexuality in itself is now no longer confined to hushed discussions in the twenty-first century. Yet, there is still anxiety and abstinence when the topic of sex comes up for discussion, especially more so between the clinician and the patient [2, 3]. This leaves a tremendous void in the delivery of complete holistic healthcare.

The WHO maintains that it is the responsibility of physicians to maintain sexual health [1]. Good sexual history taking thus becomes a core skill for clinician and this helps establish the right diagnosis of particular sexual dysfunction. However, studies have clearly shown that there seems to be a lack of comfort as well as adequate training for the clinician in taking a sexual history [4, 5]. This can lead to misdiagnosis and improper treatment of a particular sexual dysfunction. The problems are significantly amplified when a diagnosis of a sexual dysfunction has to be done for same-sex couples.

N. Reddy (✉)
Dega Institute of Sexual Medicine, Chennai, India

S. D. Khan
The Metromale Clinic and Fertility Center,
No 1, Crescent Park Street, T-Nagar, Chennai, India

© Springer Nature Singapore Pte Ltd. 2019

K. Gunasekaran, S. D. Khan (eds.), *Sexual Medicine*,
https://doi.org/10.1007/978-981-13-1226-7_2

Interestingly, only about 35% of primary care physicians report that they have ever taken a sexual history [6]. Swiss general practitioners also showed a preference to use their own diagnostic criteria which are not well validated [4, 7]. Moreover, older GPs were less likely to give a therapy for sexual dysfunction and frequently referred patients to a specialist [8, 9]. Female GPs were also less comfortable in evaluating male sexual dysfunction in general [10].

The aim of this chapter is to give the primary care physician a brief content and a structured interview outline that assist in taking a sexual history for both men and women presenting to a clinic with sexual dysfunction.

Why Are Clinicians Reluctant to Take a Sexual History?

Just as clinicians are comfortable in enquiring about the colour of stools and urine, a routine assessment of sexual health is of paramount importance. Clinicians usually look towards taking help from a psychiatrist for anything that is sex related. The truth is that sexual medicine training in residency programmes world over has ill met the current needs of the practicing specialist [11, 12] (regardless of his or her specialty). Clinicians at all levels try to rationalize and justify their avoidance in taking a sexual history by stating reasons like—'If I ask a sex related question to my patient, he will shy away'. On the contrary the truth is that the clinician is the one who is actually shying away. Other reasons include—'this is not my specialty', 'A sexologist is better person to handle this issue'. The clinician usually tends to relate his or her own sexuality with that of the patient and becomes distinctly uncomfortable in asking questions which he or she feels may be too intrusive or forward. This effect is amplified more so, when the clinician deals with patients who are twice his or her age. Sometimes, the questions are vaguely phrased in a manner that entices a very poor or apathetic patient response. This problem is understandable as the clinician has no structured framework to elicit a sexual history.

Adolescents frequently pose an altogether different challenge to the clinician [13]. Most adolescents learn about sex from peers of the same age group and also from the environment. Sex and sexuality is not a topic that is touched upon by parents. A clinician may also feel uneasy or distinctly uncomfortable to ask a specific sex health-related question to a sexually active adolescent, when he or she has children in the same age group. Table 2.1 summarizes the various difficulties the patient and doctor face when dealing with a sexual dysfunction [1–3].

Table 2.1 Factors that can affect both the patient and doctor while discussing about sex

Why are doctors reluctant to discuss sex?
1. Lack of training in medical school
2. Lack of structured tools and knowledge to assess sexual history
3. Relates his or her own sexuality with patients
4. Lack of time
5. Fear of offending the patient
6. Judgemental and making assumptions that older people or disabled people do not engage sexually
Why are patients reluctant to discuss sex?
1. Believes his or her sex problem is due to illness/age 2. Worried that he or she will be judged
3. Feels shameful to discuss about sex
4. Disturbed body image
5. Misplaced or misinformed set of sex-related beliefs and/or thoughts
6. No knowledge that treatment is actually possible

Patient Discomfort

Most patients never start out discussing their sexual health concern. They look upon the physician to start a discussion first or give them explicit permission. In a study on 887 gynaecology patients only 3% of them voluntarily raised a sexual complaint, while about 19% of them only acknowledged a problem on direct enquiry [14]. In another study of over 500 Americans aged 25 years and older, over 68% feared that their physician would be embarrassed if they raised concerns about their sexual problems. Over 71% of study participants also feared that their doctors would dismiss their sexual concern [15]. Patient discomfort primarily seems to stem from fear of a physician's response rather than their inherent avoidance to discuss on the subject.

Why to Take a Sexual History?

The main objective of taking a sexual history is to narrow down the aetio-pathogenesis of a sexual health problem without blindly labelling a man with impotence or a women with frigidity.

Diagnosis of a Sexual Dysfunction—Sexual dysfunction is estimated to affect over 43% and 31% of men and women, respectively, at least once in a lifetime [16]. A sexual dysfunction is defined as a problem that interferes with the initiation and/or

Table 2.2 Various classifications of both male and female sexual dysfunction as per the DSM-5 revised classification system

DSM-5 diagnosis
Male dysfunctions
Erectile disorder
Hypoactive sexual desire disorder
Premature ejaculation
Delayed ejaculation
Male dyspareunia
Male sexual pain
Female dysfunctions
Female sexual interest/arousal disorders
Female arousal disorder
Female orgasmic disorder
Genito-pelvic pain or genito-pelvic penetration disorders
Other causes leading to a dysfunction
Sexual dysfunction due to drug abuse

consummation and/or satisfaction with sex [17]. A sexual dysfunction can affect the male or female or both partners. A dysfunction can be recently acquired or be present lifelong or simply occur in a specific situation or sometimes be generalized [16–18].

A sexual dysfunction can also affect any one of the phases of the human sexual response cycle, namely desire, excitement, orgasm or resolution [16]. A sexual dysfunction frequently results in feelings of inadequacy for both partners. Table 2.2 contains the revised DSM-5 classification of sexual dysfunction [19]. A sexual dysfunction can frequently be caused by organic problems like diabetes, hypertension and dyslipidaemia. The use of medications like antidepressants, SSRIs and antipsychotics is also associated with sexual dysfunction [20, 21].

A sexual dysfunction can be caused due to physical/organic and/or psychological factors. A good sexual history helps in establishing the diagnosis and the root cause of the dysfunction.

Prevent STD-Related Deaths—Over 400,000 HIV-related deaths do occur year on year in the USA. Chlamydia and its associated fertility-based complications along with genital herpes simplex virus infection affect over 3 million and 45 million people annually [22]. Gonococcus infection is well known for its variable prevalence as well as antibiotic resistance with differing geographical regions. The early recognition and treatment of these conditions can drastically improve outcomes [23].

Most sexually transmitted infections (STIs) also present with varying incubation and window periods. Thus in these scenarios taking a structured sexual history that involves questions about the place of contact, patient and partner's ethnicity can help tailor appropriate investigations, treatment, contact tracing and finally follow-up. STDs have now become a global problem in both developing and developed countries despite the increased awareness of the general public.

Proper sexual history taking plays a very important role in prevention of STD, avoiding unintended pregnancies as well as unhealthy sexual practices. It also gives a relevant opportunity for vaccination where appropriate and provides patients with information, counselling, reassurance and/or contraception.

General Principles in Sexual History Taking

In sexual function assessment, most clinicians face the difficulty of when, where and how to address a given topic. Making the patient feel comfortable is of paramount importance and will ease the conversation. Patient confidentiality is even more important. Assuring the patient that he or she can speak his or her mind and that everything that transpires in terms of a conversation will be kept a secret builds tremendous trust on the clinician, from a patient's perspective. Patient rapport building is key to successful sexual history taking.

Assuring and ensuring that the conversation will not be overheard and interrupted also plays a very important role in patient comfort. Early questions addressed to the patient should be with an aim to assess the patient's sexuality and general sex-related behaviour. Later questions should become more specific as time passes. Specific questions should address the specific sexual dysfunction. Always start broad and go narrow later in the interview.

Questions should be brief and not too formal filled with medical jargon, or the clinician risks losing information from a lack of patient understanding. Questions asked should also not be judgemental in nature. It is better to ask—'How long have you been with your partner?' rather than uses terms like husband, wife or girlfriend.

The clinician should also avoid the use of slang language as this will make him or her appear untrained and unprofessional. An example would be if the patient states his or her chief complaint as 'I come to early, I am unable to control it', a clinician's response should be 'After how many minutes or seconds do you ejaculate?'. The use of appropriate terminology in a sexual medicine setting is easier said than done. Repeated practice of sexual terminology helps desensitize the clinician to the use of sexual terminology without feeling embarrassed.

Maintaining a proper body language and avoiding looking at the floor all bolster patient trust in the clinician. Maintaining a calm composure and eye contact also helps. Blushing or stammering to patient answers clearly shows that the clinician is not adequately trained to deal with sexual health-related problems. Observing the patient's language and voice hesitancy can give valuable insights into framing questions in a different way to allay apprehension. This part comes only with practice over a period of time. Table 2.3 summarizes some general principles that the clinician should bear in mind during sexual history taking.

Table 2.3 Overview of general principles in sexual history taking

General principles in sexual history taking
Ensure patient privacy plus confidentiality
Be non-judgemental and maintain eye contact
Recognize non-verbal cues
Ask questions that are appropriate with the right terminology
General question first followed by specific questions later
Explain all procedures and treatments thoroughly

In-Depth Sexual History Taking

Sexual history taking should comprehensively cover social, psychiatric, medical and surgical information comprehensively. Sexual functioning is multifaceted influenced by one's upbringing, environmental influence, past and/or current health and past and/or current sexual experiences. Human sexuality is complex and is influenced by a myriad of factors (Table 2.4). An in-depth sexual history taking should touch upon all the possible factors that can affect an individual's sexuality [24, 25].

Most of the time, eliciting a sexual history can be easily done when the patient visits a clinician for another medical problem. For example, in an infertility evaluation, patients are routinely asked briefly about their frequency of sexual intercourse and where appropriate additional questions on a male partner's erection, penetration and ejaculation are elicited. In another example, a patient may walk into the office for a diabetes workup; he can be asked if he noticed any recent changes in his sexual function, especially his erection. For women, eliciting a history about their menstrual cycles and current method of contraception itself can help probe into a specific sexual problem and/or concern.

Before actually progressing into an in-depth sexual history session, a brief set of questions as outlined below can help screen the patient for a particular sexual health problem.

Question 1—Hi, hope you are doing great! How are things going for you from a sexual viewpoint?

Question 2 (For men specifically)—Do you have any problems with your erection? Do you have any problems with ejaculation or any other aspect of sex?

Question 3 (For men again)—Many men in the age group (range) and having either diabetes/hypertension/cardiac disease/other chronic illness will have some problem with their erection. Stress can also lead to difficulties in achieving an erection. If you have a problem, feel free to tell me. The right treatment will definitely help you enjoy a better quality of life.

Table 2.4 Overview of factors that affect human sexuality

Factors that influence an individual's sexuality
Family background, culture and religion
Menarche, menopause, pregnancy, infertility, birthing and contraception, miscarriage or still birth or termination of a pregnancy
Major surgeries like mastectomy or radical prostatectomy
Colostomy and other surgeries that disturb one's body image
Illness like diabetes, hypertension and cancer
Sexual beliefs, past sexual experience and past sexual abuse history
Life events like marriage, start of a new relationship, presence of young children
Masturbation and ability to accept it
Physical set-up
Emotional connect with partner
Medication both prescribed and recreational

Question 4 (For women)—Many women who are currently experiencing a new relationship/pregnancy/post-childbirth/menopause report to have some difficulties like pain during intercourse or a lack of interest and/or arousal. You must tell me your concern if you have any; treatments are available and they can significantly improve your relationship and avoid unnecessary strain.

If the patient has a sexual health problem an appropriate clinical decision can be taken to decide whether to proceed with an in-depth history or to proceed at subsequent visit. The four questions outlined above will usually be more than sufficient for the initial sexual health screen. An in-depth sexual history also gives us a tremendous opportunity for the practice of preventive medicine especially in the context of an STD [26, 27]. Table 2.5 outlines an in-depth questionnaire along with the required physical examination and tests that can be used for taking a structured sexual history. Although sexual history taking can be subjective, the clinician should bear in mind that human behaviour is complex and can change from period to period because it is influenced by diversity of factors. Thus, using a watertight questionnaire may not be very helpful in day-to-day clinical practice. However these validated questionnaires (Table 2.5) can be used as a guide before going into a focussed assessment of the problem as suggested by Kothari and Reddy [27–30].

In a situation where the patient is a part of couple, the interview should ideally include both partners in the couple. Following a sexual history assessment, a thorough head-to-foot physical examination is recommended along with suitable blood tests relevant to the problem. In certain circumstances, a referral has to be made; this is true particularly in certain complex problems like gender identity disorder and sexual abuse. The clinician should reassure the patient for an appropriate referral, since most patients would feel that the clinician is trying to 'get rid of them'. Some sexual health issues are better managed through a multidisciplinary team-based approach to treatment [31].

Scales and Questionnaires

Questionnaires can be used to aid in the diagnosis of both male and female sexual dysfunction. The usage and choice of a questionnaire however depend on the theoretical background and rationale of use. Table 2.6 highlights a few questionnaires available in the scientific literature. Some of these questionnaires focus on the patient's sexual function and some others on the partner's sexual function and/or sexuality.

However, an important point to be borne in mind is that none of the aforementioned questionnaires can substitute an in-depth sexual history taking. Most of the questionnaires/scales can only assess a specific sexual symptom. Most of these questionnaires fail to assess the social aspect of a patient's sexuality and/or sexual function on the basis of his or her current relationship [32, 33]. Cultural and linguistic variations also diminish the accuracy of the scales. The objective of any good sexual history is to elicit a desirable patient response; scales sometimes cannot achieve that objective. This is exactly why we strongly recommend every clinician to take an in-depth structured sexual history.

Table 2.5 Sexual history taking, a structured approach

Structured sexual history questionnaire
General history
Patient's age, educational status and occupation
Patient's current relationship status (married, single, divorced, widower) Patient's medication history and lifestyle factors (smoking/alcohol/drug use) Patient's past medical and surgical history (diabetes, hypertension, cardiovascular disease, hypercholesterolaemia, any major abdominal and/or urogenital surgeries) For female patients specifically ask on pregnancy, birthing, current contraception if any *Chief complaints* For male—Assess if the patient has a problem with (a) desire, (b) erection, (c) penetration, (d) maintenance of erection, (e) ejaculation, (f) orgasm, (g) satisfaction For female—Assess if the patient has a problem with (a) desire, (b) lubrication, (c) accommodation, (d) orgasm (e) Satisfaction For both men and women assess if the current complaint is (a) situation or (b) global *Sexual profile* Are you currently actively engaging in sex? If yes, how frequently? Do you engage in sex outside your current relationship? Do you prefer men or women or both? How many partners have you had in past 6 months? Lifetime? How satisfied are you with your partner? How has the frequency of sexual intercourse changed in the last 6 months? How has your sexual desire changed in the last 6 months? Who initiates intercourse, you or your partner? When did you first masturbate? (For women ask about self-stimulation, as it is a more familiar term) When did you first have intercourse? Are you planning for a pregnancy? Have you tried oral or anal intercourse? Do you use any specific object during sex? Do you have any pain during sex? Do you have any specific sexual fantasy? What is it that you miss in sex? Are your marital expectation fulfilled? Anything specifically you dislike in your partner? Have you had any blood transfusions? Needle-stick injuries? Or partners who might have put you at a risk of contracting an STD? Have you been screened for HIV/syphilis/other STDs? (Explain and offer a pretest counsel) Have you been immunized for hepatitis A/B? (Assess risk and vaccinate if appropriate) Do you use contraception? If so what type? Examination and tests were appropriate *Examination of the male* Height, weight, BMI calculation, waist circumference, androgenization, thorough urogenital exam *Examination of the female* Monomanual and bimanual vaginal exam combined with a speculum exam; also check height, weight and BMI *Tests* Fasting and postprandial blood sugar, HBA1C, complete blood evaluation, TSH, FSH, LH, total and calculated free testosterone, oestrogen, prolactin with urinalysis, and LFT were indicated; basic STD screening (HIV, syphilis, hepatitis B); specialized tests for other STDs should be given only where appropriate

Table 2.6 Sexual function questionnaires

Questionnaires	Level of evidence
Female Sexual Function Index (FSFI)	A1
Female Sexual Distress Scale-Revised (FSDS-R)	A1
International Index of Erectile Function (IIEF)	A1
Male Sexual Health Questionnaire (MSHQ)	B2
Premature Ejaculation Profile (PEP)	B2
PROMIS Sexual Function and Satisfaction Scale	A1
Multiple Sclerosis Intimacy and Sexuality Questionnaire (MSISQ-19)	B1
Pelvic Organ Prolapse Sexual Questionnaire (PISQ)	B2
Female and Male Genital Self Image Scale (FGSIS and MGSIS)	A1

Conclusion

The importance of sexual health cannot be overemphasized enough. Sexual health is crucial for both men and women and significantly influences the quality of life. The aim of this chapter is primarily to orient clinicians to the importance of sexual health and also provide them with the necessary set of questions to help them take a sexual history in a structured way. Although elaborate treatment options have been discussed elsewhere in this textbook, one cannot treat a problem if he or she does not know whether it exists.

References

1. World Health Organization. Education and treatment in human sexuality: the training of health professionals. Report of a WHO meeting. Albany, NY: Q Corporation; 2000.
2. Alarcao V, Ribeiro S, Miranda FL, et al. GP's knowledge, attitudes, beliefs and practices in the management of sexual dysfunction. Results of the Portugese SEXOS study. J Sex Med. 2012;9(10):2508–15.
3. Goodwach R. Sex therapy: historical evolution, current practice. Part II. Aust N Z J Fam Ther. 2005;26(4):178–83.
4. Platano G, Margraf J, Alder J, Bitzer J. Frequency and focus of sexual history taking in male patients—a pilot study conducted among Swiss general practitioners and urologists. J Sex Med. 2008;5(1):47–59.
5. Sobecki JN, Curlin FA, Rasinski KA, Lindau ST. What we don't talk about when we don't talk about sex: results of a National Survey of US Obstetrician/Gynecologists. J Sex Med. 2012;9(5):1285–94.
6. Temple-Smith MJ, Mulvey G, Keogh L. Attitudes to taking a sexual history in general practice in Victoria. Aust Sex Trans Infect. 1999;75:41–4.
7. Platano G, Margraf J, Alder J, Bitzer J. Psychosocial factors and therapeutic approaches in the context of sexual history taking in men: a study conducted among Swiss general practitioners and urologists. J Sex Med. 2008;5:2533–56.
8. Skelton JR, Matthews PM. Teaching sexual history taking to health care professionals in primary care. Med Educ. 2001;35:603–8.
9. Gott M, Hinchliff S. Barriers to seeking treatment for sexual problems in primary care: a qualitative study with older people. Fam Pract. 2003;20:690–5.

10. De Berardis G, Pellegrini F, Franciosi M, Pamparana F, Morelli P, Tognoni G, Nicolucci A, EDEN study group. Management of erectile dysfunction in general practice. J Sex Med. 2009;6:1127–34.
11. Mas M, Garcia-Giralda L, Rey JR, Martinez-Salamanca JI, Guirao L, Turbi C. Evaluating a continuous medical education program to improve general practitioners awareness and practice on erectile dysfunction as a cardiovascular risk factor. J Sex Med. 2011;8:1585–93.
12. Rosen R, Kountz D, Post-Zwicker T, Leiblum S, Wiegel M. Sexual communication skills in residency training: the Robert wood Johnson model. J Sex Med. 2006;3:37–46.
13. Felice ME, Feinstein RA, Fisher M, Kaplan DW, Olmedo LF, Rome ES, et al. American Academy of Pediatrics. Committee on adolescence. Contraception in adolescents. Pediatrics. 1999;104(5 Pt 1):1161–6.
14. Bachmann GA, Leiblum SR, Grill J. Brief sexual inquiry in gynecologic practice. Obstet Gynecol. 1989;73(3 Pt 1):425–7.
15. Marwick C. Survey says patients expect little physician help on ex. JAMA. 1999;281:2173.
16. Reddy N, Swamy V, Pandiyan N, Dupesh S. Sexual dysfunction and infertility. In: Male infertility. New Delhi: Springer; 2017. p. 231–42.
17. Spector IP, Carey MP. Incidence and prevalence of the sexual dysfunctions: a critical review of the empirical literature. Arch Sex Behav. 1990;19:389–408.
18. Read S, King M, Watson J. Sexual dysfunction in primary medical care: prevalence, characteristics and detection by the general practitioner. J Public Health Med. 1997;19:387–91.
19. American Psychiatric Association. Diagnostic and statistical manual of mental disorders (DSM-5®). Arlington, VA: American Psychiatric Publishing; 2013. p. 22.
20. Pauls RN, Kleeman SD, Karram MM. Female sexual dysfunction: principles of diagnosis and therapy. Obstet Gynecol Surv. 2005;60(3):196–205.
21. Phillips NA. Female sexual dysfunction: evaluation and treatment. Am Fam Physician. 2000;62(1):127–36. 141–2
22. Weinhardt LS, Carey MP, Johnson BT, Bickham NL. Effects of HIV counseling and testing on sexual risk behavior: a meta-analytic review of published research, 1985-1997. Am J Public Health. 1999;89:1397–405.
23. Centers for Disease Control and Prevention. Trends in sexual risk behaviors among high school students, United States, 1991–1997. MMWR Morb Mortal Wkly Rep. 1998;47:749–52.
24. Brotto L, Atallah S, Johnson-Agbakwu C, et al. Psychological and interpersonal dimensions of sexual function and dysfunction. J Sex Med. 2016;13(4):538–71.
25. Bullard D, Knight S, editors. Sexuality and physical disability. Personal perspectives. St. Louis, MO: CV Mosby. p. 1981.
26. Cates W Jr, Stone C. Family planning-sexually transmitted diseases and contraceptive choice: a literature update—Part I. Fam Plan Perspect. 1992;24:122–8.
27. Kothari P. Endocrine, metabolic, physical and psychiatric evaluation of ejaculatory dysfunctions in man, Ph.D. Thesis, Bombay University; 1981.
28. Kothari P. Ejaculatory dysfunction—a new dimension. Bombay Hosp J. 1982:19–23.
29. Kothari P. Multiorgasm: psychophysiodynamics. In: Kothari P, editor. Orgasm—new dimensions. Bombay: VRP Publishers; 1989. p. 47.
30. Reddy DN. Studies on sexual disorders in human males. PhD thesis, University of Madras, p. 35–47; 1993.
31. Kingsberg SA. Just ask! Talking to patients about sexual function. Sex Reprod Menopause. 2004;2(4):1–5.
32. Hatzichristou D, Kirana PS, Banner L, Althof SE, Lonnee-Hoffmann RA, Dennerstein L, Rosen RC. Diagnosing sexual dysfunction in men and women: sexual history taking and the role of symptom scales and questionnaires. J Sex Med. 2016;13(8):1166–82.
33. Hatzichristou D, Rosen RC, Derogatis LR, et al. Recommendations for the clinical evaluation of men and women with sexual dysfunction. J Sex Med. 2010;7:337–48.

3 Erectile Dysfunction

Karthik Gunasekaran and Shah Dupesh Khan

Introduction

Erectile dysfunction (ED) is the most well publicized among all the causes of male sexual dysfunction. ED has been frequently defined as the inability to sustain or maintain an erectile function that is sufficient enough to achieve sexual intercourse that is satisfactory leading to considerable distress to one or both partners [1]. The consistency of the problem is more important since the sexual dysfunction should have been present for at least a period of 3 months before a conclusive diagnosis is made [2].

ED is predicted to affect an estimated 300 million people by the year 2025 [3]. Prevalence studies indicate that ED affects over 50% of men between the age group of 40–70 years [4]. Data from the Massachusetts male ageing study (MMAS) suggests that the prevalence of ED is about 70%, especially in men more than 70 years [5]. ED is progressive in nature, and significantly impairs both the physical and social well-being of both partners and their family members [6]. While initial studies suggested that the cause of ED is mainly psychological, recent studies have established the fact that ED is well associated with numerous physical conditions like diabetes, hypertension, dyslipidemia, metabolic syndrome, lower urinary tract symptoms, and depression [4]. Strong evidence from meta-analysis has also suggested that ED is independently as well as significantly associated with cardiovascular disease, stroke, coronary artery disease, and all-cause mortality [7].

The bigger issue with ED is that it is frequently underdiagnosed, underreported, as well as undertreated [1]. Studies suggest that patients seldom feel comfortable explicitly opening up about their sexual health problems to their primary care physician, until or unless they are given permission to discuss the same [8]. The lack of training in sexual medicine is another professional hurdle for most practicing

K. Gunasekaran, MS, FRCS (Glasgow), FECSM · S. D. Khan (✉)
The Metromale Clinic and Fertility Center,
No 1, Crescent Park Street, T-Nagar, Chennai, India

© Springer Nature Singapore Pte Ltd. 2019

K. Gunasekaran, S. D. Khan (eds.), *Sexual Medicine*,
https://doi.org/10.1007/978-981-13-1226-7_3

clinicians to properly evaluate and treat ED. Bearing this fact in mind, the primary aim of this chapter is to provide a brief clinical overview to help the practicing physician in the diagnosis and management of ED.

Comorbidities in Erectile Dysfunction

ED and Diabetes

An estimated 40% of men with diabetes also present with ED. The causal link between ED and diabetes is well established [9]. Over 12% of men with ED were found to have previous undiagnosed diabetes. The severity of ED also increases with the increasing duration of diabetes and the age of onset [10]. In general the incidence of ED is reported to be found over three times higher in diabetics versus nondiabetics [10, 11].

The pathophysiology of ED in diabetics is multifactorial with no one cause being at the forefront [12]. Normal erectile function is a complex hemodynamic and/or electrophysiological event mediated in part by nitric oxide release and other substances like Rho kinase/activation of cGMP and/or cAMP second messenger systems along with intracellular Ca^{2+} release [13]. The end result is that there is vasodilatation of the corporal vessels and cavernosal smooth muscle relaxation, thereby allowing an increased blood flow. The increasing blood flow and pressure compress the outgoing venous outflow leading to erection [13]. The whole process is further regulated by the parasympathetic, sympathetic, and somatic nervous system at the central as well as peripheral levels.

Many mechanisms are postulated for the onset of ED in diabetics [4]. In the cavernosal tissue, nitric oxide is a key molecule required for vasodilatation; in diabetes this NO is usually quenched and rendered ineffective by reactive oxygen species (ROS). In diabetic patients the ROS production occurs due to nonenzymatic glycation of proteins resulting in advanced glycation end products (AGE). This is also called the Maillard reaction [14, 15]. Human penile tissue of diabetics has shown to consist a high amount of AGE. The formation of AGE is associated with a high amount of ROS production and thereby oxidative stress; this induces damage to the endothelial cells of the corpora and ultimately results in ED [15].

The other mechanism by which diabetes impairs erection is by its action mediated by a decreased insulin-dependent transport of nitric oxide synthase (NOS) into the cell, due to insulin resistance [16]. Studies on animal models suggest that not just impaired transport but an enhanced enzymatic degradation of L-arginine may also undermine ED in diabetes. L-arginine is a cardinal molecule by which NOS exerts its vasodilatory effects [17]. In diabetic tissue, L-arginine is shown to be rapidly metabolized by overexpressed arginase, thereby impairing the action of NOS and thus its vasodilatory effect [16, 17].

Diabetes-induced erectile dysfunction (DIED) should be first managed with strict glycemic control, control of lipids, and general lifestyle modifications like abstaining from alcohol and smoking combined with regular physical activity [18]. Oral PDE-5 inhibitors are recommended when ED persists despite adequate lifestyle modifications [19].

ED and Hypertension

Arterial hypertension is a significant and vexing public health issue that is responsible for causing 7 million deaths globally year on year [20]. The prevalence of ED in patients with arterial hypertension is almost twice that of normotensive individuals [21]. Similar to diabetes, ED severity significantly increases with the duration of hypertension. Both basic and clinical studies have suggested that a combination of both structural and functional changes in the penile arteries leads to erectile dysfunction [22].

Accumulating evidence suggests that ED is more prevalent in treated versus untreated hypertensives [21, 22]. Treatment approaches to managing ED in both untreated and treated patients are slightly different [23]. In untreated hypertensive patients for a brief period of time, lifestyle modifications along with salt restriction, smoking cessation, and alcohol abstinence are advised. Lifestyle modifications definitely show significant benefit in both improving erectile function and controlling blood pressure [23]. In scenarios, where compliance to the aforementioned strategy is poor, newer antihypertensive medications like nebivolol and angiotensin receptor blockers (ARB) are recommended for men who are sexually active [24]. Studies have clearly indicated that older drugs like diuretics and beta-blockers significantly impair erectile function [24].

In treated patients already on hypertensives it is important to first rule out whether the onset of ED was before the medication was initiated or it occurred after medication was started. Sometimes, ED may occur many years after taking medication; this is probably due to progressive atherosclerosis and not due to the antihypertensive in itself [25]. In either case, the choice of changing the antihypertensive medication should be made after carefully accounting for the patient's current cardiovascular health status and associated comorbidities [25]. If the patient is on beta-blockers for cardiac failure, it may not be wise changing medication. In these scenarios, patients may be offered PDE-5 inhibitors combined with active lifestyle modifications.

Erectile Dysfunction and Atherosclerosis/Hypercholesterolemia

There is a definite association between atherosclerosis and ED [26]. The first notable mention of the same was made as early as 1920, described as Leriche's syndrome characterized by claudication of intermittent nature in the hip and buttocks along with erectile dysfunction and aorto-iliac atherosclerosis [27]. ED can thus be associated with patchy rather than extensive arterial disease that can occur anywhere between the aorta and the penile arteries. Thus any risk factor for an arterial disease is also a risk factor for ED. As discussed above, diabetes and hypertension along with dyslipidemia are strongly associated with ED [26]. On the subject of isolated dyslipidemia and its association with ED, the MMAS study found no association between total cholesterol and ED; on the contrary however, a strong correlation was seen between lower HDL levels and increased incidence of ED especially in the age group of 40–55 years [28]. At values of HDL nearing 30 mg/dL, the incidence of ED was about 16%. The mechanism of vasculogenic impotence in lipid profile disorders seems to stem partly from impaired relaxation of the corpora cavernosa at least based on findings from animal studies [29, 30].

We would thus assume that medical therapy directed to lower serum lipids would thus significantly improve erection. The findings are however conflicting [31]. Use of statins and/or fibrates has been found to be associated with erectile dysfunction as a side effect. The mechanism though is unknown. While findings definitely suggest that reversing hypercholesterolemia is associated with improved global endothelial function, whether this specifically applies to the penile arteries remains to be investigated. Further prospective clinical data and studies are required to assess the changes in erectile function after control of hypercholesterolemia [31].

ED and Cardiovascular Disease

In the context of ED, the third Princeton Consensus panel meet in 2010 defines a cardiovascular risk as the risk of a morbid event that occurs 3–5 years from the diagnosis of ED [32]. ED, just like a family history of myocardial infarction, smoking, and dyslipidemia, has a similar predictive value of future cardiovascular events. In a meta-analysis of 12 prospective studies that included over 36,744 participants, ED was found to be an independent predictor of coronary artery disease (CAD), cardiovascular disease (CVD), and stroke [33]. A diagnosis of ED provides a significant opportunity of risk prevention. ED also identifies a risk of CVD independent of the presence or absence of CVD symptoms [34]. The consensus panel currently recommends a cardiological workup for men diagnosed with ED [35]. In our clinic we routinely perform an ECG for patients diagnosed with erectile dysfunction. We also routinely check the fasting and postprandial blood sugar, total cholesterol profile, and morning testosterone.

The routine measurement of testosterone (T) has proved to be controversial in ED. The American College of Physicians does not recommend it [36], while the British Society of Sexual Medicine and the Princeton Consensus differ and recommend a routine assessment [35]. Recent evidence also suggests that low levels of testosterone and ED are linked with CVD [37]. In a large-scale cohort study of 7000 men, low T was found in about 16% of men with ED in the age group less than 50 years [38]. Studies have also suggested that in the presence of hypogonadism the efficacy of PDE-5 inhibitors is diminished, and this is reversible with T replacement therapy [39]. Lifestyle modification yet again seems to have a pleiotropic effect, not just in diabetes, hypertension, and lipid profile but also in significantly reducing the risk of CVD [40–42].

Diagnosis of ED

ED is usually diagnosed by patient self-report. ED can be broadly classified into two subtypes, organic and psychogenic [2]. A clinical diagnosis of psychogenic ED is usually a "diagnosis of exclusion," where all possible etiological factors that could lead to ED are ruled out after a thorough clinical evaluation. In most clinical scenarios though, patients will present with a mixed pattern of both organic and psychogenic ED.

The clinical evaluation of a suspected ED usually starts off with a general history taking followed by a focused psychosexual history and physical exam and/or laboratory evaluation [43]. A multidisciplinary approach with utmost respect for the patient's ethnic, cultural, and religious belief is required when evaluating ED. Partner involvement is a critical aspect of ED management and is highly recommended to have the partner from the beginning of the evaluation as this helps in stratifying treatment modalities appropriately. The patient's expectation should form the basis of the clinician's treatment goals. The patient's priorities, expectations, and needs from the treatment should be borne in mind before initiating a specific therapy [43].

The psychosocial history plays an important role in the evaluation of ED; the presence of anxiety, depression, history of past abuse, identity disorders, and partner conflicts can all significantly impair treatment outcomes. In parallel, these conditions have to be properly identified and managed concomitantly with ED [2].

Several screening tools/questionnaires like the International Index of Erectile Function (IIEF) [44], the Brief Male Sexual Function Inventory (BMSFI) [45], and the Sexual Health Inventory for Men (SHIM) [46] are available. While most of these tools are reproducible and well validated, they cannot substitute for an in-depth clinical history taking. Table 3.1 outlines a brief overview of questions that can be asked to patients who present with ED.

A focused physical exam usually follows after an in-depth history taking. A physical exam should look at the patient's androgenization and secondary sexual characteristics along with examination of the patient's penis, testis, and scrotum [47]. An assessment of the patient's BP, BMI, and heart rate is also recommended. The clinician should look out for signs of hypogonadism, prostate enlargement, and Peyronie's disease specifically. Where positive findings are found, a suitable line of management follows.

Diagnostic blood testing in men with suspected ED includes fasting and postprandial blood sugars along with a lipid profile to rule out diabetes and dyslipidemia [48]. In men with suspected hypogonadism, the clinician should assess morning total testosterone between 9:00 and 11:00 a.m. in the morning, along with SHBG, FSH, and lastly LH [47, 48]. A repeat assessment for confirmation is usually recommended in case the blood values do not fall in the reference range. Both the American Urological Association (AUA) and WHO recommend limited diagnostic assessment of men with ED [47, 49]. Additional testing using the Rigiscan (nocturnal penile tumescence and rigidity test), penile Doppler ultrasound, MRI studies of sella, and/or neurophysiological testing is only recommended when ED is refractory to standard treatment modalities.

Table 3.1 Questionnaire to assess erectile dysfunction

Questions to assess ED
General history
(1) Name. (2) Occupation. (3) Age. (4) Married. (5) Unmarried but sexually active. (6) Divorced. (7) Single
Have you been diagnosed with (a) diabetes, (b) hypertension, (c) high cholesterol
Have you had a past cardiac attack or chest pain during intercourse?
Have you had a past history of stroke?
Have you had problems like depression/anxiety or any other psychiatric illness?
Do you have any renal or thyroid disease?
Do you have any neurological disease?
Have you had any trauma or surgery done in the pelvis/perineum/testis/penis/scrotum?
Do you have any urinary symptoms like hesitancy/poor flow/burning micturition?
Do you get adequate sleep? Is it restful? Do you have any daytime sleepiness?
Have you been checked for STDs?
Medication and personal history
Do you take any medication for anxiety/sleeplessness/hypertension/cholesterol/diabetes/any other neurological problems/any other specific illness?
Do you smoke? Do you drink alcohol? Do you chew tobacco? Do you use drugs?
Psychosocial history
How is your relationship with your partner? Are you happy with her?
Have you had past partners? How was your relationship with your past partners?
Does your partner have any specific sexual difficulty? Like pain during penetration? Low sex interest or mood? Past history of traumatic abuse?
Have you had a recent change with respect to your job/finances?
Do you have conflicts with other members in your family?
Are you worried about performing well during sex?
Are you currently depressed or anxious? Are you under physical and/or emotional stress?
Do you have a past history of sexual abuse?
Focused sexual history
How long have you had your sexual problem?
How has your sexual problem affected your relationship?
What do you think is the probable reason for your sexual problem?
When do you think was the last time you achieved a satisfactory erection?
How did the problem start? Was it sudden or gradual?
Do you get early morning erections? Do you get erections in the night?
When you are stimulated are you able to initiate an erection?
When you are stimulated are you able to sustain an erection?
Is your erection hard enough for penetration?
Do you lose your erection in a specific situation or partner?
Do you lose your erection before penetration or after penetration?
If it's after penetration, do you lose your erection before orgasm?
Do you have any pain during erection?
Do you have to concentrate too much to maintain your erection?
How is your sex interest?
Do you frequently fantasize about it?
Do you have any specific sexual fantasy that is not fulfilled in your current relationship?

Treatment of ED

Lifestyle Modification

The in-depth clinical history should technically identify any potential risk factor for ED. Correcting risk factors and modifying pharmacotherapy for ED is the first step of treatment [50]. Smoking, obesity, and sedentary lifestyle which are risk factors for cardiovascular disease are also risk factors for ED. Increasing exercise and reducing body weight improve erectile function significantly [51]. However, patient compliance to only lifestyle modifications as an isolated treatment modality is usually poor.

Oral PDE-5 Inhibitors

Henry Hyde Salter first discovered the bronchodilating properties of caffeine and attributed it to cyclic AMP activation and PDE-5 inhibition [52]. It was only about 100 years later when sildenafil was first introduced with an aim to treat angina patients. Some of them reported unexpected side effect of penile erection, which was found to be extremely beneficial for them. Over 100 clinical trials have been conducted to verify both the safety and efficacy of sildenafil citrate [53]. For all types of ED both the AUA and EUA recommend oral PDE-5 inhibitors as the first line of therapeutic management [47, 48]. Currently, there are four approved PDE-5 inhibitors that are approved by most regulatory bodies worldwide for ED. They are sildenafil, tadalafil, vardenafil, and avanafil.

Numerous double-blind placebo-controlled studies have demonstrated significantly improved erections compared to placebo with sildenafil [54]. The drug has an onset of action in approximately 20 min and a plasma half-life of 4 h. The medication should not be administered with a fat-rich diet [55]. Tadalafil on the other hand is a much more selective PDE-5 inhibitor and its action does not depend on food intake or alcohol. Its plasma half-life is long at 17.5 h and duration of action goes up to 36 h [56]. Multicenter, randomized placebo-controlled trials have clearly shown that tadalafil significantly improved erectile function in over 64% of men as compared to 34% of men in the placebo arm, 36 h after drug administration [57]. Of all PDE-5 inhibitors, tadalafil has the longest duration of action [55].

Vardenafil, also approved in 2003, is another potent PDE-5 inhibitor. Its duration of action is similar to sildenafil and plasma half-life is about 4–5 h [58]. The efficacy of vardenafil also reduces after a heavy meal, but to a lesser extent as compared to sildenafil. Vardenafil has been found to be particularly effective in difficult-to-treat patient subgroups like diabetics [58]. Avanafil is the newest PDE-5 inhibitor introduced in 2012 and its plasma value peaks at 34 min with a half-life of 1.5 h [58]. As compared to other PDE-5 inhibitors, it demonstrates similar safety, efficacy, and adverse events. Table 3.2 compares the three most commonly used PDE-5 inhibitors.

Table 3.2 Key differences among different PDE-5 inhibitors

Drug	Dose (mg)	Drug duration (hours)	Onset of action (minutes)
Sildenafil	50–100	4	14–60
Tadalafil	10–20	36	16–45
Vardenafil	10–20	4	25

The commonly reported side effects of PDE-5 inhibitors are usually mild and transient. These include headaches, flushing, dyspepsia, and rhinitis. The side effects occur due to PDE-5 inhibition in other vascular beds [59]. Reported adverse events include visual disturbances probably due to concomitant PDE-6 inhibition associated with sildenafil and backache due to PDE 11 inhibition with tadalafil usage [59]. A rare but important adverse event that has been reported is non-arteritic anterior ischemic optic neuropathy (NAION), which can lead to irreversible blindness. However a causal link between the PDE-5 use and NAION is yet to be proved [60]. In general, when patients experience visual symptoms they are advised to stop taking the medication [61].

Despite the fact that PDE-5 inhibitors have a low adverse risk profile, indiscriminate use is not warranted. Nitrates and PDE-5 inhibitors should never be co-administered together, as there is a clinical risk of hypotension. Caution should also be exercised in patients taking alpha-blockers due to the risk of orthostatic hypertension [8]. Only the lowest possible dose of PDE-5 inhibitors should be given. The choice of PDE-5 inhibitors ultimately depends on the patient's preference, lifestyle factors, and sexual habits. No one PDE-5 inhibitor is superior to the other in terms of IIEF scores [62]. While a subjective preference for tadalafil has been reported in the literature, caution should be exercised while interpreting data from such sponsored studies [63, 64].

PDE-5 inhibitors should only be prescribed after proper sexual stimulation. At least 4–6 sexual attempts must be tried by the patient before dose titration or moving to another drug. The clinician should instruct the patient on the time gap that is required before starting intercourse, since this varies from drug to drug.

On-Demand and Daily Dosing

Traditional treatment regimes for ED involved on-demand dosing with PDE-5 inhibitors with good results in 60% of patients. However, recent randomized double-blind placebo-controlled trials have suggested that daily dosing with tadalafil may be as good as on-demand dosing if not superior [65]. Interestingly, studies have also suggested that long-term dosing with tadalafil may improve sexual function in the long term through a mechanism of vascular remodelling and improved endothelial function. The EMA (European Medical Agency) approved tadalafil 2.5 and 5 mg for daily-dosing regimes. Daily dosing has the advantage of achieving a steady-state plasma concentration and also improves general sexual well-being, thus presenting a very promising treatment option.

Surgical and Other Treatment Options for ED

When PDE-5 inhibitors fail, alprostadil can be used as a second-line treatment option [66]. The intracavernosal form is better tolerated and preferred over the intraurethral forms by patients. The clinician should start with the lowest possible dose and carefully titrate it till an adequate response in terms of erectile function is achieved while carefully monitoring for syncope. Intraurethral alprostadil has certain adverse events like urethral pain, bleeding, and dysuria. Intracavernosal alprostadil on the one hand may present with certain adverse events like pain, nodules, and plaques and sometimes priapism [66]. Patients should be specifically counselled on the risk of priapism where erections could last for more than 4 h, which requires management with aspiration of blood from the corpus using a local anesthetic.

Vacuum pumps are second-line noninvasive treatment strategies and involve a certain learning curve [67]. They are strictly not advisable in men with sickle cell disease or men who are on anticoagulants. Surgical treatment options like penile prosthesis are third-line treatment options that have to be performed by a urologist trained in the procedure [68]. The patient should also be clearly explained about the various risks, benefits, and outcomes of the procedure. Penile arterial or penile venous reconstructive surgeries are not recommended by the AUA and should not be offered as a therapeutic treatment option.

Conclusion

ED is complex in the sense that the natural progression of the disease can depend not only an individual's health, but also on various psychosocial factors that modify the severity of presentation. ED evaluation is best done with an in-depth medical and psychosexual history with limited diagnostic testing. All men with organic ED will invariably have some degree of psychogenic symptoms; thus strictly delineating the two in day-to-day clinical practice may not be always possible. Regardless of the cause, PDE-5 inhibitors are the mainstay of ED treatment. The clinician treating ED must combine psychosexual counselling in the context of the patient's religion, culture, and ethnicity and then treat the patient with right PDE-5 inhibitor depending on his preference. Following a structured evaluation and treatment process for ED will optimize successful return of erectile function from dysfunction.

References

1. NIH Consensus Development Panel on Impotence. Impotence: NIH consensus development panel on impotence. JAMA. 1993;270(1):83–90.
2. Lue TF, Giuliano F, Montorsi F, Rosen RC, Andersson KE, Althof S, Christ G, Hatzichristou D, Hirsch M, Kimoto Y, Lewis R. Summary of the recommendations on sexual dysfunctions in men. J Sex Med. 2004;1(1):6–23.
3. Aytac IA, McKinlay JB, Krane RJ. The likely worldwide increase in erectile dysfunction between 1995 and 2025 and some possible policy consequences. BJU Int. 1999;84:50–6.

4. Inman BA, Sauver JL, Jacobson DJ, McGree ME, Nehra A, Lieber MM, et al. A population-based, longitudinall study of erectile dysfunction and future coronary artery disease. Mayo Clin Proc. 2009;84(2):108–13.
5. Feldman HA, et al. Impotence and its medical and psychosocial correlates: results of the Massachusetts male aging study. J Urol. 1994;151:54.
6. Fugl-Meyer AR, Lodnert G, Branholm IB, Fugl-Meyer KS. On life satisfaction in male erectile dysfunction. Int J Impot Res. 1997;9:141–8.
7. Dong JY, Chang YH, Win Q. Erectile dysfunction and risk of cardiovascular disease: meta-analysis of prospective cohort studies. J Am Coll Cardiol. 2011;58(13):1378–85.
8. Baldwin K, Ginsberg P, Harkaway RC. Under-reporting of erectile dysfunction among men with unrelated urologic conditions. Int J Impot Res. 2003;15(2):87–9.
9. Koldny RC, Kahn CB, Goldstein HH, Barnett DM. Sexual function in diabetic men. Diabetes. 1973;23:306–9.
10. McCulloch DK, Campbell IW, Wu FC, Prescott RJ, Clarke BF. The prevalence of diabetic impotence. Diabetologia. 1980;18:279–83.
11. McCulloch DK, Young RJ, Prescott RJ, Campbell IW, Clarke BF. The natural history of impotence in diabetic men. Diabetologia. 1984;26:437–40.
12. Dunsmuir WD, Holmes SAV. The aetiology and management of erectile, ejaculatory and fertility problems in men with diabetes mellitus. Diabet Med. 1996;13:700–8.
13. Sáenz de Tejada I, Angulo J, Cellek S, González-Cadavid N, Heaton J, Pickard R, Simonsen U. Physiology of erectile function. J Sex Med. 2004;1(3):254–65.
14. Mullarkey CJ, Edelstein D, Brownlee M. Free radical generation by early glycation products: a mechanism for accelerated atherogenesis in diabetes. Biochem Biophys Res Commun. 1990;173:932–9.
15. Angulo J, Sanchez-Ferrer CF, Peiro C, Marin J, Rodriguez Mañas L. Impairment of endothelium- dependent relaxation by increasing percentages of glycosylated human hemoglobin. Possible mechanisms involved. Hypertension. 1996;28:583–92.
16. Pieper GM, Dondlinger LA. Plasma and vascular tissue arginine are decreased in diabetes: acute arginine supplementation restores endothelium dependent relaxation by augmenting cGMP production. J Pharmacol Exp Ther. 1997;283:684–91.
17. Bivalacqua TJ, Hellstrom WJG, Kadowitz PJ, Champion HC. Increased expression of arginase II in human diabetic corpus cavernosum: in diabetic associated erectile dysfunction. Biochem Biophys Res Commun. 2001;283:923–7.
18. Jackson G. Sexual dysfunction and diabetes. Int J Clin Pract. 2004;58(4):358–62.
19. Rendell MS, Rajfer J, Wicker PA, Smith MD. Sildenafil diabetes study group. Sildenafil for treatment of erectile dysfunction in men with diabetes: a randomized controlled trial. JAMA. 1999;281(5):421–6.
20. Lawes CM, Vander Hoorn S, Rodgers A. Global burden of blood-pressure-related disease. Lancet. 2008;371:1513–8.
21. Manolis A, Doumas M. Sexual dysfunction: the ‘prima ballerina’ of hypertension-related quality-of-life complications. J Hypertens. 2008;26:2074–84.
22. Doumas M, Douma S. Sexual dysfunction in essential hypertension: myth or reality? J Clin Hypertens. 2006;8:269–74.
23. Doumas M, Boutari C, Viigimaa M. Arterial hypertension and erectile dysfunction: an under-recognized duo. J Cardiol Pract. 2016;14(4):1–7.
24. Sharp RP, Gales BJ. Nebivolol versus other beta blockers in patients with hypertension and erectile dysfunction. Ther Adv Urol. 2017;9(2):59–63.
25. Chang HH, Chien CT, Hsu SP. The exploration of pathophysiologic mechanisms and therapeutic strategy for diabetes and hypertension related erectile dysfunction. Obes Rev. 2016;17:42.
26. Skeldon SC, Detsky AS, Goldenberg SL, Law MR. Erectile dysfunction and undiagnosed diabetes, hypertension, and hypercholesterolemia. Ann Fam Med. 2015;13(4):331–5.
27. Krane RJ, Goldstein I, Saenz de Tejada I. Impotence. N Engl J Med. 1989;321:1648–59.
28. Feldman HA, Goldstein I, Hatzchristou DG, Krane RJ, McKinlay JB. Impotence and its medical and social correlates: results of the Massachusetts Male Aging Study. J Urol. 1994;151:54–61.

29. Azadzoi KM, Goldstein I, Siroky MB, Traish AM, Krane RJ, Saenz de Tejada I. Mechanisms of ischemia-induced cavernosal smooth muscle relaxation in a rabbit model of vasculogenic erectile dysfunction. J Urol. 1998;160:2216–22.
30. Azadzoi KM, Saenz de Tejada I. Hypercholesterolemia impairs endothelium-dependent relaxation of rabbit corpus cavernosum smooth muscle. J Urol. 1991;146:238–40.
31. Elgendy AY, Elgendy IY, Mahmoud AN, Al-Ani M, Moussa M, Mahmoud A, Mojadidi MK, Anderson RD. Statin use in men and new onset of erectile dysfunction: a systematic review and meta-analysis. Am J Med. 2017;131(4):387–94.
32. Hodges LD, Kirby M, Solanki J, O'Donnell J, Brodie DA. The temporal relationship between erectile dysfunction and cardiovascular disease. Int J Clin Pract. 2007;61(12):2019–25.
33. Gupta BP, Murad MH, Clifton MM, Prokop L, Nehra A, Kopecky SL. The effect of lifestyle modification and cardiovascular risk factor reduction on erectile dysfunction: a systematic review and meta-analysis. Arch Intern Med. 2011;171(20):1797–803.
34. Greenstein A, Chen J, Miller H, Matzkin H, Villa Y, Braf Z. Does severity of ischemic coronary disease correlate with erectile function? Int J Impot Res. 1997;9(3):123–6.
35. Nehra A, Jackson G, Miner M, Billups KL, Burnett AL, Buvat J, Carson CC, Cunningham GR, Ganz P, Goldstein I, Guay AT. The Princeton III Consensus recommendations for the management of erectile dysfunction and cardiovascular disease. Mayo Clin Proc. 2012;87(8):766–78.
36. Qaseem A, Snow V, Denberg TD, et al. Hormonal testing and pharmacologic treatment of erectile dysfunction: a clinical practice guideline from the American college of physicians. Ann Intern Med. 2009;151(9):639–49.
37. Bhasin S, Cunningham GR, Hayes FJ, et al. Testosterone therapy in men with androgen deficiency syndromes: an Endocrine Society clinical practice guideline. J Clin Endocrinol Metab. 2010;95(6):2536–59.
38. Buvat J, Bou JG. Significance of hypogonadism in erectile dysfunction. World J Urol. 2006;24(6):657–67.
39. Blute M, Hakimian P, Kashanian J, Shteynshluyger A, Lee M, Shabsigh R. Erectile dysfunction and testosterone deficiency. Front Horm Res. 2009;37:108–22.
40. Thompson PD, Buchner D, Pina IL, et al. Exercise and physical activity in the prevention and treatment of atherosclerotic cardiovascular disease: a statement from the Council on Clinical Cardiology (Subcommittee on Exercise, Rehabilitation, and Prevention) and the Council on Nutrition, physical activity, and metabolism (Subcommittee on Physical activity). Circulation. 2003;107(24):3109–16.
41. Netz Y, Wu MJ, Becker BJ, Tenenbaum G. Physical activity and psychological well-being in advanced age: a meta-analysis of intervention studies. Psychol Aging. 2005;20(2):272–84.
42. Bassuk SS, Manson JE. Epidemiological evidence for the role of physical activity in reducing risk of type 2 diabetes and cardiovascular disease. J Appl Physiol. 2005;99(3):1193–204.
43. Hatzimouratidis K, Amar E, Eardley I, F. Giuliano, I. Moncada, A Salonia. Guidelines on male sexual dysfunction: erectile dysfunction and premature ejaculation. European Association of Urology website. http://uroweb.org/guideline/male-sexual-dysfunction/. Updated 2015. Eur Urol 2015;68(4):e78.
44. Rosen RC, Cappelleri JC, Gendrano Iii N. The international index of erectile function (IIEF): a state-of-the-science review. Int J Impot Res. 2002;14(4):226.
45. O'Leary MP, Fowler FJ, Lenderking WR, Barber B, Sagnier PP, Guess HA, Barry MJ. A brief male sexual function inventory for urology. Urology. 1995;46(5) 697–706.
46. Cappelleri JC, Rosen RC. The sexual health inventory for men (SHIM): a 5-year review of research and clinical experience. Int J Impot Res. 2005;17(4):307.
47. Montague DK, Jarow JP, Broderick GA, et al. For the erectile dysfunction guideline update panel. Chapter 1: the management of erectile dysfunction: an AUA update. J Urol. 2005;174(1):230–9.
48. Erectile Dysfunction Guideline Update Panel. The management of erectile dysfunction: an update. Baltimore, MD.: American Urological Association Education And Research, Inc.; 2005. http://www.ngc.gov/summary/summary.aspx?doc_id=10018&nbr=005332&string=erectile+AND+dysfunction. Accessed 9 July 2008.

49. Jardin A, Wagner G, Khoury S, et al. Recommendations of the 1st International. Consultation on Erectile Dysfunction. In: Jardin A, Wagner G, Khoury S, et al., editors. Erectile dysfunction. Plymouth: Health Publication Ltd; 2000. p. 711–26.
50. Esposito K, Giugliano F, Di Palo C, et al. Effect of lifestyle changes on erectile dysfunction in obese men: a randomized controlled trial. JAMA. 2004;291(24):2978–84.
51. Kostis JB, Jackson G, Rosen R, et al. Sexual dysfunction and cardiac risk (the second Princeton consensus conference). Am J Cardiol. 2005;96(2):313–21.
52. Rudd RM, Gellert AR, Studdy PR, Geddes DM. Inhibition of exercise-induced asthma by an orally absorbed mast cell stabilizer (M & B 22,948). Br J Dis Chest. 1983;77(1):78–86.
53. FDA approves oral therapy for erectile dysfunction. Am J Health Syst Pharm 1998;55(10):981, 984.
54. Carson CC, Burnett AL, Levine LA, Nehra A. The efficacy of sildenafil citrate (Viagra) in clinical populations: an update. Urology. 2002;60(2 Suppl 2):12–27.
55. Nichols DJ, Muirhead GJ, Harness JA. Pharmacokinetics of sildenafil after single oral doses in healthy male subjects: absolute bioavailability, food effects and dose proportionality. Br J Clin Pharmacol. 2002;53(Suppl 1):5S–12S.
56. Montorsi F, Verheyden B, Meuleman E, *et al.* Long-term safety and tolerability of tadalafil in the treatment of erectile dysfunction. Eur Urol 2004; 45(3):339-344; discussion 344-5.
57. Porst H, Padma-Nathan H, Giuliano F, et al. Efficacy of tadalafil for the treatment of erectile dysfunction at 24 and 36 hours after dosing: a randomized controlled trial. Urology. 2003;62(1):121–5; discussion 125-6
58. Doumas M, Lazaridis A, Katsiki N, Athyros V. PDE-5 inhibitors: clinical points. Curr Drug Targets. 2015;16(5):420–6.
59. Gresser U, Gleiter CH. Erectile dysfunction: comparison of efficacy and side effects of the PDE-5 inhibitors sildenafil, vardenafil and tadalafil-review of the literature. Eur J Med Res. 2002;7(10):435–46.
60. Thurtell MJ, Tomsak RL. Nonarteritic anterior ischemic optic neuropathy with PDE-5 inhibitors for erectile dysfunction. Int J Impot Res. 2008;20(6):537–43.
61. Azzouni F, Abu samra K. Are phosphodiesterase type 5 inhibitors associated with vision-threatening adverse events? A critical analysis and review of the literature. J Sex Med. 2011;8(10):2894–903.
62. Jannini EA, Isidori AM, Gravina GL, Endotrial study Group, et al. The ENDOTRIAL study: a spontaneous, open-label, randomized, multicenter, crossover study on the efficacy of sildenafil, tadalafil, and vardenafil in the treatment of erectile dysfunction. J Sex Med. 2009;6(9):2547–60.
63. von Keitz A, Rajfer J, Segal S, et al. A multicenter, randomized, double-blind, crossover study to evaluate patient preference between tadalafil and sildenafil. Eur Urol 2004; 45(4): 499-507; discussion 507-9.
64. Govier F, Potempa AJ, Kaufman J, Denne J, Kovalenko P, Ahuja S. A multicenter, randomized, double-blind, crossover study of patient preference for tadalafil 20 mg or sildenafil citrate 50 mg during initiation of treatment for erectile dysfunction. Clin Ther. 2003;69(11):2709–23.
65. Porst H, Rajfer J, Casabé A, Feldman R, Ralph D, Vieiralves LF, Esler A, Wolka AM, Klise SR. Long-term safety and efficacy of tadalafil 5 mg dosed once daily in men with erectile dysfunction. J Sex Med. 2008;5(9):2160–9.
66. Heidelbaugh JJ. Management of erectile dysfunction. Am Fam Physician. 2010;81(3):305–12.
67. Lewis RW, Witherington R. External vacuum therapy for erectile dysfunction: use and results. World J Urol. 1997;15(1):78–82.
68. Carson CC, Mulcahy JJ, Govier FE. Efficacy, safety and patient satisfaction outcomes of the AMS 700CX inflatable penile prosthesis: results of a long-term multicenter study. J Urol. 2000;164(2):376–80.

Ejaculatory Dysfunction

4

Pandiyan Natarajan and Shah Dupesh Khan

Introduction

While erectile dysfunction has received much-needed publicity, ejaculatory disorders are far more common and affect over 30% of men in the age group of 40–80 years [1–3]. Ejaculatory dysfunction encompasses a spectrum of conditions, namely, premature ejaculation (PE), delayed ejaculation (DE) and anejaculation (AE) that includes retrograde ejaculation (RE). Due to the lack of standardized definitions for these problems, the clinical diagnosis and management strategies for ejaculatory dysfunctions are somewhat arbitrary. Ejaculatory dysfunction not only affects a man's sexual health but can also interfere with his fertility when conception is desired, thereby resulting in significant distress for both partners [4].

Ejaculatory Physiology

Masters and Johnson's description of the human sexual response shows that there are four distinct phases, namely, excitement, plateau, orgasm and resolution [5]. The latency period is defined as the time period from the start of sexual stimulation to the point of ejaculation and this period can greatly vary among men depending on their sexuality, habits and other factors [6, 7]. Ejaculation in itself is a distinct emotional and/or cortical event, while erection is a spino-cerebral event [4]. This is also why ejaculation occurs without a degree of voluntary control during sleep-related erections (SRE). Orgasm on the other hand is not strictly a separate phenomenon and occurs and/or overlaps with ejaculation [8].

P. Natarajan (✉)
Department of Reproductive Medicine, Chettinad Super Speciality Hospital, Chettinad Academy of Research and Education, Chennai, India

S. D. Khan
The Metromale Clinic and Fertility Center, No 1, Crescent Park Street, T-Nagar, Chennai, India

© Springer Nature Singapore Pte Ltd. 2019

K. Gunasekaran, S. D. Khan (eds.), *Sexual Medicine*,
https://doi.org/10.1007/978-981-13-1226-7_4

Ejaculation strictly has two phases: (1) emission and (2) expulsion. During the emission phase, the peristaltic smooth muscle contraction of the seminal tract propels semen into the posterior urethra via the ejaculatory duct. This process is mediated by the sympathetic nerves (T10 to L2). The ejection phase controlled by somatic nerves (S2–S4) involves the pulsatile contractions of the pelvic floor muscles and the bulbocavernosus along with concomitant relaxation of the external urinary sphincter. There is some limited degree of voluntary control in the ejection phase. In parallel the bladder neck also closes to prevent retrograde flow along with rhythmic contractions of the pelvic floor muscles that then drives the spermatozoa suspended in the seminal fluid forward. Orgasm perceived as a pleasurable experience results from the cognitive processing of the pudendal nerve stimuli due to increased pressure in the posterior aspect of the urethra along with sensory stimuli from the accessory sex organs and/or contraction of the urethral bulb. Both orgasm and ejaculations are coordinated by separate neural mechanisms and can also occur separately from one another. Animal studies have clearly shown the importance of spinal ejaculatory center in integrating signals from both central and peripheral stimuli and coordinating the ejaculatory reflex through the pelvi-perineal musculature. Mechanism to inhibit ejaculation is located at higher centers in the brain such as the posterodorsal amygdaloid nucleus, the posteromedial nucleus of the stria terminalis and the parvocellualar nuclei of the thalamus. These higher centers control and modulate the final output from all the ejaculatory stimuli [8–13].

Neurotransmitters in Ejaculation

Neurotransmitters play an important role in the control ejaculation. Of cardinal importance are dopamine and serotonin. Other neurotransmitters like acetylcholine, oxytocin, GABA, norepinephrine and nitric oxide are also involved in coordination of the complex ejaculatory process and are of secondary importance [9, 10]. Defining the exact role of each of the neurotransmitters is difficult due to the multifactorial and complex nature of ejaculation.

Dopamine promotes ejaculation by its action on D2 receptors. Dopamine levels rise in the region of the hypothalamus, and dopamine signalling has been implicated in both arousal and orgasm. Rat studies have also shown that dopamine levels increase steadily through intercourse until the point of ejaculation [10]. Serotonin is inhibitory and exhibits its effects by its action on 5HT2C and 5HT1A receptors [14]. Serotonin is the most well-studied neurotransmitter in the neurophysiology of ejaculation. Numerous seminal animal studies have shown that 5HT2C receptor stimulation is associated with a delay in ejaculation and longer latency time of ejaculation, while 5HT1A stimulation results in shorter latency time [14, 15]. The balance between receptor stimulation and inhibition may play a role in establishing a latency time point that could vary depending on the individual's sexuality, age, illness, relationship and a host of other factors. Animal studies have also suggested that oxytocin may have an important role to play in the ejaculatory process [16]. An excess of oxytocin is associated with early ejaculation and an oxytocin deficiency is associated with delayed ejaculation [16, 17].

Premature Ejaculation

Definition and Aetiology

Premature ejaculation (PE) affects over 39% of men in the general community and data suggests that PE is the most common male sexual disorder [17]. But a certain degree of disparity exists between reported data, since the definition of PE in itself is poorly validated and/or inconsistent [18].

More importantly, PE is a self-reported symptom that occurs due to an individual distress. Thus getting exact prevalence data is difficult. The other problem is also the inconsistency of presenting symptoms.

Most previous definitions of PE are based on stopwatch studies that estimate the intravaginal ejaculation latency time (IELT), which is the time interval measured from the point of penetration till ejaculation [6]. But this data is highly inaccurate as not only does the IELT time vary between countries and study participants, but also the data is mostly based on studies done in the Western population.

The definition of PE has had numerous revisions. The first definition of PE was by Masters and Johnson; PE was defined by "the inability of a man to delay ejaculation long enough for his partner to reach orgasm in 50% of intercourse attempts" [5]. This definition was however confounded by the women's ability to reach climax.

Subsequent professional society and individual definition were more authority based rather than evidence based. The American Psychiatric Association (APA) definition was revised twice to address its vague nature and lack of standardized operational criteria. Following mounting pressure from the FDA and other regulators, the International Society of Sexual Medicine (ISSM) convened a meeting twice and a defined PE in 2008 finally as when ejaculation occurs within 1 min before or after penetration with a complete lack of control and also causing distress to one or both partners [19].

PE can be classified as either being lifelong or acquired and/or variable or subjective. The aetiology of lifelong PE is different compared to acquired PE [20, 21]. Men facing lifelong PE may have hyposensitivity at the level of the 5HT2C or hypersensitivity of the 5HT1A receptors. Genetic variations may contribute and these problems are frequently amplified by psychological factors [22]. Acquired PE on the one hand can be due to a comorbid ED or prostatitis. Many men with ED also suffer from PE; men with ED may rush through intercourse out of fear of losing erection leading to PE. These effects may also be compounded by their performance anxiety [23]. Thyroid disorders and relationship and/or psychological problems can also lead to acquired PE [24, 25].

While anxiety has been frequently stated among medical communities as a cause of PE, there is insufficient data to support the same. Authors have suggested that anxiety-induced activation of the sympathetic nervous system reduces the threshold for ejaculation leading to PE. Acquired PE can also be caused by hypoactive sexual desire and also by female sexual dysfunctions [8]. Variable PE is considered more of a normal variation in sexual performance and occurs in situational context. Subjective PE is when the patient has a false preconceived notion that he has PE [8].

Diagnosis and Treatment

PE is best diagnosed by an in-depth psychosexual history-taking session. Table 4.1 outlines a few questions that can be asked by the clinician to help establish a diagnosis. A thorough medical history to check for other systemic health conditions should also be elicited. While it is best to have the partner involved in the sexual history-taking session, for PE this is not mandatory until or unless the patient's sexual history reveals a problem in the partner [26].

In general no specific investigations are recommended for men with PE. A physical exam is mandatory though.

Treatment of PE usually involves psychosexual counselling and/or pharmacotherapy. Integrated treatment strategies usually work best. In men with situational and/or subjective PE, a simple session of psychosexual education will correct their understanding of the problem [27, 28].

Psychosexual based behavioural therapies for PE as an isolated treatment modality include the popularly used "stop-start" manoeuvre and its modification the "squeeze-pinch technique". The advantage of these techniques is that they are free from side effects and also have greater patient acceptability, with no associated pain [29, 30]. These techniques are also highly specific to the problem in hand. The disadvantages are that there is a learning curve to the techniques and these techniques also lack immediacy and also require partner co-operation. The long-term efficacy of these techniques is unknown. Few other techniques like mental imagery, utilizing different sex positions, may increase the timing of ejaculation [31, 32].

Pharmacological treatment of PE includes the use of topical anaesthetics as well as selective serotonin reuptake inhibitors (SSRI). Topical local anaesthetics like lignocaine and/or prilocaine cream are moderately efficacious in PE, but unless a condom is used they can cause vaginal numbness and also penile hypoanaesthesia

Table 4.1 Questions to assess PE

Questions to assess PE
1. How much time do you last from the time you penetrate till ejaculation?
2. Are you able to control your ejaculation?
3. When did you first experience this symptom? Do you feel upset by it?
4. Does your partner feel upset by it?
5. How is your erection? Do you have difficulties in sustaining your erection?
6. Is PE affecting your relationship?
7. Have you taken any medications for this problem?
8. Does your partner complain of any specific difficulty like pain or lack of interest in sex?

[33–37]. A study suggested that the use of a metered-dose aerosol spray containing lidocaine and prilocaine produced a 2.4-fold increase in IELT and ejaculatory control [38].

Dapoxetine, a short-acting SSRI, has received regulatory approval for the on-demand treatment of PE [39–42]. The usual dose varies between 30 and 50 mg, taken 2 h before intercourse. These drugs work by blocking the reuptake of serotonin in the synaptic cleft of both the peripheral and central serotonergic neurons, thereby resulting in enhanced 5HT neurotransmission [41, 42]. When taken 1–2 h on demand, a modest increase in the IELT time ranging from 2.5- to 3.0-fold is seen. However, as compared to on-demand dosing, daily dosing has significantly better effects in delaying ejaculation as well as reducing symptoms of interpersonal distress [43]. More controlled studies though are required to find out which is better.

Different SSRIs in different dosages have been used in PE; they are namely paroxetine 10–40 mg, sertraline 50–200 mg, citalopram 20–40 mg, and fluoxetine 20–40 mg. These doses are usually well tolerated and safe. While all of them delay ejaculation, a recent meta-analysis suggested that paroxetine exerted the strongest delay in ejaculation exerting a delay of over 8.8-fold over baseline [43–45]. However, due to the lack of regulatory approval, these drugs are only prescribed off label. On a daily dosing protocol ejaculation delay usually occurs within 5–10 days of starting a treatment, but full therapeutic benefits usually occur after 2 or 3 weeks. ED is the reported side effect but it is uncommon [21].

Patients should be specifically told not to suddenly discontinue the medication as it may lead to SSRI withdrawal syndrome. PDE-5 inhibitors have been frequently used along with SSRIs in the treatment of PE; numerous systematic reviews have failed to show any benefit. PDE-5s can be used along with SSRIs when PE presents itself with comorbid ED [21].

Delayed Ejaculation and Anejaculation

Definition and Aetiology

Delayed ejaculation (DE) is the least studied and most poorly understood sexual dysfunction. The reported prevalence of DE is 1–4% [46, 47]. The WHO defines DE as the persistent difficulty or delay or complete inability to attain an orgasm after sufficient sexual stimulation leading to personal distress [48]. A well-defined operationalized criteria for DE does not exist. Assuming that most men would ejaculate in the range of 5–10 min post-penetration, a clinician can make a diagnosis of DE when men have ejaculatory latencies beyond 20 or 30 min (twice the standard deviation of the measured IELT) [6]. Anejaculation (AE) on the other hand can be orgasmic or anorgasmic. The commonest cause of orgasmic AE is retrograde ejaculation (RE) [4]. In RE semen is propelled in a retrograde fashion towards the bladder during an orgasm, rather than antegrade.

A man can also have DE if he ceases sexual activity due to exhaustion or distress. DE is of two types: primary (lifelong) or secondary (acquired). The strict definition and/or delineation of DE into primary and secondary subtypes is difficult due to numerous external factors that play a role in causing a dysfunction. Waldinger's study on IELT found a natural variation ranging from 33 s to 44 min, and this value differed greatly across the study population [6]. This study combined with highly variable central sensitivity to both serotonin and dopamine is suggestive of DE that could be physiological rather than pathological (a type of DE that has no specific aetiology).

Congenital DE can be caused by certain malformations like Wolffian duct abnormalities, Mullerian duct remnants and prune belly syndrome [49, 50]. Although these conditions are rare, DE frequently presents with psychological and/or behavioural components. Orthodox beliefs on "spilling the seed" outside of intercourse apart from the purpose of conception may lead to a poorer probability of achieving an orgasm outside intercourse [51]. Another common cause of DE is autosexual orientation where there is a preference to masturbation over sexual intercourse. This condition is termed as "idiosyncratic masturbation". Studies suggest that men with idiosyncratic masturbation feel that they get better arousal subjectively and are able to reach their ejaculatory threshold more quickly via masturbation as when compared to penetrative intercourse [52].

Post-surgical causes of acquired DE and/or AE usually include surgeries done to the prostate, penile cancer treatment by means of partial penectomy and/or testicular cancer treatment. Surgeries that compromise the bladder neck, such as transurethral incision of the prostate, are invariably associated with RE. RE is seen in over 45% of such patients undergoing the procedure [53–56].

Common endocrine causes of DE seen in clinical practice include hypothyroidism, hypogonadism and hyperprolactinaemia. With the widespread use of SSRIs, sexual dysfunction is a well-reported side effect after prolonged drug use. DE comprises a significant portion of these sexual dysfunctions associated with SSRI use [57, 58]. Neurogenic causes of DE commonly reported include spinal cord injury, diabetes and multiple sclerosis. Men with lower motor neuron lesions do retain ejaculatory ability, but the bigger issue is erectile dysfunction and RE especially seen in men with complete spinal cord injury [59, 60]. Table 4.2 summarizes the various known causes of DE and AE.

Diagnosis and Treatment

As is with other sexual dysfunctions, a clear pathophysiology for DE is lacking and DE should be considered as an interaction between organic and psychogenic factors [61]. Both organic and psychogenic factors work in tandem and affect a man's ejaculatory latency throughout his life. The treatment of DE should encompass a thorough understanding and assessment of these interactions.

DE evaluation starts with a thorough medical history and/or psychosexual history to rule out conditions listed in Table 4.2. Next specific history should focus on (1) age of first ejaculation, (2) masturbatory practices and also (3) ascertaining whether DE occurs with partnered sex or during masturbation only. Lifelong DE will present with global sexual dysfunction in both masturbation and partnered

Table 4.2 Various causes of DE and AE

Causes of DE and AE
Congenital and anatomical causes
Wolffian duct abnormality
Prune belly syndrome
Mullerian duct cyst
Transurethral resection of prostate (TURP)
Infective causes
Urethritis
Genitourinary TB
Neurogenic causes
Diabetes mellitus
Spinal cord injuries
Prostate surgeries
Bilateral sympathectomy
Multiple sclerosis
Endocrine causes
Hyperprolactinaemia
Hypogonadism
Hypothyroidism
Medication
Thiazide diuretics
Tricyclic antidepressants and SSRIs
Alcohol abuse
Alpha-methyldopa
Antiandrogens
Phenothiazines
Psychological causes
Relationship and life stress
Negative sex beliefs
Idiosyncratic masturbatory preferences
Chronic conditions
Increasing age
Vascular disease
Chronic pain due to other illnesses

intercourse. It is also important to ascertain information about the practices or sexual preferences of the individual that would allow him to reach the ejaculatory threshold. In addition, the patient's partner relationship should also be ascertained. The presence of a female sexual dysfunction should be ruled out.

If the patient has a small-volume ejaculate or no ejaculate and if fertility is the objective, the clinician must differentiate ejaculatory duct obstruction from congenital bilateral absence of the vasa deferentia (CBAVD). Both forms are associated with small-volume ejaculate and azoospermia [62–65]. A physical exam of the testes, epididymis and palpation of the vasa on both sides combined with an ultrasound imaging usually helps in making a diagnosis [65]. The presence of spermatozoa in the first void urine after orgasmic anejaculation is suggestive of retrograde ejaculation [65].

Other investigations like blood sugars, hormonal assessment, lipid profile and appropriate imaging studies to rule out organic causes of DE are usually recommended. The primary objective of history taking and examination in DE is to rule out all probable organic causes of DE before concluding that the DE is psychogenic in nature.

Treatment for DE can be broadly classified into two types—psychological and pharmacotherapy. Depending on the individual's receptiveness to counselling, psychotherapy is usually the first-line treatment for DE [66]. While there are numerous psychotherapeutic strategies recommended for DE, none of them have been properly evaluated in terms of efficacy through large-scale studies. "Masturbation retraining" and "sensate focus" exercises are effective psychotherapeutic treatment strategies for DE [67–69].

Briefly, the objective of these interventions is to first destigmatize the dysfunction and remove the anxiety associated with "ejaculation on demand". First, the couples are given sex education. The man is then taught to identify pleasurable stimulation that increases his general ability to reach orgasm quicker through self-stimulation techniques. In the next step, the anorgasmia faced by the man should then be "non-stigmatized". This is achieved by allowing the man to ejaculate in a non-coital manner during partnered sex. This can be tried by incorporating different coital positions and also visualizing fantasies that can help the man improve his subjective arousal.

Next, the partner should then try to bring the male partner close to the brink of orgasm and then allow the penis to be inserted into the vagina, as this will break the mental barrier associated with partnered sexual intercourse. Subsequently, intravaginal ejaculation is then achieved. The couple is also taught to communicate specific sexual preferences to one another so that these needs can also be fulfilled in the act.

The most important clinical challenge with DE treatments is to ensure that the female partner does not feel mechanistic, due to the steps involved. The partner's sexual need should also be met. Maintaining a good couple rapport and therapeutic alliance is key. Masters and Johnson found a very low failure rate less than 18% when they used the strategies of sensate focus and intercourse modification combined with vigorous penile stimulation [5].

Drug treatment for DE/AE has had limited success. None of the drugs have regulatory approval for the treatment of DE and/or AE. Most drugs for DE are considered experimental at best and also carry significant side effects. Drugs like amantadine and cyproheptadine have been used to reverse anorgasmia induced by SSRIs. Success has been reported anecdotally. In one study on patients with spinal cord injury (SCI) and AE, daily midodrine given in doses of 7.5–12 mg helped only 50% of study participants achieve ejaculation. These drugs also cause side effects like restlessness, elevated BP and sedation which may further reduce the efficacy of treatments [70–73].

Due to the lack of randomized controlled studies, pharmacotherapy cannot be recommended for the first-line management of AE and/or DE. The scenario is different with RE though.

For RE, the aim of medical therapy is to increase sympathetic tone in the bladder neck and thus achieve antegrade ejaculation [74]. Different types and combination of medications like antihistamines, anticholinergics and alpha 1 agonists have been used. Success rates in the aforementioned medications are highly variable in terms of achieving an antegrade ejaculation.

In an RCT that involved diabetic patients with RE, the combination use of pseudoephedrine 120 mg and imipramine 25 mg twice daily helped achieve antegrade ejaculation in 62% of study participants as compared to 0% in the placebo group [75]. While there is a limited role of medical therapy in RE, where a clinical diagnosis is established, drug treatment for RE may be tried.

Where medical therapy fails and when fertility is the primary objective, the next line of treatment for RE is using a technique of sperm retrieval from the bladder [76]; here the patient is first asked to void and empty the bladder. After this, he can then proceed to collect a semen sample by masturbation; after masturbation the patient should immediately void the residual urine into a sterile container that contains physiological medium for sperm harvesting. Sperm harvested this way can then be used for fertility treatments. When this technique fails, a penile vibrostimulator (PVS) can be used. The final line of management would be resorting to use electroejaculation (EEJ) and/or direct sperm retrieval from the testis [77]. In men with spinal cord injury, prostatic massage (PM) may help in achieving antegrade ejaculation [78].

Conclusion

PE and DE significantly impair the quality of life for both the partner and the afflicted individual. The importance of a proper history taking and physical exam cannot be stressed enough. All potential organic causes of ejaculatory dysfunctions must be ruled out before coming to a conclusion. While psychotherapies and/or sex education have an important role to play in managing ejaculatory dysfunctions, the use of pharmacotherapy cannot be ignored. In the case of PE, SSRIs along with psychosexual therapies can definitely be used while in case of DE and/or RE medications have a limited role to play. Where fertility is the primary objective of the patient, efforts should be made to harvest sperm for relevant fertility-based treatments. In these scenarios, alternate methods of inducing an antegrade ejaculation with the penile vibrostimulator (PVS) and/or electroejaculation (EEJ) can be tried with medications.

References

1. Laumann E, Nicolosi A, Glasser D, Paik A, Gingell C, Moreira E, Wang T. Sexual problems among women and men aged 40–80 y: prevalence and correlates identified in the global study of sexual attitudes and behaviors. Int J Impot Res. 2005;17:39–57.
2. Nicolosi A, Laumann EO, Glasser DB, Moreira ED Jr, Paik A, Gingell C. Sexual behavior and sexual dysfunctions after age 40: the global study of sexual attitudes and behaviors. Urology. 2004;64:991–7.
3. Montorsi F. Prevalence of premature ejaculation: a global and regional perspective. J Sex Med. 2005;2(suppl 2):96–102.

4. Khan SD, Pandiyan N. Ejaculatory dysfunction—a mini review. Adv Sex Med. 2015;5:39–42.
5. Masters WH, Johnson VE. Reproductive biology research foundation (US). Human sexual response. 1st ed. Boston: Little, Brown; 1966.
6. Waldinger MD, Quinn P, Dilleen M, Mundayat R, Schweitzer DH, Boolell M. A multinational population survey of intravaginal ejaculation latency time. J Sex Med. 2005;2:492–7.
7. Waldinger M, Zwinderman A, Olivier B, Schweitzer D. Proposal for a definition of lifelong premature ejaculation based on epidemiological stopwatch data. J Sex Med. 2005;2:498–507.
8. Donatucci CF. Etiology of ejaculation and pathophysiology of premature ejaculation. J Sex Med. 2006;3(4 suppl):303–8.
9. Kimura Y, Kisaki N, Sakurada S, Tadano T. On the brain monoaminergic systems relating to ejaculation. II. Brain serotonin and ejaculation. Andrologia. 1977;9:50–4.
10. Hull EM, Du J, Lorrain DS, Matuszewich L. Extracellular dopamine in the medial preoptic area: implications for sexual motivation and hormonal control of copulation. J Neurosci. 1995;15:7465–71.
11. Peroutka SJ, Snyder SH. Multiple serotonin receptors: differential binding of [3H]5-hydroxytryptamine, [3H]lysergic acid diethylamide and [3H]spiroperidol. Mol Pharmacol. 1979;16:687–99.
12. Ahlenius SLK, Svensson L, Hjorth S, Carlsson A, Lindberg P, Wikström H, Sanchez D, Arvidsson LE, Hacksell U, Nilsson JL. Effects of a new type of 5-HT receptor agonist on male rat sexual behavior. Pharmacol Biochem Behav. 1981;15:785–92.
13. Meisel RL, Sachs BD. The physiology of male sexual behavior. In: Knobil E, Neill JD, editors. The physiology of reproduction. 3rd ed. New York: Raven Press; 2005. p. 3–105.
14. Olivier B, van Oorschot R, Waldinger MD. Serotonin, serotenergic receptors, selective serotonin reuptake inhibitors and sexual behaviour. Int Clin Psychopharmacol. 1998;13(suppl 6):S9–S14.
15. Mos J, Mollet I, Tolbloom JT, et al. A comparison of the effects of different serotonin reuptake blockers on sexual behaviour of the male rat. Eur Neuropsychopharmacol. 1999;9:123–35.
16. Argiolas A, Melis MR. The role of oxytocin and the paraventricular nucleus in the sexual behaviour of male mammals. Physiol Behav. 2004;83:309–17.
17. Andersson KE. Pharmacology of penile erection. Pharmacol Rev. 2001;53:417–50.
18. Patrick DL, Althof SE, Pryor JL, Rosen R, Rowland DL, Ho KF, et al. Premature ejaculation: an observational study of men and their partners. J Sex Med. 2005;2:58–367.
19. McMahon CG, Althof SE, Waldinger MD, et al. An evidence-based definition of lifelong premature ejaculation: report of the International Society for Sexual Medicine (ISSM) ad hoc committee for the definition of premature ejaculation. J Sex Med. 2008;5:1590–606.
20. Schapiro B. Premature ejaculation, a review of 1130 cases. J Urol. 1943;50:374–9.
21. Waldinger MD. Premature ejaculation: definition and drug treatment. Drugs. 2007;67:547–68.
22. Janssen PKC, Bakker SC, Rethelyi J, Zwinderman AH, Touw DJ, Olivier B, et al. Serotonin transporter promoter region (5-HTTLPR) polymorphism is associated with the intravaginal ejaculation latency time in Dutch men with lifelong premature ejaculation. J Sex Med. 2009;6:276–84. Early-on-line.
23. Corona G, Petrone L, Mannucci E, Jannini EA, Mansani R, Magini A, et al. Psycho-biological correlates of rapid ejaculation in patients attending an andrologic unit for sexual dysfunctions. Eur Urol. 2004;46:615–22.
24. Sharlip ID. Guidelines for the diagnosis and management of premature ejaculation. J Sex Med. 2006;3(4 suppl):309–17.
25. Atkinson RL, Dahms WT, Fisher DA, Nichols AL. Occult thyroid disease in an elderly hospitalized population. J Gerontol. 1978;33:372–6.
26. Althof SE, Abdo CH, Dean J, Hackett G, McCabe M, McMahon CG, Rosen RC, Sadovsky R, Waldinger M, Becher E, Broderick GA, Buvat J, Goldstein I, El-Meliegy AI, Giuliano F, Hellstrom WJ, Incrocci L, Jannini EA, Park K, Parish S, Porst H, Rowland D, Segraves R, Sharlip I, Simonelli C, Tan HM. International Society for Sexual Medicine. International Society for Sexual Medicine's guidelines for the diagnosis and treatment of premature ejaculation. J Sex Med. 2010;7:2947–69.

27. McMahon CG. The etiology and management of premature ejaculation. Nat Clin Pract Urol. 2005;2:426–33.
28. Jannini EA, Lenzi A, Wagner G. Behavioural therapy and counselling. In: Schill WB, Comhaire FH, Hargreave TB, editors. Andrology for the clinician. Berlin: Springer; 2006. p. 598–607.
29. McCarthy B. Cognitive-behavioral strategies and techniques in the treatment of early ejaculation. In: Leiblum SR, Rosen RC, editors. Principles and practice of sex therapy: update for the 90s. New York: Guilford Press; 1990. p. 141–67.
30. Metz M, McCarthy B. Coping with premature ejaculation: how to overcome PE, please your partner and have great sex. Oakland, CA: New Harbinber Publications; 2003.
31. Zilbergeld B. The new male sexuality. New York: Bantam; 1992.
32. Lowe JC, Mikulas WL. Use of written material in learning self-control of premature ejaculation. Psychol Rep. 1975;37:295–8.
33. Berkovitch M, Keresteci AG, Koren G. Efficacy of prilocaine-lidocaine cream in the treatment of premature ejaculation. J Urol. 1995;154:1360–1.
34. Xin ZC, Choi YD, Lee SH, Choi HK. Efficacy of a topical agent SS-cream in the treatment of premature ejaculation: preliminary clinical studies. Yonsei Med J. 1997;38:91–5.
35. Busato W, Galindo CC. Topical anaesthetic use for treating premature ejaculation: a double-blind, randomized, placebo controlled study. BJU Int. 2004;93:1018–21.
36. Choi H, Xin ZC, Cho IR. The local therapeutic effect of SS-cream on premature ejaculation. Korean J Androl Soc. 1993;11:99–106.
37. Atikeler MK, Gecit I, Senol FA. Optimum usage of prilocaine-lidocaine cream in premature ejaculation. Andrologia. 2002;34:356–9.
38. Dinsmore WW, Hackett G, Goldmeier D, et al. Topical eutectic mixture for premature ejaculation (TEMPE): a novel aerosol-delivery form of lidocaine-prilocaine for treating premature ejaculation. BJU Int. 2007;99(2):369–75.
39. Hellstrom WJ, Althof S, Gittelman M, et al. Dapoxetine for the treatment of men with premature ejaculation (PE): dose finding analysis. J Urol. 2005;173:238; abstract 877
40. Buvat J, Tesfaye F, Rothman M, Rivas DA, Giuliano F. Dapoxetine for the treatment of premature ejaculation: results from a randomized, double-blind, placebo-controlled phase 3 trial in 22 countries. Eur Urol. 2009;55:957–67.
41. Pryor JL, Althof SE, Steidle C, et al. Efficacy and tolerability of dapoxetine in treatment of premature ejaculation: an integrated analysis of two double-blind, randomised controlled trials. Lancet. 2006;368:929–37.
42. McMahon C, Kim S, Park N, et al. Treatment of premature ejaculation in the Asia-Pacific region: results from a phase iii double-blind, parallel-group study of dapoxetine. J Sex Med. 2010;7:256–68.
43. Waldinger M. Towards evidenced based drug treatment research on premature ejaculation: a critical evaluation of methodology. J Impot Res. 2003;15:309–13.
44. Haensel SM, Klem TM, Hop WC, Slob AK. Fluoxetine and premature ejaculation a double-blind, crossover, placebocontrolled study. J Clin Psychopharmacol. 1998;18:72–7.
45. Biri H, Isen K, Sinik Z, Onaran M, Kupeli B, Bozkirli I. Sertraline in the treatment of premature ejaculation: a double-blind placebo controlled study. Int Urol Nephrol. 1998;30:611–5.
46. Jannini E, Lenzi A. Ejaculatory disorders: epidemiology and current approaches to definition, classification and subtyping. World J Urol. 2005;23:68–75.
47. Jern P, Santtila P, Witting K, Alanko K, Harlaar N, Johansson A, Sandnabba K. Premature and delayed ejaculation: genetic and environmental effects in a population based sample of Finnish twins. J Sex Med. 2007;4:1739–49.
48. McMahon C, Abdo C, Incrocci L, Perelman M, Rowland D, Waldinger M, Xin Z. Disorders of orgasm and ejaculation in men. J Sex Med. 2004;1:58–65.
49. Harley LM, Chen Y, Rattner WH. Prune belly syndrome. J Urol. 1972;108:174–6.
50. Zugor V, Schott G, Labanaris A. The prune belly syndrome: urological aspects and long-term outcomes of a rare disease. Pediatr Rep. 2012;4:e20.
51. Rowland D, McMahon C, Abdo C, Chen J, Jannini E, Waldinger M, Ahn T. Disorders of orgasm and ejaculation in men. J Sex Med. 2010;7(Pt 2):1668–86.

52. Perelman MA, Rowland DL. Retarded ejaculation. World J Urol. 2006;24:645–52.
53. Pettus J, Carver B, Masterson T, Stasi J, Sheinfeld J. Preservation of ejaculation in patients undergoing nerve-sparing postchemotherapy retroperitoneal lymph node dissection for metastatic testicular cancer. Urology. 2009;73:328.
54. Coogan C, Hejase M, Wahle G, Foster R, Rowland R, Bihrle R, Donohue J. Nerve sparing post-chemotherapy retroperitoneal lymph node dissection for advanced testicular cancer. J Urol. 1996;156:1656–8.
55. Romero F, Romero K, Mattos M, Garcia C, Fernandes R, Perez M. Sexual function after partial penectomy for penile cancer. Urology. 2005;66:1292–5.
56. Rosen R, Altwein J, Boyle P, Kirby R, Lukacs B, Meuleman E, Giuliano F. Lower urinary tract symptoms and male sexual dysfunction: the multinational survey of the aging male (MSAM-7). Eur Urol. 2003;44:637–49.
57. Carani C, Isidori A, Granata A, Carosa E, Maggi M, Lenzi A, Jannini E. Multicenter study on the prevalence of sexual symptoms in male hypo- and hyperthyroid patients. J Clin Endocrinol Metab. 2005;90:6472–9.
58. Corona G, Mannucci E, Petrone L, Fisher A, Balercia G, De Scisciolo G, Maggi M. Psychobiological correlates of delayed ejaculation in male patients with sexual dysfunctions. J Androl. 2006;27:453–8.
59. Bors E, Comarr AE. Neurological disturbances of sexual function with special reference to 529 patients with spinal cord injury. Urol Surv. 1960;10:191–221.
60. Comarr AE. Sexual function among patients with spinal cord injury. Urol Int. 1970;25:134–68.
61. Hendry WF, Altof SE, Benson GS, et al. Male orgasmic and ejaculatory disorders. In: Jardin A, Wagner G, Khoury S, Giuliano F, Padma-Hathan H, Rosen R, editors. Erectile dysfunction. Paris: Health Publication, Ltd. Distributed by Plymbridge, Plymouth; 2000. p. 477–506.
62. Schlegel PN, Shin D, Goldstein M. Urogenital anomalies in men with congenital absence of the vas deferens. J Urol. 1996;155:1644–8.
63. Mickle J, Milunsky A, Amos JA, Oates RD. Congenital unilateral absence of the vas deferens: a heterogeneous disorder with two distinct subpopulations based upon aetiology and mutational status of the cystic fibrosis gene. Hum Reprod. 1995;10:1728–35.
64. McCarthy B. Strategies and techniques for the treatment of ejaculatory inhibition. J Sex Ed Ther. 1981;7:20–3.
65. Pandiyan N, Khan SD. A clinical approach to male infertility. In: Gunasekaran K, Pandiyan N, editors. Male infertility. New Delhi: Springer; 2017.
66. McMahon CG, Waldinger M, Rowland DL, et al. Ejaculatory disorders. In: Porst H, Buvat J, editors. Standard practice in sexual medicine. Oxford: Blackwell Publishing; 2006. p. 188–209.
67. Kaplan H. The evaluation of sexual disorders: psychological and medical aspects. New York: Brunner/Mazel; 1995.
68. Barbach LG. For yourself: a guide to female orgasmic response. New York: Doubleday; 1974.
69. Heiman JR, Meston CM. Empirically validated treatment for sexual dysfunction. Annu Rev Sex Res. 1997;8:148–94.
70. McCormick S, Olin J, Brotman AW. Reversal of fluoxetine induced anorgasmia by cyproheptadine in two patients. J Clin Psychiatry. 1990;51:383–4.
71. Ashton K, Hamer R, Rosen R. Serotonin reuptake inhibitor induced sexual dysfunction and its treatment: a large-scale retrospective study of 596 psychiatric outpatients. J Sex Marital Ther. 1997;23:165–75.
72. Feder R. Reversal of antidepressant activity of fluoxetine by cyproheptadine in three patients. J Clin Psychiatry. 1991;52:163–4.
73. Lauerma H. Successful treatment of citalopram-induced anorgasmia by cyproheptadine. Acta Psychiatr Scand. 1996;93:69–70.
74. Kamischke A, Nieschlag E. Treatment of retrograde ejaculation and anejaculation. Hum Reprod Update. 1999;5(5):448–74.
75. Safarinejad MR. Midodrine for the treatment of organic anejaculation but not spinal cord injury: a prospective randomized placebo-controlled double-blind clinical study. Int J Impot Res. 2009;21(4):213–20.

76. Pandiyan N, Pandiyan R, Muthiah S, Moorthy PS, Kanakaraj S. Sperm retrieval from the bladder-A simple non-invasive technique. Fertil Steril. 1998;70:1187.
77. Brackett NL, Ibrahim E, Iremashvili V, Aballa TC, Lynne CM. Treatment for ejaculatory dysfunction in men with spinal cord injury: an 18-year single center experience. J Urol. 2010;183(6):2304–8.
78. Arafa MM, Zohdy WA, Shamloul R. Prostatic massage: a simple method of semen retrieval in men with spinal cord injury. Int J Androl. 2007;30(3):170–3.

Sexual Dysfunction and Infertility

5

Pandiyan Natarajan and Shah Dupesh Khan

"Sex is a natural function.
You cannot make it happen, but you can teach people
to let it happen".

William H. Masters

Introduction

Human sexuality is an enigma, regulated by a byzantine interplay between vascular, endocrine, and neurological systems. Both fertility and sexuality share the same anatomical structures, and a problem in one center may lead to a problem in another. They have independent but interdependent physiological pathways. Human sexuality is woven into the very fabric of human existence; for some, sexual interest and encounters may be brief, and for others it may lead to a start of new relationship, culminating in the start of a new family and reproduction [1]. Sexuality is also influenced by an individual's societal, religious, personal, and cultural beliefs and undergoes significant change with the health status of the concerned individual. Each partner of a couple brings in diverse sexual needs, attitudes, and beliefs; hence a breakdown in any one of these areas ultimately would result in sexual dysfunction.

Giving a comprehensive update on all management strategies for the various sexual dysfunctions in an infertility setting is beyond the scope of this review, but

P. Natarajan
Department of Reproductive Medicine, Chettinad Super Speciality Hospital,
Chettinad Academy of Research and Education, Chennai, India

S. D. Khan (✉)
The Metromale Clinic and Fertility Center,
No 1, Crescent Park Street, T-Nagar, Chennai, India

© Springer Nature Singapore Pte Ltd. 2019

K. Gunasekaran, S. D. Khan (eds.), *Sexual Medicine*,
https://doi.org/10.1007/978-981-13-1226-7_5

on the other hand the aim of this chapter is to briefly highlight the complexities involved in managing a patient with sexual dysfunction and to also give the reader a few basic treatment strategies that could be utilized in a primary care setting.

A recent interest and upsurge of research into the field of sexual medicine can be attributed to the earlier pioneering work of Masters and Johnson, who are frequently considered as pioneers in the field of sexual dysfunction. They studied 10,000 complete cycles of sexual response, by observing close to 790 couples including homosexuals [2]. In their book titled "Human Sexual Inadequacy," these authors describe in depth the diverse presentations of the various sexual dysfunctions, along with their management [3].

Sexual Dysfunctions: Definition and Classification

Sexual dysfunctions are becoming increasingly common; a lack of large-scale epidemiological studies to accurately assess the exact prevalence of sexual dysfunctions is seen in the scientific literature. However, perusal of data from numerous smaller studies suggests that, in the age groups between 18 and 59 years including both men and women, approximately 43 and 31% of men and women experienced at least one symptom of sexual dysfunction. Disparate patterns of sexual dysfunction are also seen among different ethnic groups. The severity of dysfunction also varies as a function of the patient's age and educational attainment [4].

A sexual dysfunction is a problem that can potentially interfere with the initiation, and/or consummation, and/or satisfaction with sex. They can afflict either the male or the female partner in a coupling. Disorders of sexual function are independent of sexual orientation and can potentially impede any of the four phases that encompass the human sexual response cycle, i.e., the phases of desire, excitement, orgasm, and finally resolution. These disorders can ultimately lead to anxiety, depression, and feelings of inadequacy for both partners. A dysfunction can be stratified as being either lifelong and always present, recently acquired, or generalized or situational. The popularly used DSM-4 (Diagnostic and Statistical manual of Mental disorders) criteria for the classification of dysfunction was modeled along the lines of the work done by Masters and Johnson [5] and further by Kaplan [6]. The manual was published in 1994 and reflected the general scientific knowledge and thinking generated in publications at that point in time [7]. However recent findings have questioned the validity and general applicability of the DSM-4 classification of sexual dysfunction. The latest DSM-5 manual published in May 2013 clearly states that a diagnosis of sexual dysfunction should only be made if the dysfunction has lasted for a *minimum of 6 months* and if the frequency of dysfunction is seen in *75–100% of sexual encounters*. Furthermore the dysfunction should have caused *considerable distress* to the couple [8]. In addition to the scale of classifying a sexual dysfunction disorder as lifelong, generalized, or situational; the disorder is also classified as being mild, moderate, or severe [8]. Revised classification of various disorders is given in Table 5.1.

A very significant change in the revised classification of sexual dysfunction as per the DSM-5 is the inclusion of dyspareunia and vaginismus as a single entity titled

Table 5.1 Various changes in the classification of both male and female sexual dysfunction as per the DSM-5 revised classification system

DSM-4 diagnosis	Revised DSM-5 diagnosis
Male dysfunctions	
Male erectile disorder	Now listed as erectile disorder
Hypoactive sexual desire disorder	Unchanged
Premature ejaculation	Unchanged
Male orgasmic disorder	Now changed to delayed ejaculation
Male dyspareunia	Not listed
Male sexual pain	Not listed
Female dysfunctions	
Female hypoactive desire	Integrated into female sexual interest/ arousal disorder
Female arousal disorder	Integrated into female sexual interest disorders
Female orgasmic disorder	No changes
Dyspareunia	Now called genito-pelvic pain or genito-pelvic penetration disorder
Vaginismus	Now called genito-pelvic pain or genito-pelvic penetration disorder
Other causes leading to a dysfunction	
Sexual aversion disorder and sexual dysfunction attributable to a general medical condition	Deleted because of a lack of evidence
Sexual dysfunction due to drug abuse	Unchanged

genito-pelvic pain disorder, since there is a remarkable degree of similarity in the way these dysfunctions manifest, as suggested by a large body of empirical evidence [9]. The diagnosis of male dyspareunia has been scrapped due to the extreme rarity of the condition. Not much change has taken place in the classification of male sexual dysfunction. Sexual aversion disorders as a separate classification has been deleted, since these aversion disorders frequently coincide symptomatically with phobias and/or anxiety disorders.

Diagnosing a Sexual Dysfunction in an Infertility Setting

Sexual dysfunction can have an organic or a psychogenic etiology; however caution is advised, as all organically induced dysfunction would have some degree of overlap involving a psychological component. Most of the time in a clinical setting, finding a mixed etiology is not uncommon. In an interesting case-control study on 119 women with infertility, using 99 women (age group 18–45 years) of proven fertility as controls, patients with infertility were found to have significantly ($p < 0.05$) lower scores, in not just the desire and/or arousal responses, but also in the lower frequency of intercourse and masturbation. Scores from sex life satisfaction were also reduced after a diagnosis of infertility was made, while the scores were equal to control before the diagnosis [10]. In another study, where a demographic survey was done among 121 infertile couples presenting to an infertility setting, about 22% of men reported mild-to-moderate erectile dysfunction and about 23% reported some degree of depression [11]. What this means is that infertility can lead to some form of sexual dysfunction, *but* the vice versa is also true since about 10% of patients presenting to an infertility clinic suffer from primary infertility due to sexual dysfunction [12]. In our clinic, of the 544 male partners of couples who presented for an infertility evaluation between February 2014 and January 2015, about 13% of the men suffered from some form of sexual dysfunction (Table 5.2). *Infertility can be both a cause and a consequence of a sexual dysfunction*, although much larger studies are required to validate this statement.

Infertility can create a situation of "sex on demand" and can drain the patient of their satisfaction in their sex lives (Fig 5.1). "Sex-on-demand" situations arising in an infertility setting include collecting a semen sample for sperm preparation and

Table 5.2 72 of 544 patients, between February 2014 and January 2015, presented with sexual dysfunction at our clinic

Sexual dysfunction	No. of patients
Erectile dysfunction only (ED)	27
Anejaculation with ED	2
Premature ejaculation (PE) with ED	2
Decreased libido with ED	9
Infertility with ED	6
Dyspareunia	2
Sexual concern	6
Ejaculatory disorders	18
Total	**72**

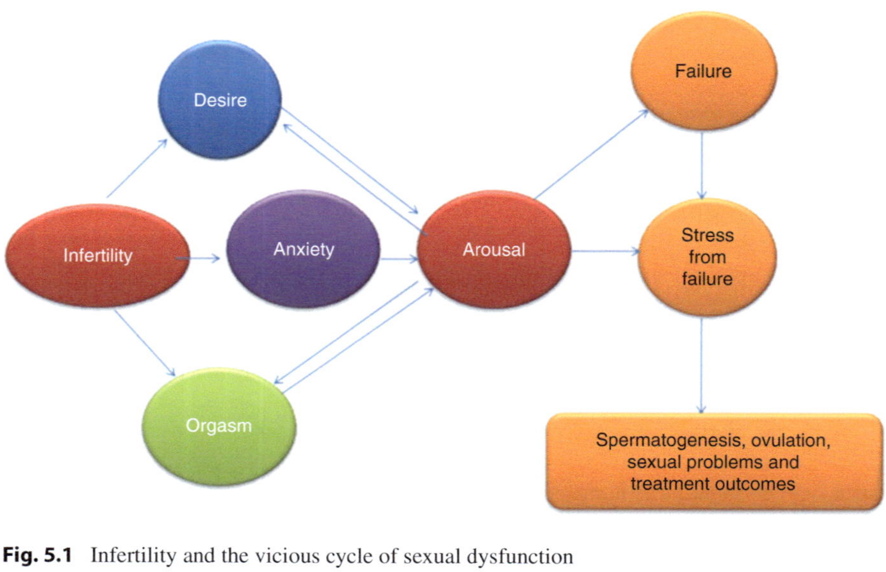

Fig. 5.1 Infertility and the vicious cycle of sexual dysfunction

Table 5.3 Various possible causes of both male and female sexual dysfunctions

Male sexual dysfunction: associated medical conditions	Female sexual dysfunction: associated medical conditions
Cardiovascular disease	Genito-pelvic pain syndrome
Diabetes mellitus	Recurrent cystitis
Dyslipidemia	Vulvar dystrophy
Metabolic syndrome	Vulvar vestibulitis
Obesity	Bartholinitis
Smoking/alcohol consumption/recreational drug use	Episiotomy scars and strictures
Hypogonadotropic hypogonadism	Endometriosis
Hyperprolactinemia	Chemotherapy and/or radiotherapy
Hyper- and hypothyroidism	Hyperprolactinemia
Surgeries like radical prostatectomy	Neurogenic disease
Radiotherapy and/or chemotherapy	Obesity
Neurogenic disease	Surgeries like hysterectomies
Spinal cord injury	Breast cancer
Stroke	
Chronic renal failure	
Surgery of the urethra	
Drug-induced sexual dysfunction	**Drug-induced sexual dysfunction**
Psychotropic medications	*Psychotropic medications*
Neuroleptics	Antipsychotics
Barbiturate and benzodiazepines	Barbiturate and benzodiazepines
SSRI	SSRI
Antidepressants	Antidepressants
Cardiovascular and antihypertensive drugs	*Cardiovascular and antihypertensive drugs*
Statins	Statins
Fibrates	Fibrates
Beta-adrenergic blocking agents	Beta-adrenergic blocking agents
Clonidine	Clonidine
Digoxin	Digoxin
Diuretics	Diuretics
H2 receptor antagonist	
Proton pump inhibitors	*Hormonal preparations*
	Danazol
	GnRH agonists
	Oral contraceptive pill

consequent intrauterine insemination (I.U.I.) on a specific day (i.e., if the said patient has difficulty in collecting a sample by masturbation), or having intercourse during a monitored natural cycle on a particular day of expected ovulation, or collecting a semen sample on demand for a simple semen analysis. Procreation in these cases then becomes the order of the day. The treating specialist should understand the situation and should be empathic and sensitive to the needs of the patient. Questions asked to elicit a sexual history should be direct but not repulsive; a careful choice of words and being empathetic at all times is the key to a successful history taking.

A proper history should elucidate responses pertaining to the couple's frequency of intercourse in the number of days per week and also the frequency after the dysfunction occurred; moreover the couple's sexual response cycle should also be completely assessed and charted, independently for both the male and female. A history of any associated medical illness and their treatment, substance abuse, and pattern of work hours including sleep should be elucidated by the treating physician (Table 5.3). A complete physical examination should follow the history taking. One must also assess if the sexual dysfunction in question is specific to a particular partner, a particular situation, or a circumstance. If this is the case, it is called situational dysfunction. An example would be this: Masturbation is normally a pleasurable exercise but it becomes a ritual and embarrassing when it has to be done in the hospital, laboratory, or toilet. The effect is confounded, when the male patient has to collect the entire ejaculate into a container. In another example, as a part of an infertility management, the couple has to be in a constant state of vigilance regarding ovulation to correctly time intercourse. The female partner then may lose interest in intercourse outside of the fertile period, and then male partner may develop an erectile dysfunction due to the *stress on demand situation* created on the day of ovulation. Another important point of clinical interest is that, one sexual dysfunction may frequently mask or exacerbate another dysfunction due to an interdependence seen between sexual dysfunctions. For example, a women who may be primarily diagnosed with genito-pelvic pain disorder (previously called vaginismus) could affect her partner's erection leading to secondary erectile dysfunction that occurs because the male is afraid that he may cause his partner pain during attempted penetration. In another example, a patient may complain of decreased desire, but this could have secondarily developed due to inadequate foreplay leading to inadequate lubrication resulting in unsatisfactory sex. The primary problem here lies in the male partner who had not adequately aroused his female partner.

One must direct questions in such a way so as to elucidate what he/she thinks/assumes could be causing the problem. Some other useful questions are given below:

- Has your fertility problems afflicted your sexual life?
- What has changed in your sexual life since you started trying for a pregnancy?
- How best can you describe your sex life/sexual activity?
- How frequently do you have penetrative sex?
- How is your interest in sex?
- Do you have any problems with erection and ejaculation?
- Do you feel guilty about having sex?
- Do you feel sex is a sin?
- Do you engage in sex outside your marriage?
- Have you experienced any trauma during sex?

Medical conditions can concomitantly affect sexual function either directly or indirectly [13–17]. For the couple, an in-depth history taking should comprehensively investigate the associated conditions listed in Table 5.2. Numerous large-scale epidemiological studies have established a causal link between cardiovascular and metabolic status with sexual health for both men [18] and women [19]. The appropriate treatment and management of comorbid medical conditions with respect to their sexual implication may improve sexual performance. Numerous medications affect both male and female sexual function; appropriate dose adjustments, change in medications, and stopping substance abuse may also significantly improve sexual function.

Basic Treatment Strategies for the Female

Management of a sexual dysfunction in an infertility setting involves utilizing an "amalgamated therapeutic strategy" which brings in a combination of an appropriate medical and surgical management, sex therapy, counseling, and marital therapy. Educating the patient on what is normal sexual function, sexual response cycle, and basic anatomy of the female genital tract would by itself allay certain doubts and the phobic fear of pain in certain patients presenting with genito-pelvic pain syndrome. Education followed by encouragement of nonsexual behavior will sensitize the patient with her partner. Advising patients to eliminate routine sexual behavior and encouraging the use of explicit sexual materials like books ands videos may also be of some benefit for a few patients [20].

The physician must assess whether the patient is comfortable in discussing her issues, and must also respect the patient's decision in the event she declines treatment. For some patients presenting with sexual dysfunction and infertility, the management of infertility is of more considerable importance than the sexual dysfunction itself. Appropriate counseling and support must be extended to such patients. Other treatment strategies for the female include the usage of lubricants, adopting different sex positions, and finally, but most importantly, Kegel's exercise which if done regularly would improve the strength of the pubococcygeus muscle and also improve the vaginal muscle tone [21]. The role of testosterone replacement therapies in women presenting with sexual desire disorders remains unproven and is not a recommended line of management [22].

Basic Treatment Strategies for the Male

Basic treatment strategies for the male should also follow an amalgamated approach. The patient should be advised to stop smoking and alcohol consumption and is also advised strict weight reduction regime. Patients are also advised strict weight reduction along with lifestyle modifications because from a fertility viewpoint weight reduction has a positive impact on sperm and semen parameters [23] and also loss of body weight is associated with a counter rise in free testosterone, sex hormone-binding globulin, total testosterone, and FSH. This rise in endogenous hormones displays a robust reciprocal dose-response relationship with the degree of weight loss and weight gain as verified through extensive, large-scale interventional studies [24]. An increase in endogenous testosterone would improve erection in obese patients presenting at baseline with erectile dysfunction [25]. Regardless of the etiology of erectile dysfunction, PDE-5 inhibitors have been advocated as the first-line therapy of choice for the management of erectile dysfunction by the European Medical Agency (EMA) [26]. All PDE-5 inhibitors require sexual arousal for erection to be achieved. Sildenafil is the most commonly used drug with a recommended starting dose of 25 mg. Adverse events reported are generally not severe and self-limiting with continuous use [27]. In a dose-response study, a significant improvement was documented in the erectile function among 56% of men who received 25 mg of sildenafil, 77% of men who received 50 mg of sildenafil, and about 84% of men who were started on 100 mg of sildenafil, following 24 weeks of therapy as compared to about 25% of men who were on placebo [28]. This study used standardized questionnaires to assess outcomes. The safety profile and the efficacy of sildenafil are well established in all subtypes of erectile dysfunction [29]. A cardiovascular assessment must be done before prescribing PDE-5 inhibitors. If the patient is on organic nitrate therapy, PDE-5 inhibitors are absolutely contraindicated. PDE-5s are absolutely contraindicated in the following conditions: (1) patients with a history of myocardial infarction, arrhythmia, or stroke in the preceding 6 months; (2) patients presenting with a resting blood pressure less than 90/50 mm of Hg or with diagnosed primary hypertension with blood pressure greater than 170/100 mmHg; and (3) patients with a past history of congestive cardiac failure, angina, or an attack of angina during sexual intercourse [26].

Although the medical management of erectile dysfunction is inveterate, the role of placebo in significantly improving erectile function deserves a special mention and cannot be ignored. In a randomized single-blind, prospective parallel group study, done on 123 patients with diagnosed ED, patients were randomly assigned into three groups and all three groups were given different forms of a placebo and the study reported a significant ($p < 0.001$) improvement in erectile function after 8 weeks of therapy [30].

The next most common dysfunction seen in an infertility setting is premature ejaculation (PE). No global concordance has been reached on the exact definition of PE; the European Urology Association (EUA) defines PE as the inability to control ejaculation for a sufficient length of time before vaginal penetration is achieved [31]. Selective serotonin reuptake inhibitors (SSRI) have been frequently used for the management of PE. Recommended management is by sexual counseling and behavioral techniques like start-stop and the squeeze-pinch method [32]. SSRIs are frequently combined with psychosexual techniques for managing PE.

An important mention must also be made of orgasmic anejaculation; here the commonest cause is retrograde ejaculation, where the semen instead of moving in an antegrade direction moves retrograde back into the bladder [32]. Common etiologies include diabetes mellitus, surgeries to the spinal cord, use of alpha-1 antagonist, and a few psychotropics; other causes include RPLND (retroperitoneal lymph node dissection) and bladder neck surgery [32]. Management would include a simple noninvasive technique of attempting to harvest the sperm from the postcoital urine from a fertility viewpoint [33], but from sexual dysfunction perspective the aim of treatment would be to help the patient achieve an antegrade ejaculation. Use of a mechanical penile vibrostimulation (PVS), either single PVS or dual PVS, can be tried for these patients [34, 35]. While a choice of devices are commercially available, it would be prudent to use a device that offers an amplitude of vibration rated at 2.5 mm; these devices are also called high-amplitude vibrators. Sperm collection and success of antegrade ejaculation are best with these devices. The lower amplitude vibrators commercially available in the market are called "massagers" and offer an amplitude that is much lesser than 2.5 mm [36]. Where PVS fails, the use of electroejaculation (EEJ) with the help of an electroejaculator can be tried; when EEJ also fails and where fertility becomes the primary objective sperm retrieval from the testis is recommended [37].

Conclusion

Sexual dysfunction in an infertility setting represents a complex problem. "Infertility is a race against time." The very diagnosis of a male factor infertility and/or female factor infertility causes a loss of self-esteem, distress, and marital conflicts, all of which could potentially affect sexual function in either one or both of the partners. Patients presenting to an infertility clinic with both infertility and concomitant sexual dysfunction require specialized care and/or treatment using a multidisciplinary team-based approach. The most important point is that the couple must be advised and counseled to view the odyssey towards a normal sexual function and the quest for fertility as two separate and distinct issues.

References

1. Bachmann GA, Phillips NA. Sexual dysfunction. In: Steege JF, Metzger DA, Levy BS, editors. Chronic pelvic pain: an integrated approach. Philadelphia: Saunders; 1998. p. 77–90.
2. Phillips NA. Female sexual dysfunction: evaluation and treatment. Am Fam Physician. 2000;62(1):127–48.
3. Frank E, Anderson C, Rubinstein D. Frequency of sexual dysfunction in normal couples. N Engl J Med. 1978;299(3):111–5.
4. Laumann EO, Paik A, Rosen RC. Sexual dysfunction in the United States: prevalence and predictors. JAMA. 1999;281(6):537–44.
5. Masters WH. Human sexual response. WH Masters & VE Johnson.
6. Kaplan HS, Fyer AJ, Novick A. The treatment of sexual phobias: the combined use of antipanic medication and sex therapy. J Sex Marital Ther. 1982;8(1):3–28.
7. Widiger TA, Samuel DB. Diagnostic categories or dimensions? A question for the diagnostic and statistical manual of mental disorders. J Abnorm Psychol. 2005;114(4):494.
8. American Psychiatric Association. Diagnostic and statistical manual of mental disorders (DSM-5®). Arlington, VA: American Psychiatric Publishing; 2013.
9. Binik YM. The DSM diagnostic criteria for vaginismus. Arch Sex Behav. 2010;39(2):278–91.
10. Millheiser LS, Helmer AE, Quintero RB, Westphal LM, Milki AA, Lathi RB. Is infertility a risk factor for female sexual dysfunction? A case-control study. Fertil Steril. 2010;94(6):2022–5.
11. Shindel AW, Nelson CJ, Naughton CK, Ohebshalom M, Mulhall JP. Sexual function and quality of life in the male partner of infertile couples: prevalence and correlates of dysfunction. J Urol. 2008;179(3):1056–9.
12. Irvine DS. Epidemiology and aetiology of male infertility. Hum Reprod. 1998;13(suppl 1):33–44.

13. Phillips NA. The clinical evaluation of dyspareunia. Int J Impot Res. 1998;10(suppl 2):S117–20.
14. Gratzke C, et al. Anatomy, physiology, and patho-physiology of erectile dysfunction. J Sex Med. 2010;7(1 Pt 2):445–75.
15. Weiner DN, Rosen RC. Medications and their impact. In: Sipski ML, Alexander CJ, eds. Sexual function in people with disability and chronic illness: a health professional's guide. Gaithersburg, MD: Aspen, 1997.
16. Drugs that cause sexual dysfunction: an update. Med Lett Drugs Ther. 1992;34:73–8.
17. Thranov I, Klee M. Sexuality among gynaecologic cancer patients—a cross-sectional study. Gynecol Oncol. 1994;52:14–9.
18. Laumann EO, et al. The epidemiology of erectile dysfunction: results from the National Health and Social Life Survey. Int J Impot Res. 1999;11(Suppl 1):S60–4.
19. Miner M, et al. Cardiometabolic risk and female sexual health: the Princeton III summary. J Sex Med. 2012;9(3):641–51.
20. Striar S, Bartlik B. Stimulation of the libido: the use of erotica in sex therapy. Psych Annals. 1999;29:60–2.
21. Kaplan HS. The illustrated manual of sex therapy. 2d ed. New York: Brunner; 1987. p. 72–98.
22. Gelfand MM, Wiita B. Androgen and estrogen–androgen hormone replacement therapy: a review of the safety literature, 1941 to 1996. Clin Ther. 1997;19:383–404; discussion 367–8
23. Jensen TK, Andersson AM, Jørgensen N, Andersen AG, Carlsen E, Skakkebæk NE. Body mass index in relation to semen quality and reproductive hormones among 1,558 Danish men. Fertil Steril. 2004;82(4):863–70.
24. Camacho EM, Huhtaniemi IT, O'neill TW, Finn JD, Pye SR, Lee DM, Tajar A, Bartfai G, Boonen S, Casanueva FF, Forti G. Age-associated changes in hypothalamic–pituitary–testicular function in middle-aged and older men are modified by weight change and lifestyle factors: longitudinal results from the European male ageing study. Eur J Endocrinol. 2013;168(3):445–55.
25. Esposito K, Giugliano F, Di Palo C, Giugliano G, Marfella R, D'Andrea F, D'Armiento M, Giugliano D. Effect of lifestyle changes on erectile dysfunction in obese men: a randomized controlled trial. JAMA. 2004;291(24):2978–84.
26. Yuan J, et al. Comparative effectiveness and safety of oral phosphodiesterase type 5 inhibitors for erectile dysfunction: a systematic review and network meta-analysis. Eur Urol. 2013;63(5):902–12.
27. Goldstein I, et al. Oral sildenafil in the treatment of erectile dysfunction. Sildenafil Study Group. J Urol. 1998;167(2 Pt 2):1197–203; discussion 1204
28. Moncada I, et al. Efficacy of sildenafil citrate at 12 hours after dosing: re-exploring the therapeutic window. Eur Urol. 2004;46(3):357–60; discussion 360–1
29. Giuliano F, et al. Safety of sildenafil citrate: review of 67 double-blind placebo-controlled trials and the postmarketing safety database. Int J Clin Pract. 2010;64(2):240–55.
30. De Araujo AC, Da Silva FG, Salvi F, Awad MC, Da Silva EA, Damião R. The management of erectile dysfunction with placebo only: does it work? J Sex Med. 2009;6(12):3440–8.
31. Waldinger MD. The neurobiological approach to premature ejaculation. J Urol. 2002;168(6):2359–67.
32. Khan SD, Pandiyan N. Ejaculatory dysfunction—a mini review. Adv Sex Med. 2015;5(02):39.
33. Pandiyan N, et al. Sperm retrieval from the bladder—a simple non-invasive technique. Fertil Steril. 1998;70:492.
34. Ohl DA, Quallich SA, Sonksen J, Brackett NL, Lynne CM. Anejaculation and retrograde ejaculation. Urol Clin North Am. 2008;35:211–22.
35. Sonksen J, Ohl DA. Penile vibratory stimulation and electro-ejaculation in the treatment of ejaculatory dysfunction. Int J Androl. 2002;25:324–32.
36. Brackett NL. Semen retrieval by penile vibratory stimulation in men with spinal cord injury. Hum Reprod Update. 1999;5(3):216–22.
37. Pandiyan N, Khan SD. A clinical approach to male infertility. In: Male infertility. New Delhi: Springer; 2017. p. 41–54

Female Sexual Dysfunction

6

Manu Lakshmi and Shah Dupesh Khan

Introduction

Female sexual dysfunction (FSD) represents an enigmatic yet complex set of disorders in this millennia, wherein significant changes have been implemented in defining, categorizing and managing these conditions. FSD is best viewed through a biopsychosocial modelled approach that integrates the ever-changing scenarios that can affect a woman's health [1]. This includes a woman's psychological issues, interpersonal factors, her current health status and other sociocultural factors. Women's sexuality is highly complex and the association between various factors like society, family, relationship and health is strictly non-linear in nature [2]. A problem in any one of these areas can ultimately result in a sexual dysfunction. The aim of this chapter is to briefly overview the female sexual interest/arousal disorder and orgasmic disorder and also outline the management of the same. Female pain disorders now reclassified as the genito-pelvic pain disorder have been comprehensively reviewed separately in the textbook.

Nosological Reclassification

FSDs were reclassified in the DSM-5 manual [3]. The categories of hypoactive sexual desire disorder (HSDD) were merged with the categories of female sexual arousal disorder (FSAD) and were renamed as a single entity as female sexual interest/arousal disorder (FSIAD) [3]. The separate diagnosis of dyspareunia and vaginismus was merged into a single category called the genito-pelvic pain disorder.

M. Lakshmi (✉)
Department of Reproductive Medicine, The Metromale Clinic & Fertility Center, Chennai, India

S. D. Khan
The Metromale Clinic and Fertility Center, No 1, Crescent Park Street, T-Nagar, Chennai, India

© Springer Nature Singapore Pte Ltd. 2019

K. Gunasekaran, S. D. Khan (eds.), *Sexual Medicine*,
https://doi.org/10.1007/978-981-13-1226-7_6

Sexual aversion disorder has been removed due to lack of data supporting its existence. Lastly a criterion for frequency and severity was also introduced [4].

Both DSM-4 and DSM-5 have major limitations in the sense that they suffer from a high degree of false negatives [5]. Both the old and new classification systems significantly fail to identify all patients presenting with a sexual dysfunction. Lumping two separate diagnostic categories into one single category only serves to further reduce the specificity and/or precision of the classification [5]. Moreover the DSM-4 criteria were based on the linear model of the human sexual response cycle, which in itself is a limitation [6]. We know for a fact that not all individuals fit into the linear model of the sexual response cycle as proposed by Masters and Johnson [7].

Furthermore experts in field of sexual medicine explicitly state that criterion change was not supported by field trials. In an interesting study, which was a survey done via phone interviews it was found that over 92% of female respondents who had a sexual problem did not fit the DSM-5 diagnosis, and over 75% of respondents did not fit the DSM-4 diagnosis as well [8]. The clinical criteria that require the dysfunction to be present for a period of 4–6 months and in over 75–100% of encounters further lowered the number of respondents who would fit in a diagnosis. Those in support of the nosology change state that women cannot distinguish between subjective arousal and genital arousal and thus the unification of the categories is justified [9]. No consensus in general has been made about the DSM-5 revised classification [10].

Key Points in Diagnosing an FSD

Studies have suggested that FSD can be present anywhere between 19 and 50% of outpatient population [11–14]. Physician chart notes on the other hand point to a 2% incidence [13]. Part reason for this discrepancy can stem from a lack of clinical training in this field. Patients also seldom report their problems with sexual intercourse until or unless they are given explicit permission. In a recent observational study on 819 oncology patients, only 29% of them had ever asked their oncology consultant about sex [15]. In the PRESIDE study that involved 50,000 US women of whom 63% were respondents, HSDD was found to be 8.9% in the age group of 18–44 years [16]. In another Finnish study, 70–80% of women in the age group of 55–75 years reported a decrease in sexual desire [17]. Regardless of the varying epidemiological data, sexual desire disorders seem to be the most commonly reported FSD.

The proper diagnosis of an FSD requires the clinician to take a thorough history about the patient's medical and/or gynaecological conditions combined with a psychosexual assessment. Use of validated questionnaires can ease history taking and allay anxiety among patients. The questionnaires can be given to the patient before the actual clinical consultation and/or exam. Different questionnaires like the Female Sexual Function Index (FSFI) [18], the Sexual Function Questionnaires (SFQ) [19], and the Sexual Function and Satisfaction Brief Profile measure (PROMIS) [20] are well validated in terms of assessing sexual desire, arousal (subjective and genital), and/or orgasm. The problem with using these questionnaires though arises when dealing with geographies where sexual literacy is poor and/or language is a barrier. In general, although these questionnaires have demonstrated psychometric validity, these questionnaires are no substitute for an in-depth sexual history taking.

When diagnosing a sexual dysfunction, questions directed to the patient should be non-judgemental and direct. Identifying the patient's sexual orientation and gender identity is the first step in the workup of an FSD. The onset of an FSD, its duration and context of occurrence, i.e. situational or global, should be elicited. A situational FSD is a dysfunction that occurs with a specific partner and/or circumstance. A global FSD on the other hand occurs with all partners/circumstance. FSDs are frequently interdependent in nature; for example a woman may complain of decreased desire secondary to pain during intercourse. The clinician should not treat the desire but should treat the pain that led to the decreased desire [21].

Sometimes, it is wise to ask the patient on 'what motivates her to take the treatment'. A woman's motivational factor for sex can help guide appropriate treatment. For example, some women may complain of decreased desire and when questioned they may reveal that they want to engage in more sex for their partners' sake [22]. Some others may state that they want to feel close to their partner. Either way, the motivational component can help the clinician tailor individual treatment strategies for the patient based on her goals.

Another commonly asked question in the assessment of an FSD is 'what she thinks is causing the problem'. This may reveal important information such as a fear of pain during penetration or lack of partner intimacy non-sexually that is making her avoid and/or lose interest in sexual intercourse.

Female Sexual Interest/Arousal Disorder

Due to the limited data on FSIAD and due to the lack of peer-reviewed validated studies on prevalence and clinical interventions, this diagnosis in itself has not much clinical applicability [23]. For the sake of better understanding we have listed all the possible organic and psychosocial factors that can affect a woman's sexual interest and/or desire in Table 6.1. The clinician should do a thorough assessment that involves history taking combined with a sexological gynaecological physical exam. The exam should involve both a mono-manual and bimanual palpation. In general limited blood tests are recommended for sexual arousal and interest disorders and there is no uniform prescribed testing criteria. Interpersonal factors as outlined in Table 6.1 are highly crucial in identifying a possible aetiology to the FSD [24]. Sexual abuse and partner conflicts impair desire. A death of loved one, domestic misunderstanding and/or financial problems along with religious taboos/beliefs can also affect a woman's desire and concomitantly her arousal. Numerous medications like antidepressants, antipsychotic medications, antilipid drugs and oral contraceptives can also significantly impair desire and arousal and their usage should be ruled out with an in-depth clinical history [24].

Table 6.1 Various gynaecological, interpersonal factors and drugs associated with FSAID

FSIAD-associated conditions
Gynaecological conditions
Pregnancy
Childbirth
Infertility
Menopause
Hysterectomy
Cervical malignancy
Breast surgery
Imperforate hymen
Vaginal septum
Lichen sclerosus and lichen planus
Interstitial cystitis
Pelvic organ prolapse
HPV infections
Fistulas
Candidal yeast infections
Vaginal atrophy
Vulvodynia
Endometriosis
Pelvic inflammatory disease
Hemorrhoids
Chronic pelvic pain
Vaginitis
Interpersonal factors
Religious beliefs
Past history of sexual abuse
Partner conflicts
Sexual orientation
Other conflicting relationships
Financial stressors
Family stress
Depression/anxiety and other mental illnesses
Medications
Antihypertensives
Antipsychotics
Antilipids
Barbiturates
Benzodiazepines
SSRI
OCPs
Danazol
Other hormonal preparations
Beta-blockers

Menopause that occurs with increasing age can also hinder desire and/or arousal. However what is striking is that the 'distress' over the sexual dysfunction also decreases as age advances. With increasing age, especially between 40s and 80s the attrition of relationships and partners and poor erectile function in the partner are all different contributory factors to decreased desire/arousal during partnered intercourse [25].

Some questions that can be used to assess desire/arousal disorders during a clinical evaluation are as follows:

1. How long have this problem been bothering you?
2. How often do you think of sex? How has it changed since the occurrence of the problem?
3. Out of ten, how many times do you initiate partnered sex? How has this changed since the problem?
4. Do you masturbate frequently?
5. What turns you on? Reading erotica? Sex scenes in movies? Anything specific?
6. During intercourse do you experience intense mental pleasure?
7. Do you have any pain during sex?
8. How has your relationship changed since the problem?
9. Why do you think you have this problem?
10. How frequently do you achieve an orgasm?
11. How do you think this treatment will help you?
12. What would it mean to you if this problem goes away?

Female Orgasmic Disorder

A female orgasmic disorder (FOD) is defined as the inability and/or difficulty of the individual to experience an orgasm during partnered sex. A study on 866 women suggested that an FOD is experienced by over 48% of the time in at least 50% of all sexual encounters. Interestingly, over 50% of participants voiced difficulties with arousal and about 57% suffered from distress [26]. A diagnosis of FOD is not made when symptoms occur due to usage of certain medications like SSRIs and other psychotropic drugs or when there is another mental disorder, interpersonal distress and/or any other medical condition that could have a contributory role to play in causing the symptom [24].

Female orgasms have always been a difficult entity to operationally define. 'Clitoral orgasm' is different from 'vaginal orgasm' [27]. A majority of women are capable of experiencing an orgasm during clitoral stimulation with masturbation but not during vaginal intercourse. An FOD diagnosis is given to women only when they are unable to experience orgasm during both clitoral and vaginal intercourse [24].

Women with primary anorgasmia are defined to have never experienced an orgasm even once in their lifetime. They tend to be of a younger age and less sexually experienced. Poor socioeconomic factors, restrictive beliefs and anxiety disorders are all associated with lesser frequency of experiencing an orgasm and these should be systematically ruled out by the clinician [28]. On the other end of spectrum studies have suggested that women can experience orgasm even in their sleep [29] and even after a spinal cord injury [30].

Management of FSD

Female Sexual Arousal/Interest Disorders

Treatment of desire/arousal disorders can be broadly categorized into psychotherapeutic (loosely called behavioural or cognitive) techniques or medical management with hormonal and non-hormonal therapy. Psychoeducation is probably the first step in the managing of all FSDs [31]. Educating the distressed patient and her partner about the normal sexual anatomy/physiology call help allay misconceptions and wrong beliefs.

Directed masturbation or masturbation training can be done for patients, where in a series of steps the patient explores different parts of her body that arouses her and allows her to reach orgasm [32]. Multiple RCTs support the use of masturbation training in the management of FSD [33]. Other treatment strategies used include the implementation of sensate focus exercises, coital alignment techniques and use of erotica and vibrators [34]. Recent studies have suggested that use of vibrators is associated with greater sexual satisfaction among couples despite the claimed fears that women may become dependent on it to reach orgasm [35].

A Cochrane review on the use of combined oestrogens and progestogens in peri- and postmenopausal women to improve sexual function found a small-to-moderate benefit [36]. Androgens have been linked with desire disorders and anecdotal evidence suggests that androgens are safe in postmenopausal women. Although not FDA approved, androgens are used off label for treating sexual desire disorders. Among all preparations, transdermal testosterone combined with oestrogens seems to have some clinical benefits in postmenopausal women. Dosing recommendation has not yet been standardized through trials though. When on testosterone therapy monitoring of testosterone levels, liver function tests, lipids and symptoms of androgenization is recommended [37].

Ospemifene is a 19-nortestosterone derivative and a selective oestrogen receptor modulator (SERM). This drug has received clearance for use in genito-pelvic pain syndrome. In a 12-week RCT, daily 60 mg of ospemifene was found to improve domains of desire, arousal and pain significantly [38].

Flibanserin is non-hormonal medication approved for the treatment of desire disorders. It acts by agonistic action on 5HT1A receptors while simultaneously antagonizing 5HT2A receptors. At a daily dose of 100 mg bedtime, flibanserin was found to significantly improve desire symptoms after 24 weeks compared to placebo and also concomitantly reduce distress. No serious adverse effects or withdrawal symptoms were reported after discontinuing the medication [39].

PDE-5 inhibitors have been used empirically in treating sexual arousal disorders. Data on efficacy however is conflicting [40]. The biggest hurdle seems to be the discordance between subjective and genital arousal. While numerous studies on heterogeneous population of women report genital response after 50 or 100 mg sildenafil dosing, a subjective sense of pleasure was not elicited by the drug [41, 42].

Nutritional supplements like L-arginine, ginseng and damiana have been evaluated in women with sexual desire/arousal disorders and in one study on 108 women after 4 weeks of therapy over 72% of participants reported increased desire/arousal and satisfaction with sexual relationship [43].

Female Orgasmic Disorder

Treatment options for FOD seem highly limited. Most of the previous discussion on desire and arousal management would work with an aim to increase arousal and thus help the women reach orgasm. However in some women with primary anorgasmia where desire and arousal is not a problem, intranasal oxytocin may be tried although much larger clinical studies are required to confirm efficacy [44, 45]. Eros, a wearable clitoral suction device, has received FDA approval and can be tried to improve the ability of a woman to reach orgasm [24]. Other management options include the use of sensate focus, psychoeducation, bibliotherapy and mindfulness-based exercises.

Conclusion

Female sexual dysfunction is complex in the sense numerous physical, hormonal and other known/unknown psychosexual factors interplay among another in causing the dysfunction. Current classification systems are also not robust enough to completely encompass to a wide spectrum of reported sexual dysfunctions. The clinician should thus use his/her clinical acumen in properly diagnosing and assessing a symptom before branding the patient with a sexual dysfunction. This is possible with simple yet effective clinical history taking and focussed physical examination. The clinician should also remember the interpersonal factors that contribute to a dysfunction. Where possible the treating clinician should combine behavioural treatment strategies along with medical therapy for managing an FSD.

References

1. Althof S, Leiblum S, Chevret-Meason M, et al. Psychological and interpersonal dimensions of sexual function or dysfunction. J Sex Med. 2005;26:793–800.
2. Rosen RC, Barsky JL. Normal sexual response in women. Obstet Gynecol Clin N Am. 2006;33:515–26.

3. American Psychiatric Association. Diagnostic and statistical manual of mental disorders (DSM-5®). Arlington, VA: American Psychiatric Publishing; 2013.
4. Sungur MZ, Gunduz A. A comparison of DSM-IV-TR and DSM-5 definitions for sexual dysfunctions: critiques and challenges. J Sex Med. 2014;11(2):364–73.
5. Clayton AH, Hamilton DV. Female sexual dysfunction. Obstet Gynecol Clin. 2009;36(4):861–76.
6. Giles KR, McCabe MP. Conceptualizing women's sexual function: linear vs. circular models of sexual response. J Sex Med. 2009;6(10):2761–71.
7. Masters WH, Masters VJ. Human sexual inadequacy. New York City, New York: Bantam Books; 1980.
8. Sarin S, Amsel RM, Binik YM. Disentangling desire and arousal: a classificatory conundrum. Arch Sex Behav. 2013;42:1079–100.
9. Graham CA, Brotto LA, Zucker KJ. Response to Balon and Clayton (2014): female sexual interest/arousal disorder is a diagnosis more on firm ground than thin air. Arch Sex Behav. 2014;43:1231–4.
10. Balon R, Clayton AH. Female sexual interest/arousal disorder: a diagnosis out of thin air. Arch Sex Behav. 2014;43:1227–9.
11. Bachmann GA, Leiblum S, Grill J. Brief sexual inquiry in gynecologic practice. Obstet Gynecol. 1989;73(3 pt 1):425–7.
12. Angst J. Sexual problems in healthy and depressed persons. Int Clin Psychopharmacol. 1998;13(suppl 6):S1–4.
13. Read S, King M, Watson J. Sexual dysfunction in primary medical care: prevalence, characteristics and detection by the general practitioner. J Public Health Med. 1997;19:387–91.
14. Michael RT. Sex in America: a definitive survey. Boston: Little, Brown; 1994. p. 111–31.
15. Flynn KE, Reese JB, Jeffery DD, et al. Patient experiences with communication about sex during and after treatment for cancer. Psychooncology. 2012;21:594–601.
16. Shifren JL, Monz BU, Russo PA, et al. Sexual problems and distress in United States women: prevalence and correlates. Obstet Gynecol. 2008;112:970–8.
17. Kontula O, Haavio-Mannila E. Sexual pleasures. Enhancement of sex life in Finland 1971–1992. Dartmouth (NH): Aldershot Publishing; 1995.
18. Rosen C, Brown J, Heiman S, Leiblum C, Meston R, Shabsigh D, Ferguson R, D'Agostino R. The female sexual function index (FSFI): a multidimensional self-report instrument for the assessment of female sexual function. J Sex Marital Ther. 2000;26(2):191–208.
19. Quirk FH, Heiman JR, Rosen RC, Laan E, Smith MD, Boolell M. Development of a sexual function questionnaire for clinical trials of female sexual dysfunction. J Womens Health Gend Based Med. 2002;11(3):277–89.
20. Flynn KE, Lin L, Cyranowski JM, et al. Development of the NIH PROMIS® sexual function and satisfaction measures in patients with cancer. J Sex Med. 2013;10:43–52.
21. Phillips NA. Female sexual dysfunction: evaluation and treatment. Am Fam Physician. 2000;62(1):127–48.
22. Meston C, Buss D. Why women have sex: sexual motivation from adventure to revenge—and everything in between. London: The Bodley Head; 2009.
23. Clayton AH, Juarez EM. Female sexual dysfunction. Psychiatr Clin. 2017;40(2):267–84.
24. Kingsberg SA, Althof S, Simon JA, Bradford A, Bitzer J, Carvalho J, Flynn KE, Nappi RE, Reese JB, Rezaee RL, Schover L. Female sexual dysfunction—medical and psychological treatments, committee 14. J Sex Med. 2017;14(12):1463–91.
25. Graziottin A, Leiblum SR. Biological and psychosocial pathophysiology of female sexual dysfunction during the menopausal transition. J Sex Med. 2005;2(s3:133–45.
26. Rowland DL, Kolba TN. Understanding orgasmic difficulty in women. J Sex Med. 2016;13(8):1246–54.
27. Clark L. Is there a difference between a clitoral and a vaginal orgasm? J Sex Res. 1970;6(1):25–8.
28. Barbach LG. Group treatment of preorgasmic women. J Sex Marital Ther. 1974;1:139–45.
29. Wylie K, Levin R, Hallam-Jones R, et al. Sleep exacerbation of persistent sexual arousal syndrome in a postmenopausal woman. J Sex Med. 2006;3:296–302.

30. Komisaruk BR, Whipple B, Crawford A, et al. Brain activation during vaginocervical self-stimulation and orgasm in women with complete spinal cord injury: fMRI evidence of mediation by the vagus nerves. Brain Res. 2004;1024:77–88.
31. Bradford A. Inhibited sexual desire in women. In: Grossman L, Walfish R, editors. Translating psychological research into practice. New York: Springer; 2014. p. 515–8.
32. Nairne KD, Hemsley DR. The use of directed masturbation training in the treatment of primary anorgasmia. Br J Clin Psychol. 1983;22:283–94.
33. Riley AJ, Riley EJ. A controlled study to evaluate directed masturbation in the management of primary orgasmic failure in women. Br J Psychiatry. 1978;133:404–9.
34. American Psychiatric Association. Training in and dissemination of empirically-validated psychological treatments: report and recommendations. Clin Psychol. 1995;48:3–24.
35. Schick V, Herbenick D, Rosenberger JG, et al. Prevalence and characteristics of vibrator use among women who have sex with women. J Sex Med. 2011;8:3306–15.
36. Melnik T, Hawton K, McGuire H. Interventions for vaginismus. Cochrane Database Syst Rev. 2012;12:CD001760.
37. Davis SR, Worsley R, Miller KK, et al. Androgens and female sexual function and dysfunction- findings from the fourth international consultation of sexual medicine. J Sex Med. 2016;13(2):168–78.
38. Bachmann GA, Komi JO. Ospemifene Study Group. Ospemifene effectively treats vulvovaginal atrophy in postmenopausal women: results from a pivotal phase 3 study. Menopause. 2010;17(3):480–6.
39. Gao Z, Yang D, Yu L, et al. Efficacy and safety of flibanserin in women with hypoactive sexual desire disorder: a systematic review and meta-analysis. J Sex Med. 2015;12:2095–104.
40. Berman JR, Berman LA, Toler SM, et al. Safety and efficacy of sildenafil citrate for the treatment of female sexual arousal disorder: a double-blind placebo controlled study. J Urol. 2003;170(6 Pt 1):2333–8.
41. Basson R, McInnes R, Smith MD, et al. Efficacy and safety of sildenafil citrate in women with sexual dysfunction associated with female sexual arousal disorder. J Womens Health Gend Based Med. 2002;11(4):367–77.
42. Caruso S, Intelisano G, Lupo L, et al. Premenopausal women affected by sexual arousal disorder treated with sildenafil: a double-blind, cross-over, placebo controlled study. BJOG. 2001;108(6):623–8.
43. Ito TY, Polan ML, Whipple B, et al. The enhancement of female sexual function with ArginMax, a nutritional supplement, among women differing in menopausal status. J Sex Marital Ther. 2006;32(5):369–78.
44. Magon N, Kalra S. The orgasmic history of oxytocin: love, lust and labor. Indian J Endocrinol Metab. 2011;15(Suppl 3):S156–61.
45. Behnia B, Heinrichs M, Bergmann W, et al. Differential effects of intranasal oxytocin on sexual experiences and partner interactions in couples. Horm Behav. 2014;65:308–18.

Sexual Pain Disorders in Women

7

Manu Lakshmi and Shah Dupesh Khan

Introduction

The Problem

Sexual pain disorders in women are extremely distressing and significantly impact a large population of women and their partners from an emotional, social and physical context of a relationship. Pain during sex was defined as early as the 1800s, long before current medical terminologies of dyspareunia and vaginismus even came into the practice [1, 2]. Studies indicate that the prevalence of sexual pain disorders (3–46%) seems to vary from culture to culture and also with respect to the setting in which a diagnosis is made. Several authors found discrepancies in the reported incidence of sexual pain disorders, which depended on whether the patient was self-reporting a particular problem or whether the clinician was actively questioning the patient on the sexual dysfunction [3, 4]. This is not surprising, since data indicates that only 52% of women actually ever receive a formal diagnosis of a sexual pain disorder [5]. Sexual pain disorders have been frequently underdiagnosed and undertreated.

Clinicians for years have frequently avoided actively pursuing research into this field, due to uncertainties and difficulties in conceptualizing these disorders. Much basic information is definitely missing, thus making clinical care extremely difficult.

M. Lakshmi (✉)
Department of Reproductive Medicine, The Metromale Clinic & Fertility Center, Chennai, India

S. D. Khan
The Metromale Clinic and Fertility Center, No 1, Crescent Park Street, T-Nagar, Chennai, India

© Springer Nature Singapore Pte Ltd. 2019

K. Gunasekaran, S. D. Khan (eds.), *Sexual Medicine*,
https://doi.org/10.1007/978-981-13-1226-7_7

Nosological Variances in Classifying Sexual Pain Disorders

Apart from the clinically well-recognized sexual pain disorders of vaginismus and dyspareunia, numerous labels and classification systems have come in the recent past that describes pain during intercourse without an identifiable pathology. These are namely clitorodynia, vulvodynia, vulvar vestibulitis and provoked/unprovoked vestibulodynia. Vulvodynia is defined as chronic unexplained pain during sexual intercourse localized to the vulval region along with dysfunction of the pelvic floor muscles. The pain may be localized to one specific point in the vulva or throughout the vulval region. The International Society for the Study of Vulvovaginal disease (ISSVD) classifies vulvodynia based on the location of pain as well as the temporal pattern of pain distribution [6]. Provoked vestibulodynia (PVD) is the most commonest cause of vulvodynia and dyspareunia especially in premenopausal women [7].

Nosological confusions are not uncommon in medical sciences and these terminologies have been a major hindrance in clinical communication as well as research progress. While the DSM-4 manual classified sexual pain disorders into separate categories namely 'dyspareunia' and 'vaginismus', the recent DSM-5 manual classified both these conditions under genito-pelvic pain/penetration disorders [8, 9]. A patient is said to have the aforementioned disorder if she has (1) persistent or recurrent difficulties with vaginal penetration, (2) severe pain during attempts at penetration and also pain during sexual intercourse, (3) marked anxiety and fear in anticipation of vaginal penetration and (4) marked tightening of the pelvic floor muscles during vaginal penetration. The duration of symptoms should have lasted for at least 6 months before making a diagnosis [9].

Sexual pain disorders are an excellent example of a mind-body blended problem [10]. In most clinical scenarios the exact aetiology of these sexual pain disorders remains a mystery. One fact to bear in mind is that all sexual pain disorders are frequently associated with disorders of arousal, interest and difficulties in achieving an orgasm [11, 12].

Dyspareunia is defined as recurrent or persistent pain that is associated with sexual intercourse. The pain can be classified as superficial or deep [13]. Table 7.1 highlights the various causes of dyspareunia.

Vaginismus on the other hand is defined as persistent or recurrent involuntary spasm of outer one-third of the vaginal musculature that interferes with vaginal penetrative intercourse leading to personal distress. It is exceedingly difficult to actually delineate and differentiate these two conditions [13]. A great deal of overlap in terms of symptoms is seen especially in superficial dyspareunia and vaginismus; women do not differ greatly in pain scales and assessments and clinicians also find it difficult in reliably making an accurate diagnosis [14–17].

For the sake of this chapter we will use the traditional terms of 'dyspareunia' and 'vaginismus', and where appropriate we will use vulvodynia to describe vulvar pain.

Table 7.1 Common conditions that are seen with dyspareunia

Dyspareunia-associated conditions
Superficial
Imperforate hymen
Vaginal septum
Lichen sclerosus and lichen planus
Interstitial cystitis
Pelvic organ prolapse
HPV infections
Fistulas
Candidal yeast infections
Vaginal atrophy
Arousal difficulties
Vulvodynia
Deep
Endometriosis
Pelvic inflammatory disease
Pelvic floor dysfunction
Haemorrhoids
Chronic pelvic pain
Vaginitis

Consequences of Sexual Pain Disorders

Women suffering from sexual pain disorders suffer from low self-esteem, anxiety and/or depression and disturbed body image [18]. Women also feel a sense of isolation and these disorders affect every aspect of a woman's sexuality. Sexual pain disorders cause lower arousal, desire, frequency of intercourse and/or sexual satisfaction as compared to women without these conditions [19]. Women with pain disorders also tend to perceive negative cognitions about sexual penetration as compared to controls [20].

Male partners of women with sexual pain also report lowered sexual satisfaction and erectile dysfunction compared to men whose partners had no dysfunction. In one particular study, over 70% of participating men reported that their partners' pain had a negative impact on their relationship [21]. Women also frequently show feelings of shame and guilt and also fear losing their partners due to pain [19–22]. This clearly shows that clinical effort should be directed towards understanding the cause of these disorders, bearing in mind the negative impact these disorders can create in a couple's relationship.

Physiology of Pain in Sexual Pain Disorders

There is some consensus today suggesting that neuropathic pain mechanisms may be involved in sexual pain disorders. Both the central and peripheral nervous systems play a role in neuropathic pain [23–26]. The vulval and/or vaginal region has a rich neural network (rather than discrete nerves) that is capable of responding to a wide range of stimuli ranging from pleasure to pain [25]. The exact functional and anatomical correlates of this mechanism are unknown. What we do know though is that even in women with complete spinal cord injuries, the vagus nerve is still capable of conveying sensory genital inputs directly to the brain bypassing the spinal cord [27–29].

Information from the vulva, vagina and cervix is conveyed to large areas of the CNS showing that stimulation of these regions results in a wide range of physiological functions and/or perceptions. Pain is a multidimensional experience that involves affective, discriminative, motivational, cognitive and sensory aspects. Thus in essence pain can be caused directly from neural network activity without any sensory input evoked by local tissue injury and/or inflammation or any other pathology [30].

In most normal conditions, A delta fibres or C fibres convey nociceptive stimulus to the brain; it is hypothesized that in sexual pain disorders, peripheral tissue injury can lead to release of inflammatory mediators and thereby the slow but constant release of inflammatory mediators lowers the pain threshold of these receptors. This is called *peripheral sensitization*. When this occurs, these sensitized nociceptors will start responding to weak non-noxious stimuli—a condition called as allodynia (for example a simple act of even touching or probing the vulval region may trigger severe pain). With subsequent stimulus, the pain response is highly exaggerated (hyperalgesia). In the CNS, the pain signals may also be amplified abnormally, a condition called *central sensitization*. Pain signals may also be conveyed to the CNS via non-nociceptive A-β touch afferents. Over a period of time, the primary receptors as well as the secondary sensitized receptors along with the central sensitization cause changes in the plasticity of the modulatory pain pathways leading to chronic pain [23]. Brain imaging studies have shown morphological alteration in pain-processing areas of women suffering from vulvodynia. Qualitative sensory testing (QST) also shows pain hypersensitivity of the vestibule at lower pain thresholds [31]. Enhanced hypersensitivity to touch also extended to areas far away from the primary area of complaint; this suggests that both neurogenic pain and neuropathic pain mechanisms at both the central and peripheral level are involved [32]. Women with sexual pain frequently demonstrate hypervigilance and also give an exaggerated report about the pain as compared to control women when exposed to a neutral stimulus [32, 33].

The Pelvic Floor in Sexual Pain Disorders

Pelvic floor rehabilitation is a widely utilized treatment option for sexual pain. Howard Glazer first used EMG biofeedback to treat sexual pain in 33 women diagnosed with PVD. After 6 months, over 79% of women had resumed sexual intercourse [34]. Moreover, 50% of participants were pain free. Bergeron et al. had published a 2.5-year follow-up study of women diagnosed with PVD who were randomized to receive either biofeedback, vestibulectomy or cognitive behavioural therapy. For all the three arms, results showed that pain intensity was reduced [35]. Another study also compared biofeedback to lidocaine for PVD treatment; a significant improvement of 66% was seen at the end of 1 year [36]. A study by Saulnier et al. that was prospective involved 11 women who underwent comprehensive physical therapy programme including biofeedback. All participants reported a significant reduction in pain both during vaginal palpation and during sexual intercourse [37]. While there have been numerous other uncontrolled small series studies, a comprehensive randomized controlled trial is the need of the hour.

All previous definitions of vaginismus are based on vaginal spasm, but there is insufficient scientific evidence to suggest that women with vaginismus specifically attribute difficulties in sex due to muscle spasm [38, 39]. EMG data from studies shows that there is some difference in muscle tone at rest when comparing vaginismus and dyspareunia. But this difference could itself occur simply because of the expectation of pain in itself [39]. Individual clinician palpation of muscle tone is also not an accurate way to elicit muscle tone. This makes the differential diagnosis of vaginismus from dyspareunia exceedingly difficult and inaccurate. Women with vaginismus do not also show different EMG readings as compared to controls when subjected to threatening sexual and non-sexual stimuli [40].

Genital Infections in Sexual Pain Disorders

Sexual pain disorders that involve the genital skin are usually transient and can be caused by infections that are acute in nature, namely candidiasis, trichomoniasis, bacterial vaginosis, herpes and/or greater vestibular gland infection [41]. Herpes caused by human papilloma virus (HPV) can cause chronic irritation of the vulvar skin leading to dyspareunia. Treatment of the infection usually resolves the problem. Mucocutaneous disorders like lichen planus and/or lichen sclerosus can also affect the vulvar skin and lead to chronic inflammation due to constant scratching and breaks induced in the skin. Both lichen planus and lichen sclerosus respond well to topical corticosteroid application [42].

Vulvodynia—Vulvodynia is usually a diagnosis of exclusion. The exact cause of vulvodynia is unknown. There is some evidence to suggest that untreated candida infection can lead to vulvodynia; however the histopathological (HPE) findings do not seem very conclusive. The usage of combined hormonal contraception (CHC) is associated with changes in the morphology of the vestibular mucosa but large-scale population studies have shown that use of CHC does not lead to an increased risk of developing vulvodynia [43, 44]. Patients with vulvodynia have severe burning pain localized to the vulval region and topical treatment of any kind is usually not effective. Some degree of pelvic floor dysfunction is also associated with vulvodynia. QST testing also shows that patients with vulvodynia usually report lower pain thresholds as compared to normal women [45, 46].

Relationship and Psychological Factors in Sexual Pain Disorders

Numerous psychological factors are involved in the aetiology of sexual pain disorders. A study on adolescent sexual abuse found that these women were more likely to experience pain in adulthood versus women who never had a history of abuse [47]. A community study also found that vulvovaginal pain was more likely to occur in women who had antecedent anxiety or depression compared to women who did not report such symptoms [48].

There is also some evidence to suggest that cognitive beliefs or attributions about pain increased pain intensity. Hypervigilance, fear of pain and exaggerated response to neutral stimulus all correlate extremely well with increased pain in patients with vulvodynia. These symptoms also predict worse treatment outcomes [49]. Relationship factors like partner cooperation, reduced partner hostility and sympathy were associated with lower pain and better sexual function. Partner hostility and non-facilitative behaviour were associated with greater sexual pain. Underestimation of pain by the partner and ambivalent behaviour were associated with lower sexual satisfaction, greater psychological distress and more frequent relationship conflicts [50]. These findings clearly show the importance of the dyadic context of sexual pain.

Assessment and Examination of Sexual Pain Disorders

Numerous medical conditions are associated with dyspareunia and a proper history taking along with a structured physical exam is usually the key to establishing a diagnosis. The clinician should be non-judgemental about the patient's sexual preferences, sex and sexuality when asking questions. This is one of the core principles of taking a sexual history. The following questions as outlined in Table 7.2 may be asked.

Education Sexological Gynaecological Exam

The educational sexological gynaecological exam can be a highly valuable therapeutic tool for the assessment of sexual pain disorders. This exam is not a routine gynaecology exam and is easier said than done. First the patient should be thoroughly counselled about the exam; the patient should be told that no devices will be used in the internal exam. The date and time of exam should be fixed prior to the exam. The patient should also be told that she can interrupt the exam whenever she wants. The patient is also given the choice to see the examination being performed with a mirror. Patient comfort is key and lays the foundation for all meaningful future discussions [51].

The clinician should clarify to the patient about the patient's anatomy and structure where necessary. Periodically checking if the patient is doing well with the exam will also help the patient cope with the exam. This in itself will correct

Table 7.2 Questions that can be used to assess female sexual pain disorders

Structured questionnaire
General history
Patient's age, educational status and occupation
Patient's current relationship status (married, single, divorced, widower)
Patient's medication history and lifestyle factors (smoking/alcohol/drug use)
Patient's past medical and surgical history
Questions to assess pain
Describe the pain. Where is the exact site of pain?
Is the pain localized to a particular region/point? Or do you feel it distributed over a larger region?
Do you get pain
(1) When the tip of the penis touches the opening of your vagina? (2) After the penis has penetrated the vagina?
(3) During thrusting?
Do you feel tensed when your partner tries penetration?
What thoughts run through your mind when your partner tries penetration?
Do you feel pain when riding a bicycle? Or wear tight clothes? Or during any other specific activity?
Questions to assess arousal
Do you feel excited when attempting intercourse?
Do you feel your vaginal region getting wet?
Additional questions
How does this pain affect your sexual relationship?
How frequently do you attempt at intercourse?
When you get pain, do you stop intercourse or continue?
When did you first notice this pain?
Have you had any past treatments for the pain?

misplaced beliefs and misinformation. The clinician should carefully inspect the vulva, labia majora and minora, clitoris and clitoral hood, vestibule, fourchette, hymen and its edges. Using a cotton swab, sites of pain should be investigated by the application of light pressure along the hymen's outer edge. While doing the cotton swab test, application of the swab should be randomized; the clinician should also specifically ask if the patient feels pain [52, 53]. The patient's verbal and physical responses are also noted. The vulvalgesiometer can be used to accurately quantify the pain felt while applying different degrees of pressure [53].

In case there is vaginal discharge, samples for pH and bacterial cultures can be taken. Before doing an internal exam, it is highly recommended that the patient is bearing down before the physician inserts a finger; during this time involuntary pelvic muscle contraction is a common occurrence; offering information can help allay anxiety making the exam easier. Physician assessment of the pelvic muscle floor tone is not accurate, but has some clinical value. The clinician's finger should be well lubricated and inserted while keeping the finger dorsally curved and at the same time asking the patient to bear down. The pelvic floor muscles are felt and then the finger is slowly withdrawn.

Therapeutic Intervention in Sexual Pain Disorders

Regardless of the treatment option that is being chosen, the most important principle to bear in mind is that the treatment should be *individualized* to every patient. The importance of using a multidisciplinary and multidimensional treatment approach to the problem cannot be emphasized enough due to the complexity of these disorders.

Medical Management

Topical lidocaine 5% is a commonly prescribed medication for sexual pain; the medication is applied 30 min before sexual activity. However, in a recent placebo-controlled RCT, lidocaine cream was found to be no better than placebo [54]. Similarly another placebo-controlled RCT found no benefits of using topical cromolyn 4% as compared to placebo [55]. Oestrogen creams have been used, but the results are variable. Oral medications like selective serotonin reuptake inhibitors (SSRI) and tricyclic antidepressants (TCAs) have also been used but success rates are highly variable [56, 57]. Botulinum toxin A injections have been used for treating vulvodynia, but a recent placebo-controlled RCT found no benefits in terms of pain reduction, after 6 months of follow-up. In fact pain was better reduced in the saline injection group [58]. One of the biggest confounding factors with all medical based management is that placebo or no treatment in itself shows a symptom improvement of over 40%; this clearly shows that higher cognitive functions from a psychological perspective are involved in the pain pathology [59].

Hygiene Measures

Avoiding tight inner wear and potentially irritating fabric may help. Patients can also be recommended to avoid the use of vaginal douches and other potentially irritating substances where appropriate. Maintaining proper hydration with ample fluid intake also helps.

Surgical Measures

The principle of surgery is to remove the hypersensitive tissue. Vestibulectomy though is never a first-line treatment option. The success rate of vestibulectomy is also variable and ranges from 49 to 95% across studies [60]. Although a recent RCT suggested that vestibulectomy may be superior to biofeedback and psychological interventions, the extent of its treatment effect is unknown [61].

Cognitive Behavioural Therapy

Bearing in mind that sexual pain disorders are multifaceted, CBT can target the emotional, psychological and relationship aspects of pain as compared to other therapies. A recent RCT suggested the beneficial effect of group CBT that lasted for eight sessions that included pain journaling, sex education and exposure exercises. Participants felt more satisfied after this treatment as compared to biofeedback [62]. The improvements in pain although no better than the other treatment arms lasted for 2.5 years.

Physical Therapy

Physical therapy that involves retraining the pelvic floor muscles is a well-accepted treatment modality for sexual pain disorders. Education, EMG biofeedback and myofascial release techniques along with manual and/or guided insertion all play an important role in improving symptoms [63, 64]. The aim of these therapies is to desensitize pain areas, improve muscle relaxation, normalize the muscle tone and allow vaginal penetration. These exercises though have not been standardized.

Conclusion

Most research in the area of sexual pain disorders has focussed only on women without including the partners. Most studies in terms of therapeutic interventions are poorly designed and/or uncontrolled. There is an urgent need for more robust RCTs in this field that will prospectively explore combined multimodal treatment strategies for women with sexual pain disorders. More basic studies are definitely required to understand the exact physiology of pain and its effects on human sexuality. Vaginal penetration is frequently defined as the goal of treatment; however future research should look at much broader treatment definitions and treatment bearing in mind the dyadic context in which these disorders occur.

References

1. Barnes R. A clinical history of the medical and surgical diseases of women. Philadelphia: Henry C Lea; 1874.
2. Sims JM. On vaginismus. Trans Obstet Soc London. 1861;3:356–67.
3. Bachmann GA, Leiblum SR, Grill J. Brief sexual inquiry in gynecologic practice. Obstet Gynecol. 1989;73:425–7.
4. Wijma B, Schei B, Swahnberg K, Hilden M, Offerdal K, Pikarinen U, Sidenius K, Steingrimsdottis T, Stoum H, Halmesmäki E. Emotional, physical, and sexual abuse in patients visiting gynecology clinics: a Nordic cross-sectional study. Lancet. 2003;361:2107–13.
5. Harlow BL, Kunitz CG, Nguyen RH, Rydell SA, Turner RM, MacLehose RF. Prevalence of symptoms consistent with a diagnosis of vulvodynia: population-based estimates from 2 geographic regions. Am J Obstet Gynecol. 2014;210(1):40.e1–8.
6. Moyal-Barracco M, Lynch PJ. 2003 ISSVD terminology and classification of vulvodynia: a historical perspective. J Reprod Med. 2004;49:772–7.

7. Bergeron S, Rosen NO, Morin M. Genital pain in women: beyond interference with intercourse. Pain. 2011;152(6):1223–5.
8. American Psychiatric Association. Diagnostic and statistical manual for mental disorders. 4th edition (text revised) ed. Washington, DC: American Psychiatric Press; 2000.
9. Regier DA, Kuhl EA, Kupfer DJ. The DSM-5: classification and criteria changes. World Psychiatry. 2013;12(2):92–8.
10. Reissing ED, Binik YM, Khalifé S. Does vaginismus exist? A critical review of the literature. J Nerv Ment Dis. 1999;187:261–74.
11. Meana M, Binik YM, Khalifé S, Cohen D. Dyspareunia. Sexual dysfunction or pain syndrome? J Nerv Ment Dis. 1997;185:561–9.
12. Van Lankveld JJ, Brewaeys AM, Ter Kuile MM, Weijenborg PTM. Difficulties in the differential diagnosis of vaginismus, dyspareunia and mixed sexual pain disorder. J Psychosom Obstet Gynaecol. 1995;16:201–9.
13. Kruiff de MD, Ter Kuile MM, Weijenborg PTM, Van Lankveld JJDM. Vaginismus and dyspareunia: is there a difference in clinical presentation? J Psychosom Obstet Gynaecol. 2000;21:149–55.
14. Reissing ED, Binik YM, Khalife S, Cohen D, Amsel R. Vaginal spasm, pain, and behavior: an empirical investigation of the diagnosis of vaginismus. Arch Sex Behav. 2004;33:5–17.
15. Binik YM. The DSM diagnostic criteria for vaginismus. Arch Sex Behav. 2010;39:278–91.
16. Basson R, Althof S, Davis S, Fugl- Meyer K, Goldstein I, Leiblum S, Meston C, Rosen R, Wagner G. Summary of the recommendations on sexual dysfunctions in women. J Sex Med. 2004;1:24–34.
17. Abramov L, Wolman I, David MP. Vaginismus: an important factor in the evaluation and management of vulvar vestibulitis syndrome. Gynecol Obstet Investig. 1994;38:194–7.
18. Meana M, Binik YM, Khalife S, Cohen DR. Biopsychosocial profile of women with dyspareunia. Obstet Gynecol. 1997;90(4 Pt 1):583–9.
19. Cherner RA, Reissing ED. A comparative study of sexual function, behavior and cognitions of women with lifelong vaginismus. Arch Sex Behav. 2013;42:1605–14.
20. Masheb RM, Lozano-Blanco C, Kohorn EI, Minkin MJ, Kerns RD. Assessing sexual function and dyspareunia with the Female Sexual Function Index (FSFI) in women with vulvodynia. J Sex Marital Ther. 2004;3(5):315–24.
21. Smith KB, Pukall CF. Sexual function, relationship adjustment, and the relational impact of pain in male partners of women with provoked vulvar pain. J Sex Med. 2014;11(5):1283–93.
22. Reed BD, Advincula AP, Fonde KR, Gorenflo DW, Haefner HK. Sexual activities and attitudes of women with vulvar dysesthesia. Obstet Gynecol. 2003;102(2):325–31.
23. Devor M, Seltzer Z. Pathophysiology of damaged nerves in relation to chronic pain. In: Wall PD, Melzack R, editors. Textbook of pain. 4th ed. New York: Churchill Livingstone; 1999. p. 129–64.
24. McKay M. Dysesthetic (essential) vulvodynia. Treatment with amytriptilyne. J Reprod Med. 1993;37:9–13.
25. Hilliges M, Falconer C, Ekman-Ordeberg G, Johansson O. Innervation of the human vaginal mucosa as revealed by PGP 9.5 immunohistochemistry. Acta Anat (Basel). 1995;153:119–26.
26. Krantz KE. Innervation of the human vulva and vagina; a microscopic study. Obstet Gynecol. 1958;12:382–96.
27. Weijmar Schultz WC, van deWiel HB, Klatter JA, Sturm BE, Nauta J. Vaginal sensitivity to electric stimuli: theoretical and practical implications. Arch Sex Behav. 1989;18:87–95.
28. Komisaruk BR, Whipple B. Functional MRI of the brain during orgasm in women. Annu Rev Sex Res. 2005;16:62–86.
29. Berkley KJ, Benoist JM, Gautron M, Guilbaud G. Responses of neurons in the caudal intralaminar thalamic complex of the rat to stimulation of the uterus, vagina, cervix, colon and skin. Brain Res. 1995;695:92–5.
30. Melzack R. Evaluation of the neuromatrix theory of pain. The Prithvi Raj Lecture: presented at the third World Congress of World Institute of Pain, Barcelona, 2004. Pain Pract. 2005;5:85–94.

31. Giesecke J, Reed BD, Haefner HK, Giesecke T, Clauw DJ, Gracely RH. Quantitative sensory testing in vulvodynia patients and increased peripheral pressure pain sensitivity. Obstet Gynecol. 2004;104:126–33.
32. Granot M, Friedman M, Yarnitsky D, Zimmer EZ. Enhancement of the perception of systemic pain inwomen with vulvar vestibulitis. BJOG. 2002;109:863–6.
33. Pukall CF, Strigo IA, Binik YM, Amsel R, Khalife S, Bushnell MC. Neural correlates of painful genital touch in women with vulvar vestibulitis syndrome. Pain. 2005;115:118–27.
34. Glazer HI, Rodke G, Swencionis C, Hertz R, Young AW. Treatment of vulvar vestibulitis syndrome with electromyographic biofeedback of pelvic floor musculature. J Reprod Med. 1995;40(4):283–90.
35. Bergeron S, Brown C, Lord MJ, Oala M, Binik YM, Khalife S. Physical therapy for vulvar vestibulitis syndrome: a retrospective study. J Sex Marital Ther. 2002;28(3):183–92.
36. Danielsson I, Torstensson T, Brodda-Jansen G, Bohm-Starke N. EMG biofeedback versus topical lidocaine gel: a randomized study for the treatment of women with vulvar vestibulitis. Acta Obstet Gynecol Scand. 2006;85(11):1360–7.
37. Gentilcore-Saulnier E, McLean L, Goldfinger C, Pukall CF, Chamberlain S. Pelvic floor muscle assessment outcomes in women with and without provoked vestibulodynia and the impact of a physical therapy program. J Sex Med. 2010;7(2 Pt 2):1003–22.
38. van der Velde J, Everaerd W. Voluntary control over pelvic floor muscles in women with and without vaginistic reactions. Int Urogynecol J Pelvic Floor Dysfunct. 1999;10:230–6.
39. van der Velde J, Everaerd W. The relationship between involuntary pelvic floor muscle activity,muscle awareness and experienced threat in women with and without vaginismus. Behav Res Ther. 2001;39:395–408.
40. van der Velde J, Laan E, Everaerd W. Vaginismus, a component of a general defensive reaction. An investigation of pelvic floor muscle activity during exposure to emotion-inducing film excerpts in women with and without vaginismus. Int Urogynecol J Pelvic Floor Dysfunct. 2001;12:328–31.
41. Sideri M, Jones RW, Wilkinson EJ, et al. Squamous vulvar intraepithelial neoplasia: 2004 modified terminology, ISSVD Vulvar Oncology Subcommittee. J Reprod Med. 2005;50:807–10.
42. Willhite LA, O'Connell MB. Urogenital atrophy: prevention and treatment. Pharmacotherapy. 2001;21:464–80.
43. Bouchard C, Brisson J, Fortier M, Morin C, Blanchette C. Use of oral contraceptive pills and vulvar vestibulitis: a case-control study. Am J Epidemiol. 2002;156(3):254–61.
44. Harlow BL, Vitonis AF, Stewart EG. Influence of oral contraceptive use on the risk of adult-onset vulvodynia. J Reprod Med. 2008;53(2):102–10.
45. Bohm-Starke N, Hilliges M, Falconer C, Rylander E. Increased intraepithelial innervation in women with vulvar vestibulitis syndrome. Gynecol Obstet Investig. 1998;46(4):256–60.
46. Pukall CF, Binik YM, Khalifé S, Amsel R, Abbott FV. Vestibular tactile and pain thresholds in women with vulvar vestibulitis syndrome. Pain. 2002;96(1–2):163–75.
47. Payne KA, Binik YM, Amsel R, Khalifé S. When sex hurts, anxiety and fear orient attention towards pain. Eur J Pain. 2005;9(4):427–36.
48. Desrochers G, Bergeron S, Khalife S, Dupuis MJ, Jodoin M. Fear avoidance and self-efficacy in relation to pain and sexual impairment in women with provoked vestibulodynia. Clin J Pain. 2009;25(6):520–7.
49. Rosen NO, Bergeron S, Glowacka M, Delisle I, Baxter ML. Harmful or helpful: perceived solicitous and facilitative partner responses are differentially associated with pain and sexual satisfaction in women with provoked vestibulodynia. J Sex Med. 2012;9(9):2351–60.
50. Rosen NO, Bergeron S, Sadikaj G, Glowacka M, Delisle I, Baxter ML. Impact of male partner responses on sexual function in women with vulvodynia and their partners: a dyadic daily experience study. Health Psychol. 2014;33(8):823–31.
51. Carter J, Fowler L, Carlson J, Twiggs LB. How accurate is the pelvic examination as compared to transvaginal sonography? A prospective, comparative study. J Reprod Med. 1994;39:32–4.
52. Basson R. Sexuality and sexual disorders. Clin Updates Women's Health Care. 2003;11:1–94.

53. Pukall CF, Payne KA, Binik YM, Khalifé S. Pain measurement in vulvodynia. J Sex Marital Ther. 2003;29(Suppl 1):111–20.
54. Foster DC, Kotok MB, Huang LS, Watts A, Oakes D, Howard FM, et al. Oral desipramine and topical lidocaine for vulvodynia: a randomized controlled trial. Obstet Gynecol. 2010;116(3):583–93.
55. Nyirjesy P, Sobel JD, Weitz MV, Leaman DJ, Small MJ, Gelone SP. Cromolyn cream for recalcitrant idiopathic vulvar vestibulitis: results of a placebo controlled study. Sex Transm Infect. 2001;77:53–7.
56. McKay M. Dysesthetic ("essential") vulvodynia. Treatment with amitriptyline. J Reprod Med. 1993;38:9–13.
57. Munday PE. Response to treatment in dysaesthetic vulvodynia. J Obstet Gynaecol. 2001;21:610–3.
58. Petersen CD, Giraldi A, Lundvall L, Kristensen E. Botulinum toxin type A-a novel treatment for provoked vestibulodynia? Results from a randomized, placebo controlled, double blinded study. J Sex Med. 2009;6(9):2523–37.
59. Enck P, Benedetti F, Schedlowski M. New insights into the placebo and nocebo responses. Neuron. 2008;59:195–206.
60. Landry T, Bergeron S, Dupuis MJ, Desrochers G. The treatment of provoked vestibulodynia: a critical review. Clin J Pain. 2008;24(2):155–71.
61. Bergeron S, Khalife S, Glazer HI, Binik YM. Surgical and behavioral treatments for vestibulodynia: two-and-one-half year followup and predictors of outcome. Obstet Gynecol. 2008;111(1):159–66.
62. Brotto LA, Basson R, Carlson M, Zhu C. Impact of an integrated mindfulness and cognitive behavioral treatment for provoked vestibulodynia (IMPROVED): a qualitative study. Sex Relat Ther. 2013;28(1–2):3–19.
63. Rosenbaum TY, Owens A. The role of pelvic floor physical therapy in the treatment of pelvic and genital pain-related sexual dysfunction (CME). J Sex Med. 2008;5(3):513–23.
64. Friedrich EG Jr. Vulvar vestibulitis syndrome. J Reprod Med. 1987;32:110–5.

Testosterone Replacement Therapy

8

G. Rastrelli, Y. Reisman, S. Ferri, O. Prontera, A. Sforza, M. Maggi, and G. Corona

Introduction

The male gonadal gland produces sex steroids and sperms under the regulation of a complex network including intratesticular factors and extra-testicular trophic hormones. The pituitary gland regulates gonadal activity, through the secretion of luteinizing hormone (LH), which mainly regulates testosterone (T) production in Leydig cells (micromoles/day), and follicular stimulating hormone (FSH), which mainly controls sperm production in seminiferous tubules (millions/day) [1, 2]. The production and secretion of gonadotropins by the pituitary gland are stimulated by the gonadotropin-releasing hormone (GnRH) produced by the hypothalamus and inhibited by a negative feedback mediated by the central action of sex steroids and inhibin B [1, 2]. Male hypogonadism (HG) is a clinical condition due to a partial or total communication breakdown of the hypothalamus-pituitary-testis (HPT) axis. Hence, HG is a condition characterized by the impairment of testicular production of both sex steroids and sperms. The term, however, is rarely used to identify abnormalities in sperm production, while it is often applied to describe T deficiency [3].

Based on a pathogenetic classification, HG can be considered as primary (pHG) when caused by any diseases affecting the testes, and as secondary (sHG) when

G. Rastrelli · M. Maggi
Sexual Medicine and Andrology Unit, Department of Experimental, Clinical and Biomedical Sciences, University of Florence, Florence, Italy

Y. Reisman
Department of Urology, Amstelland Hospital, Amsterdam, The Netherlands

S. Ferri · O. Prontera · A. Sforza · G. Corona (✉)
Endocrinology Unit, Medical Department, Maggiore-Bellaria Hospital, Bologna, Italy

© Springer Nature Singapore Pte Ltd. 2019

K. Gunasekaran, S. D. Khan (eds.), *Sexual Medicine*,
https://doi.org/10.1007/978-981-13-1226-7_8

due to a pituitary or hypothalamic dysfunction. In the former condition, both sex steroids and sperms are impaired despite a super-stimulation of the pituitary (hypergonadotropic hypogonadism), whereas in sHG the testis is normal, but inadequately stimulated by gonadotropins (hypogonadotropic hypogonadism). In addition, another condition, known as compensated hypogonadism (normal T serum levels and elevated LH), has also been described, although its clinical significance is still debated [4, 5].

The aforementioned classification of HG, based on its etiology, presents a practical utility for didactic and treatment purposes. In fact, patients with sHG can be successfully treated by removing the precipitating cause (for example: prolactinoma) and/or by appropriate endocrine therapy (i.e., gonadotropins or GnRH if fertility is an issue or T for virilization, if fertility is not desired). Conversely, only T treatment can be offered to patients with pHG [1, 2]. However, it is important to recognize that the phenotype of the hypogonadal patient is more often affected by the age of hypogonadism onset regardless of the site of origin. If the problem occurs very early on in fetal life, symptoms can be dramatic, spanning from an almost complete female phenotype to various defects in virilization. When the problem manifests during pre- or peripubertal age, symptoms and signs are milder including a delay in the onset of puberty with an overall eunuchoidal phenotype [6, 7]. Finally, when hypogonadism develops after puberty and especially with aging (adult-onset or late-onset hypogonadism, LOH), symptoms will be relatively mild, insidious and difficult to recognize. The European Male Aging Study (EMAS), a population-based survey performed on more than 3400 men recruited from eight European centers, clearly showed that sexual symptoms—particularly erectile dysfunction (ED) and decreased frequency of sexual thoughts and morning erections—are the most sensitive and specific symptoms in identifying adulthood patients with low T [8]. Similar results were recently reported by us in a large cohort ($n = 4890$) of subjects consulting for ED [9]. In contrast, psychological and physical symptoms were less informative [8].

Finally, more recently the concept of *organic* versus *functional* HG has been introduced [10]. The former is an irreversible condition due to congenital or acquired perturbation to the HPT axis [10]. Conversely, *functional* HG is a potentially reversible condition characterized by "no recognizable structural intrinsic HPT axis problems," frequently associated with an age-dependent accumulation of morbidities impairing the HPT axis function [10]. In particular, metabolic disturbances such as type 2 diabetes mellitus (T2DM), obesity, and metabolic syndrome (MetS) are the conditions most frequently associated with functional HG [10–13]. Interestingly, we recently reported that in a large series ($n = 4220$) of subjects seeking medical care at our unit for sexual dysfunctions only a minority of patients satisfied the criteria of organic hypogonadism (15%) whereas the majority, i.e., 85%, were allocated to the functional category. In the latter group, metabolic impairment was present in 2/3 of the subjects [14].

In the following sections, the criteria defining LOH and the available T formulations along with their outcomes are analyzed in detail.

Criteria for Starting Testosterone Replacement Therapy (TRT)

Although there is no general agreement among the different andrological societies on T thresholds for initiating TRT in LOH, the most widely shared consensus is that TRT may be beneficial when total T is below 8 nmol/L (231 ng/dL) in two different measurements [15–17]. In addition, there is also general agreement that a total T level above 12 nmol/L (346 ng/dL) does not require substitution. When T levels are in the "gray area," between 8 and 12 nmol/L, TRT should be offered only to symptomatic men [15–17]. As previously reported, sexual symptoms of erectile dysfunction and decreased mood/libido and/or decreased sexual thoughts are the most specific indicators for TRT [8, 9].

Available Testosterone Preparations

The first androgenetic steroid, *androsterone*, was chemically isolated and purified from urine by Butenandt in 1931. Some years later, in 1935, Karoly Gyula David and Ernst Laqueur extracted and purified a stronger androgenic steroid from bull testes and termed it as T. In the same year, Butenandt group in Gottingen and Ruzicka and Wettstein in Basel simultaneously published the T chemical synthesis [18]. Soon after its synthesis, it became apparent that T could not be given effectively by oral or parenteral route, because of a prompt hepatic metabolism causing only a small portion of the hormone to reach systemic circulation. Hence, a series of chemical modifications were introduced to improve T bioavailability and pharmacokinetics, essentially retarding the rate of liver catabolism or enhancing its availability. The first T ester introduced on the market was a very-short-acting formulation (T propionate) which requires two to three injections per week to maintain normal T levels (see below [18]). In 1935, a 17α-methyl-T was also synthesized for oral use. However, now it is clear that this compound along with all other T-methyl derivatives is associated with an increased liver toxicity and for these reasons these formulations are no longer recommended for clinical use [18]. Unfortunately, these products are still present on the black market and abused as anabolic steroids [19]. In the mid-1950s a longer acting T formulation (T-enanthate) became available and has remained the major T preparation for more than half a century. In the late 1970s a new orally effective T formulation based on esterification of T ring in position 17β with undecancic acid (oral T undecanoate, TU) was introduced on the market. This chemical modification allows absorption via lymphatic system avoiding the first-pass effect in the liver [18]. In the mid-1990s, transdermal scrotal and non-scrotal T patches became available and in 2000 the more manageable transdermal T preparations (T gels) were approved for the treatment of male hypogonadism, first in the USA and later on also in other countries. In 2004, the injectable long-acting TU entered the market allowing a dosing regimen of 1000 mg every 12 weeks following a 6-week loading dose [18].

The specific characteristics of all the aforementioned T preparations are analyzed in detail (Table 8.1).

Table 8.1 Testosterone preparations

Formulation	Trade names	Chemical structure	T 1/2	Standard dosage
		Oral		
Testosterone undecanoate	Andriol®	17-α-Hydroxyl-ester	4 h	120–240 mg 2–3 times daily
	Andriol Testocaps®			
Mesterolone	Proviron®	1α-Methyl-4,5α-dihydrotestosterone	NA	50–100 mg 2–3 times daily
		Parental		
Testosterone enanthate	Testoviron Depot®	17-α-Hydroxyl-ester	4–5 days	250 mg every 2–3 weeks
	Delatestryl®			
	Testoenant®			
Testosterone cypionate	Delatestryl®	17-α-Hydroxyl-ester	8 days	200 mg every 2–3 weeks
Testosterone propionate	Testovis®	17-α-Hydroxyl-ester	20 h	100 mg every 2 days
Testosterone undecanoate in castor oil	Nebido®	17-α-Hydroxyl-ester	34 days	1000 mg every 10–14 weeks
	Aveed®(USA)[a]			750 mg every 10 weeks[a]
Surgical implants	Testopel®	Native testosterone	–	4–6200 mg implants lasting up to 6 months
	Testoimplant®			
		Transdermal		
Testosterone patches	*Not scrotal:*	Native testosterone	10 h	50–100 mg/day
	Androderm®			
	Andropatch®			
	Testopatch®			
Testosterone gel 1–2%	*1% Gel:*	Native testosterone	6 h	50–100 mg/day
	Androgel®			
	Testogel®			
	Testim®			
	2% Gel:			
	Testostop®			
	Tostrex® (also known as Fortesta®, Tostran®, and Itnogen® available only in Europe)			
	1.6% Gel			
	Androgel (available only in the USA)			
Dihydrotestosterone gel 2.5%	Andractim®	5α-Dihydrotestosterone		5 or 10 g/day
Underarm testosterone (testosterone solution 2%)	Axiron®	Native testosterone	NA	60–120 mg/day
		Transmucosal		
Buccal testosterone	Striant®	Native testosterone	12 h	30 mg/twice daily
Intranasal testosterone	Natesto®[b]	Native testosterone	NA	11 mg 2–3 times daily

[a]Available only in the USA
[b]Available only in the USA and Canada
NA not available

Oral Testosterone Preparations

Testosterone Undecanoate

As reported above, T undecanoate (TU) is a long-chain fatty acid ester of T absorbed by the intestines into lymphatic system lacteals, therefore bypassing the liver and enabling T delivery into the systemic circulation. The recommended dosage is one or two 40 mg caps twice or thrice daily during meals (Table 8.1). However, it is important to recognize that this formulation is characterized by an unpredictable absorption depending on the dietary fat content of food intake limiting its clinical use [15–17, 20].

Mesterolone

Mesterolone is a 1α methyl derivative of 5α-dihydrotestosterone (DHT). This chemical modification allows resistance to hepatic metabolism. Mesterolone is prescribed at a daily dose of 50–100 mg and should be taken in two to three spaced dosages [15–17, 20] (Table 8.1). However, as DHT, mesterolone cannot be converted to estrogen strongly limiting its attractiveness.

Injectable Testosterone Preparations

Subdermal Implantation of T Pellets

The subdermal implantation of T pellets was introduced on the market in the first half of the last century. This formulation is still available for clinical use only in few countries, such as the USA, the UK, and Australia. The pellets consist of pure crystals of T compressed into short rods, which are implanted under local anesthesia into the subdermal fat layer of the skin. Recommended dosage includes two to six pellets (150–450 mg) subcutaneously every 3–6 months (Table 8.1) [15–17, 20]. This formulation is still the T preparation with the longest duration of action; however, the procedure is invasive and may be unattractive to patients.

Intramuscular Injectable Preparations

According to their half-lives these formulations can be classified into short-, mid-, and long-lasting preparations (Table 8.1) [15–17, 20].

T propionate is a short-acting T formulation requiring the administration of two to three fractionated doses weekly (usually 50 mg every 2–3 days) which limits its attractiveness, although it is still present on the market worldwide (Table 8.1) [15–17, 20]. In addition, the use of this preparation determines a wide fluctuation of circulating T levels often reaching supraphysiologic levels after 24 h, followed by a gradual decline to hypogonadal levels before the following administration [15–17, 20]. This phenomenon can be recognized as unpleasant by the patients who complain of variations in well-being and also increasing the risk of erythrocytosis [21].

The longer aliphatic chain in 17β-position allows *T cypionate and enanthate* to have a longer half-life requiring it to be injected every 2–4 weeks at a dose of 200–250 mg (Table 8.1) [15–17, 20]. However, the two compounds present similar limitations as previously described for T *propionate* including wide plasma fluctuation and higher risk of erythrocytosis.

In 2004, a new, long-lasting injectable formulation of T undecanoate (TU) was introduced [15–17, 20]. In the majority of countries, this preparation is available as a depot of 1000 mg in 4 mL requiring it to be administered every 12 weeks following a booster 6-week loading dose. In the USA, a 3 mL ampoule containing 750 mg is available. The latter formulation is recommended to be injected once at initiation of therapy, at 4 weeks, and then every 10 weeks thereafter [15–17, 20]. A recent meta-analysis of all available evidence documented that this preparation shows a very good safety and benefit profile [22].

Transdermal Testosterone Preparations

Testosterone Gels

Transdermal T gels are available at different concentrations (1%, 1.62%, and 2%) and nowadays represent the most popular T formulations for the treatment of LOH along with long-acting TU (Table 8.1) [15–17, 20]. The applied gel is quickly absorbed by the skin that forms a sort of reservoir for continuous delivery to the systemic circulation. Only about 8–14% of the applied gel is usually transdermally absorbed. Considering the T production rate of 5–8 mg/day the recommended dosage of T gels is 50–100 mg daily. Local side effects such as skin irritation and erythema are seldom observed. However, the most important side effect related to the use of T gels is the possibility to transfer some amount of T to others during contact with the skin's surface. In order to overcome this possibility, newer T gel formulations at higher concentrations (1.62–2%) have been developed [15–17]. Similar effects can be obtained using the *alcohol-based T (2%) solution* which requires a daily underarm application [15–17, 20]. Unfortunately, this formulation is available only in a limited number of countries.

Testosterone Patches

Self-adherent skin patches were the first T transdermal formulation introduced on the market, firstly using scrotal systems and, later on, through non-scrotal ones (Table 8.1) [15–17, 20]. These formulations, however, are frequently associated with adverse skin reactions at the application site limiting their use [15–17, 20].

DHT Gels

In some European countries, DHT is available as a hydroalcoholic 2.5% gel requiring a dosage of 5 or 10 g/day (Table 8.1) [15–17, 20]. The gel is rapidly absorbed by the skin reaching a steady state in 2–3 days. However, similar to what was reported for mesterolone, this preparation cannot be aromatized and works as a partial androgen. Hence, this formulation can be used only for limited periods in particular conditions, such as gynecomastia and microphallus [23–25].

Transmucosal Testosterone Preparations

Transbuccal Testosterone Preparations

A T transbuccal formulation is available in several countries. This administration allows avoiding intestinal pass and liver inactivation providing the absorption of T through the oral mucosa (Table 8.1) [15–17, 20]. The system adheres to the gum or inner cheek gradually releasing medication. However, this formulation does not dissolve completely and requires removal after 12 h. This formulation is able to restore physiological T levels with minimal or transient local problems, including gum edema, blistering, and gingivitis [15–17, 20].

Transnasal Testosterone Preparations

A gel containing 5.5 mg of T in 122.5 mg for intranasal administration has been developed and available in some countries, including the USA and Canada (Table 8.1) [15–17, 20]. The recommended dosage is 11 mg of T administered intranasally three times daily (Table 8.1) [1–3, 5, 26]. The nasal gel is available as a metered-dose pump containing 11 g of gel dispensed as 60 metered pump actuations. The application is rapid, noninvasive, and convenient, and avoids secondary transference.

Testosterone Preparation Outcomes

Sexual Function

From 2005 to today, six systematic meta-analyses evaluating the effect of TRT versus placebo on sexual function have been published [26–31]. By considering all the studies reporting outcome data as effect size [29–31] and limiting the analysis only to hypogonadal patients, TRT was associated with an improvement of all sexual parameters evaluated (Table 8.2) [32]. Conversely, no effect was observed when eugonadal patients were considered (Table 8.2). According to Cohen [33], a small treatment-effect size is considered to be about 0.2, a medium effect size to be about 0.5, and a large effect size to be about 0.8. Only our study reported data categorized according to the T preparation used [29]. Interestingly, when the data on erectile function and libido outcomes were considered and studies enrolling only eugonadal patients were excluded, oral preparations did not show a positive effect, when compared to placebo, on erectile function whereas only a small effect on libido was detected (Table 8.2) [32]. Conversely, no difference in the positive efficacy of both transdermal and parental testosterone preparations was documented (Table 8.2) [32]. Finally, no sufficient data were available to evaluate possible differences among specific transdermal and parenteral preparations (not shown).

Table 8.2 Standardized mean [95% CI] for different sexual function parameters as derived from available meta-analyses

Meta-analyses considered	Overall			
	Erectile function	*Libido*	*Orgasmic function*	*Sexual satisfaction*
Isidori et al. [31]	1.87 [0.31;3.43]	1.60 [0.29;2.92]	–	1.16 [0.04;2.29]
Bolona et al. [30]	0.80 [−0.10;1.60]	1.31 [0.4;2.22]	–	–
Corona et al. [29]	1.21 [0.65;1.78]	0.95 [0.41;1.50]	0.74 [0.35;1.21]	0.86 [0.40;1.32]
	Data according to testosterone formulations (Corona et al. [29])			
	Erectile function		*Libido*	
Oral	1.77 [−0.19;3.73]		1.41 [0.14;2.68]	
Transdermal	0.31 [0.04;0.59]		0.32 [0.14;0.51]	
Injectable	0.46 [0.18;0.74]		0.81 [0.31;1.32]	

Body Composition and Glycometabolic Control

Much evidence has documented a possible association between low T and metabolic impairment [34–36]. Since 2005, four systematic meta-analyses have evaluated the effect of TRT on different parameters related to body composition and glycometabolic profile [37–40]. The meta-analyses differed in body composition and metabolic outcomes considered [37–40]. By comparing all the available data and when only hypogonadal patients were considered, TRT caused similar modifications in fat mass and lean mass without any changes in BMI (Table 8.3) [32]. Similar results were observed when fasting glycemia was considered (Table 8.3) [32]. Conversely, more conflicting results were detected when lipid profile was analyzed (Table 8.3) [32]. Finally, when body composition and metabolic profile outcomes were evaluated according to the use of the different T preparations, oral preparations did not show a positive effect on lean mass and glycometabolic profile whereas no difference in the positive efficacy of both transdermal and parental testosterone preparations on the other outcomes considered was documented (Table 8.3) [32].

Osteoporosis

The specific role of T in the regulation of bone health and its contribution to the development of male osteoporosis are conflicting [41]. Only two independent meta-analyses evaluated the effect of TRT versus placebo in RCTs [37, 42]. Both studies reported a positive effect of TRT on bone mineral density at lumber site but the effect was not documented at the femoral site [37, 42]. However, insufficient data are available to evaluate the contribution of TRT on the risk of bone fractures [41].

Table 8.3 Mean [95% CI] for different body composition parameters as derived from available meta-analyses

Meta-analyses considered	Overall							
	BMI	*Fat mass*	*Lean mass*	*Fasting glycemia (mmol/L)*	*Total cholesterol (mmol/L)*	*Triglycerides (mmol/L)*	*HDL (mmol/L)*	*LDL (mmol/L)*
Isidori et al. [37]	–	−1.46 [−3.01;0.09]	1.16 [−0.49;2.80]	–	−0.42 [−0.65;−0.19]	–	0.01 [−0.05;0.07]	−0.33 [−0.80;0.14]
Haddad et al. [47]	–	–	–		−0.22 [−0.71;0.27]	−0.27 [−0.61;0.01]	−0.04 [−0.39;0.30]	0.06 [−0.30;0.42]
Fernandez-Balsells et al. [48]	–	–	–	–	–	–	–	–
Corona et al. [49]	−0.01 [−0.45;0.42]	−0.39 [−0.61;−0.17]	0.45 [0.26;0.73]	−0.37 [−0.65;−0.09]	−0.35 [−0.61;−0.01]	−0.18 [−0.33;−0.04]	0.03 [−0.05;0.11]	–
	Data according to testosterone formulations (Corona et al. [29]**)**							
	Fat mass		*Lean mass*		*Fasting glycemia (mmol/L)*	*Total cholesterol (mmol/L)*		
Oral	−0.26 [−0.47; 0.04]		1.28 [0.28;2.67]		−1.19 [−2.76;0.37]	−1.19 [−2.76;0.37]		
Transdermal	−0.14 [−0.25;−0.03]		0.31 [0.21;0.41]		−0.22 [−0.40;−0.04]	−0.22 [−0.40;−0.04]		
Injectable	−0.65 [−0.96;−0.34]		0.61 [0.37;0.86]		−0.36 [−0.62;−0.10]	−0.36 [−0.62;−0.10]		

BMI body mass index, *HDL* high-density lipoprotein, *LDL* low-density lipoprotein

Mood and Cognition

Much evidence suggests a possible relationship between depressive symptoms and LOH; however, the relationship between low T levels and incidence of clinical depression and the effect of TRT on depressive symptoms are still unclear [43]. Similar considerations can be drawn for the relationship between reduced levels of T and age-dependent cognition deterioration or the risk of developing Alzheimer's disease [44, 45].

Potential Side Effects

Cardiovascular Risk

CV risk is still a hot topic regarding TRT safety. Interestingly, the major problems related to this issue come from limited evidence including one RCT [46], two retrospective pharmaco-epidemiological papers [47, 48], and one meta-analysis [49] published between 2013 and 2014. All these studies present important methodological limitations, which have been discussed elsewhere [50–53]. In addition, it is important to recognize that the largest observational study published so far, including almost 45,000 male patients, showed a protective effect and not an increased risk related to TRT after a median follow-up of 3.4 years [54]. In addition, besides the Xu et al.'s [49] meta-analysis, seven other meta-analyses [38, 39, 55–59] published either before or after Xu et al. [49] did not support an increased CV risk related to TRT either when aggregated or disaggregate CV events were evaluated. Similar consideration can be drawn when venous thromboembolism risk was considered [60].

Prostate Safety

Among the scientific and nonscientific community, prostate cancer (PC) or a possible exacerbation of symptoms due to benign prostatic hyperplasia (BPH) has been considered the worst complication of TRT for a long time. However, data published in the two last decades has substantially modified this position [61–63]. Accordingly, the available meta-analyses [39, 55, 64–68] showed that TRT is associated with a short-term (<12 months) increase in PSA levels, which has not been confirmed in longer trials. Conversely, no risk of prostate cancer or BPH symptoms has been documented [39, 55, 64–66]. Accordingly, almost 10 years ago, Morgentaler and Traish speculated that ("saturation hypothesis") in a physiological condition, the human prostate androgen receptors are "saturated" by the circulating androgens and therefore rather insensitive to further T increase [69]. This hypothesis was later on confirmed in both preclinical [62] and clinical studies [70–72].

Erythrocytosis

Erythrocytosis is the most common side effect related to TRT [21]. Several mechanisms could be underlying this phenomenon. First of all, T plays a direct action in stimulating endogenous erythropoietin (EPO) secretion and bone marrow erythroid progenitor cells [21]. In addition, more recent evidence suggests that T can be involved in the regulation of hepcidin metabolism resulting in an increased iron absorption, increased systemic iron transport, and erythropoiesis [21]. Finally, a possible role of T metabolites such as estradiol or dihydrotestosterone, as well as the contribution of genetic factors (androgen receptor CAG repeats), has also been considered [21]. However, it is important to recognize that several uncontrolled studies have documented that the risk of polycythemia related to TRT is higher in subjects treated with short-acting T formulations [21]. Conversely, the use of transdermal T preparations or long-acting injectable TU is associated with lower risk [21].

Conclusion

In conclusion, the treatment of hypogonadal subjects requires adequate preparation and skill. Available evidence has documented that TRT in hypogonadal subjects is able to improve sexual function and ameliorate body composition. When prescribed according to current guidelines no CV risk or risk of prostate health has been reported. Older injectable preparations are associated with a higher risk of polycythemia.

References

1. Corona G, Rastrelli G, Vignozzi L, Maggi M. Emerging medication for the treatment of male hypogonadism. Expert Opin Emerg Drugs. 2012;17:239–59.
2. Corona G, Rastrelli G, Vignozzi L, Mannucci E, Maggi M. How to recognize late-onset hypogonadism in men with sexual dysfunction. Asian J Androl. 2012;14:251–9.
3. Lenzi A, Balercia G, Bellastella A, Colao A, Fabbri A, Foresta C, Galdiero M, Gandini L, Krausz C, Lombardi G, Lombardo F, Maggi M, Radicioni A, Selice R, Sinisi AA, Forti G. Epidemiology, diagnosis, and treatment of male hypogonadotropic hypogonadism. J Endocrinol Investig. 2009;32:934–8.
4. Corona G, Maseroli E, Rastrelli G, Sforza A, Forti G, Mannucci E, Maggi M. Characteristics of compensated hypogonadism in patients with sexual dysfunction. J Sex Med. 2014;11:1823–34.
5. Giannetta E, Gianfrilli D, Barbagallo F, Isidori AM, Lenzi A. Subclinical male hypogonadism. Best Pract Res Clin Endocrinol Metab. 2012;26:539–50.
6. Corona G, Rastrelli G, Maggi M. Diagnosis and treatment of late-onset hypogonadism: systematic review and meta-analysis of TRT outcomes. Best Pract Res Clin Endocrinol Metab. 2013;27:557–79.
7. Corona G, Rastrelli G, Maggi M. The pharmacotherapy of male hypogonadism besides androgens. Expert Opin Pharmacother. 2015;6:369–87.
8. Wu FC, Tajar A, Beynon JM, Pye SR, Silman AJ, Finn JD, O'Neill TW, Bartfai G, Casanueva FF, Forti G, Giwercman A, Han TS, Kula K, Lean ME, Pendleton N, Punab M, Boonen S, Vanderschueren D, Labrie F, Huhtaniemi IT. Identification of late-onset hypogonadism in middle-aged and elderly men. N Engl J Med. 2010;363:123–35.

9. Rastrelli G, Corona G, Tarocchi M, Mannucci M, Maggi M. How to define hypogonadism? Results from a population of men consulting for sexual dysfunction. J Endocrinol Investig. 2016;39:473–84.
10. Grossmann M, Matsumoto AM. A perspective on middle-aged and older men with functional hypogonadism: focus on holistic management. J Clin Endocrinol Metab. 2017;102:1067–75.
11. Corona G, Maseroli E, Rastrelli G, Francomano D, Aversa A, Hackett GI, Ferri S, Sforza A, Maggi M. Is late-onset hypogonadotropic hypogonadism a specific age-dependent disease, or merely an epiphenomenon caused by accumulating disease-burden? Minerva Endocrinol. 2016;41:196–210.
12. Corona G, Bianchini S, Sforza A, Vignozzi L, Maggi M. Hypogonadism as a possible link between metabolic diseases and erectile dysfunction in aging men. Hormones (Athens). 2015;14:569–78.
13. Corona G, Vignozzi L, Sforza A, Mannucci E, Maggi M. Obesity and late-onset hypogonadism. Mol Cell Endocrinol. 2015;418:120–33.
14. Corona G, Maggi M. Perspective: regulatory agencies' changes to testosterone product labeling. J Sex Med. 2015;12:1690–3.
15. Wang C, Nieschlag E, Swerdloff R, Behre HM, Hellstrom WJ, Gooren LJ, Kaufman JM, Legros JJ, Lunenfeld B, Morales A, Morley JE, Schulman C, Thompson IM, Weidner W, Wu FC. Investigation, treatment and monitoring of late-onset hypogonadism in males. Int J Androl. 2009;32:1–10.
16. Khera M, Adaikan G, Buvat J, Carrier S, El-Meliegy A, Hatzimouratidis K, McCullough A, Morgentaler A, Torres LO, Salonia A. Diagnosis and treatment of testosterone deficiency: recommendations from the fourth International Consultation for Sexual Medicine (ICSM 2015). J Sex Med. 2016;13:1787–804.
17. Lunenfeld B, Mskhalaya G, Zitzmann M, Arver S, Kalinchenko S, Tishova Y, Morgentaler A. Recommendations on the diagnosis, treatment and monitoring of hypogonadism in men. Aging Male. 2015;18:5–15.
18. Nieschlag E, Nieschlag S. Testosterone deficiency: a historical perspective. Asian J Androl. 2014;16:161–8.
19. Nieschlag E, Vorona E. Mechanisms in endocrinology: medical consequences of doping with anabolic androgenic steroids: effects on reproductive functions. Eur J Endocrinol. 2015;173:R47–58.
20. Nieschlag E. Current topics in testosterone replacement of hypogonadal men. Best Pract Res Clin Endocrinol Metab. 2015;29:77–90.
21. Ohlander SJ, Varghese B, Pastuszak AW. Erythrocytosis following testosterone therapy. Sex Med Rev. 2018;6:77–85.
22. Corona G, Maseroli E, Maggi M. Injectable testosterone undecanoate for the treatment of hypogonadism. Expert Opin Pharmacother. 2014;15:1903–26.
23. Wang C, Swerdloff RS. Should the nonaromatizable androgen dihydrotestosterone be considered as an alternative to testosterone in the treatment of the andropause? J Clin Endocrinol Metab. 2002;87:1462–6.
24. Swerdloff RS, Wang C. Dihydrotestosterone: a rationale for its use as a non-aromatizable androgen replacement therapeutic agent. Bailliere Clin Endocrinol Metab. 1998;12:501–6.
25. Choi SK, Han SW, Kim DH, et al. Transdermal dihydrotestosterone therapy and its effects on patients with microphallus. J Urol. 1993;150:657–60.
26. Jain P, Rademaker AW, McVary KT. Testosterone supplementation for erectile dysfunction: results of a meta-analysis. J Urol. 2000;164:371–5.
27. Corona G, Rastrelli G, Morgentaler A, Sforza A, Mannucci E, Maggi M. Meta-analysis of results of testosterone therapy on sexual function based on international index of erectile function scores. Eur Urol. 2017;72:1000–11.
28. Tsertsvadze A, Fink HA, Yazdi F, MacDonald R, Bella AJ, Ansari MT, Garritty C, Soares-Weiser K, Daniel R, Sampson M, Fox S, Moher D, Wilt TJ. Oral phosphodiesterase-5 inhibitors and hormonal treatments for erectile dysfunction: a systematic review and meta-analysis. Ann Intern Med. 2009;151:650–61.

29. Corona G, Isidori AM, Buvat J, Aversa A, Rastrelli G, Hackett G, Rochira V, Sforza A, Lenzi A, Mannucci E, Maggi M. Testosterone supplementation and sexual function: a meta-analysis study. J Sex Med. 2014;11:1577–92.
30. Boloña ER, Uraga MV, Haddad RM, Tracz MJ, Sideras K, Kennedy CC, Caples SM, Erwin PJ, Montori VM. Testosterone use in men with sexual dysfunction: a systematic review and meta-analysis of randomized placebo-controlled trials. Mayo Clin Proc. 2007;82:20–8.
31. Isidori AM, Giannetta E, Gianfrilli D, Greco EA, Bonifacio V, Aversa A, Isidori A, Fabbri A, Lenzi A. Effects of testosterone on sexual function in men: results of a meta-analysis. Clin Endocrinol. 2005;63:381–94.
32. Rastrelli G, Maggi M, Corona G. Pharmacological management of late onset hypogonadism. Expert Rev Clin Pharmacol. 2018;11:439–58.
33. Cohen J. Statistical power analysis for the behavioral sciences. New York: Academic Press; 1977.
34. Corona G, Rastrelli G, Filippi S, Vignozzi L, Mannucci E, Maggi M. Erectile dysfunction and central obesity: an Italian perspective. Asian J Androl. 2014;16:581–9.
35. Corona G, Giagulli VA, Maseroli E, Vignozzi L, Aversa A, Zitzmann M, Saad F, Mannucci E, Maggi M. Testosterone supplementation and body composition: results from a meta-analysis of observational studies. J Endocrinol Investig. 2016;39:967–81.
36. Kelly DM, Jones TH. Testosterone and obesity. Obes Rev. 2015;16:581–606.
37. Isidori AM, Giannetta E, Greco EA, Gianfrilli D, Bonifacio V, Isidori A, Lenzi A, Fabbri A. Effects of testosterone on body composition, bone metabolism and serum lipid profile in middle-aged men: a meta-analysis. Clin Endocrinol. 2005;63:280–93.
38. Haddad RM, Kennedy CC, Caples SM, Tracz MJ, Boloña ER, Sideras K, Uraga MV, Erwin PJ, Montori VM. Testosterone and cardiovascular risk in men: a systematic review and meta-analysis of randomized placebo-controlled trials. Mayo Clin Proc. 2007;82:29–39.
39. Fernández-Balsells MM, Murad MH, Lane M, Lampropulos JF, Albuquerque F, Mullan RJ, Agrwal N, Elamin MB, Gallegos-Orozco JF, Wang AT, Erwin PJ, Bhasin S, Montori VM. Clinical review 1: adverse effects of testosterone therapy in adult men: a systematic review and meta-analysis. J Clin Endocrinol Metab. 2010;95:2560–75.
40. Corona G, Giagulli VA, Maseroli E, Vignozzi L, Aversa A, Zitzmann M, Saad F, Mannucci E, Maggi M. Therapy of endocrine disease: testosterone supplementation and body composition: results from a meta-analysis study. Eur J Endocrinol. 2016;174:R99–116.
41. Golds G, Houdek D, Arnason T. Male hypogonadism and osteoporosis: the effects, clinical consequences, and treatment of testosterone deficiency in bone health. Int J Endocrinol. 2017;2017:4602129. https://doi.org/10.1155/2017/4602129. Epub 2017 Mar 16
42. Tracz MJ, Sideras K, Boloña ER, Haddad RM, Kennedy CC, Uraga MV, et al. Testosterone use in men and its effects on bone health. A systematic review and meta-analysis of randomized placebo-controlled trials. J Clin Endocrinol Metab. 2006;91:2011–6.
43. Smith JB, Rosen J, Colbert A. Low serum testosterone in outpatient psychiatry clinics: addressing challenges to the screening and treatment of hypogonadism. Sex Med Rev. 2018;6:69–76.
44. Lv W, Du N, Liu Y, Fan X, Wang Y, Jia X, Hou X, Wang B. Low testosterone level and risk of Alzheimer's disease in the elderly men: a systematic review and meta-analysis. Mol Neurobiol. 2016;53:2679–84.
45. Wahjoepramono EJ, Asih PR, Aniwiyanti V, Taddei K, Dhaliwal SS, Fuller SJ, Foster J, Carruthers M, Verdile G, Sohrabi HR, Martins RN. The effects of testosterone supplementation on cognitive functioning in older men. CNS Neurol Disord Drug Targets. 2016;15:337–43.
46. Basaria S, Coviello AD, Travison TG, Storer TW, Farwell WR, Jette AM, Eder R, Tennstedt S, Ulloor J, Zhang A, Choong K, Lakshman KM, Mazer NA, Miciek R, Krasnoff J, Elmi A, Knapp PE, Brooks B, Appleman E, Aggarwal S, Bhasin G, Hede-Brierley L, Bhatia A, Collins L, LeBrasseur N, Fiore LD, Bhasin S. Adverse events associated with testosterone administration. N Engl J Med. 2010;363:109–22.
47. Vigen R, O'Donnell CI, Barón AE, Grunwald GK, Maddox TM, Bradley SM, Barqawi A, Woning G, Wierman ME, Plomondon ME, Rumsfeld JS, Ho PM. Association of testosterone

therapy with mortality, myocardial infarction, and stroke in men with low testosterone levels. JAMA. 2013;310:1829–36.
48. Finkle WD, Greenland S, Ridgeway GK, Adams JL, Frasco MA, Cook MB, Fraumeni JF Jr, Hoover RN. Increased risk of non-fatal myocardial infarction following testosterone therapy prescription in men. PLoS One. 2014;9:e85805.
49. Xu L, Freeman G, Cowling BJ, Schooling CM. Testosterone therapy and cardiovascular events among men: a systematic review and meta-analysis of placebo-controlled randomized trials. BMC Med. 2013;11:108.
50. Isidori AM, Balercia G, Calogero AE, Corona G, Ferlin A, Francavilla S, Santi D, Maggi M. Outcomes of androgen replacement therapy in adult male hypogonadism: recommendations from the Italian society of endocrinology. J Endocrinol Investig. 2015;38:103–12.
51. Corona G, Sforza A, Maggi M. Testosterone replacement therapy: long-term safety and efficacy. World J Mens Health. 2017;35:65–76.
52. Corona G, Vignozzi L, Sforza A, Maggi M. Risks and benefits of late onset hypogonadism treatment: an expert opinion. World J Mens Health. 2013;31:103–25.
53. Elagizi A, Köhler TS, Lavie CJ. Testosterone and cardiovascular health. Mayo Clin Proc. 2018;93:83–100.
54. Sharma R, Oni OA, Gupta K, Chen G, Sharma M, Dawn B, Sharma R, Parashara D, Savin VJ, Ambrose JA, Barua RS. Normalization of testosterone level is associated with reduced incidence of myocardial infarction and mortality in men. Eur Heart J. 2015;36:2706–15.
55. Calof OM, Singh AB, Lee ML, Kenny AM, Urban RJ, Tenover JL, Bhasin S. Adverse events associated with testosterone replacement in middle-aged and older men: a meta-analysis of randomized, placebo-controlled trials. J Gerontol A Biol Sci Med Sci. 2005;60:1451–7.
56. Corona G, Maseroli E, Rastrelli G, Isidori AM, Sforza A, Mannucci E, Maggi M. Cardiovascular risk associated with testosterone boosting medications: a systematic review and meta-analysis. Expert Opin Drug Saf. 2014;13:1327–51.
57. Borst SE, Shuster JJ, Zou B, Ye F, Jia H, Wokhlu A, Yarrow JF. Cardiovascular risks and elevation of serum DHT vary by route of testosterone administration: a systematic review and meta-analysis. BMC Med. 2014;12:211.
58. Albert SG, Morley JE. Testosterone therapy, association with age, initiation and mode of therapy with cardiovascular events: a systematic review. Clin Endocrinol (Oxf). 2016;85:436–43.
59. Alexander GC, Iyer G, Lucas E, Lin D, Singh S. Cardiovascular risks of exogenous testosterone use among men: a systematic review and meta-analysis. Am J Med. 2017;130:293–305.
60. Corona G, Dicuio M, Rastrelli G, Maseroli E, Lotti F, Sforza A, Maggi M. Testosterone treatment and cardiovascular and venous thromboembolism risk: what is 'new'? J Investig Med. 2017;65:964–73.
61. Corona G, Gacci M, Baldi E, Mancina R, Forti G, Maggi M. Androgen deprivation therapy in prostate cancer: focusing on sexual side effects. J Sex Med. 2012;9(3):887–902.
62. Corona G, Baldi E, Maggi M. Androgen regulation of prostate cancer: where are we now? J Endocrinol Investig. 2011;34:232–43.
63. Lopez DS, Advani S, Tsilidis KK, Wang R, Canfield S. Endogenous and exogenous testosterone and prostate cancer: decreased-, increased- or null-risk? Transl Androl Urol. 2017;6:566–79.
64. Cui Y, Zhang Y. The effect of androgen-replacement therapy on prostate growth: a systematic review and meta-analysis. Eur Urol. 2013;64:811–22.
65. Cui Y, Zong H, Yan H, Zhang Y. The effect of testosterone replacement therapy on prostate cancer: a systematic review and meta-analysis. Prostate Cancer Prostatic Dis. 2014;17:132–43.
66. Guo C, Gu W, Liu M, Peng BO, Yao X, Yang B, Zheng J. Efficacy and safety of testosterone replacement therapy in men with hypogonadism: a meta-analysis study of placebo-controlled trials. Exp Ther Med. 2016;11:853–63.
67. Kang DY, Li HJ. The effect of testosterone replacement therapy on prostate-specific antigen (PSA) levels in men being treated for hypogonadism: a systematic review and meta-analysis. Medicine (Baltimore). 2015;94:e410.

68. Boyle P, Koechlin A, Bota M, d'Onofrio A, Zaridze DG, Perrin P, Fitzpatrick J, Burnett AL, Boniol M. Endogenous and exogenous testosterone and the risk of prostate cancer and increased prostate-specific antigen (PSA) level: a meta-analysis. BJU Int. 2016;118:731–41.
69. Morgentaler A, Traish AM. Shifting the paradigm of testosterone and prostate cancer: the saturation model and the limits of androgen-dependent growth. Eur Urol. 2009;55:310–20.
70. Rastrelli G, Corona G, Vignozzi L, Maseroli E, Silverii A, Monami M, Mannucci E, Forti G, Maggi M. Serum PSA as a predictor of testosterone deficiency. J Sex Med. 2013;10:2518–28.
71. Corona G, Boddi V, Lotti F, Gacci M, Carini M, De Vita G, Sforza A, Forti G, Mannucci E, Maggi M. The relationship of testosterone to prostate-specific antigen in men with sexual dysfunction. J Sex Med. 2010;7(1 Pt 1):284–92.
72. Gacci M, Corona G, Apolone G, Lanciotti M, Tosi N, Giancane S, Masieri L, Serni S, Maggi M, Carini M. Influence of serum testosterone on urinary continence and sexual activity in patients undergoing radical prostatectomy for clinically localized prostate cancer. Prostate Cancer Prostatic Dis. 2010;13:168–72.

Psychotherapy for Sexual Dysfunctions 9

A. Sathyanarayana Reddy

Introduction

Sexual relationships are influenced by individual's sexuality, biology, and psychological markup. Society, culture, and religious factors also significantly influence sexual function. Sexual medicine denotes the study of the biological and/or psychological components of both normal sexual function and sexual dysfunction in both the individual and the partner.

Organic and psychogenic factors play a significant role in the causation of sexual dysfunctions. The relation between sexual dysfunction and psychological disturbances in an individual is bidirectional and complex in nature.

Psychological disturbances can be the cause of the sexual dysfunctions or the effect of the sexual dysfunctions and in some clinical scenarios both. Even in sexual dysfunctions of biological origin, some psychological component exist. All the indices of sexual function and dysfunction assess the genital organ functions and consequently good sex is considered to be a good physical response. It is now clear that good body function alone does not mean good sex [1]. Sexual desire, sexual pleasure, and sexual satisfaction are more important than genital function, especially in women as compared to men. Erectile dysfunction management involves the use of PDE5 inhibitors which give robust sex in about 70% of men. But it may not be satisfactory sex. So, in such men psychological counseling and psychotherapy have a role to play.

A. Sathyanarayana Reddy
Leo Institute of Sexual Medicine, Hyderabad, Telangana, India

Apollo Fertility, Hyderabad, Telangana, India

© Springer Nature Singapore Pte Ltd. 2019

K. Gunasekaran, S. D. Khan (eds.), *Sexual Medicine*,
https://doi.org/10.1007/978-981-13-1226-7_9

Psychological Basis of Sexual Dysfunctions

Sexual dysfunction is frequently influenced by a variety of precipitating and/or predisposing factors along with maintaining and/or contextual factors [2].

Predisposing Factors

Predisposing factors normally include both constitutional and prior life experiences that contribute to a person's vulnerability for developing a dysfunction. However these factors alone are rarely sufficient to cause sexual dysfunction. Constitutional factors include congenital anatomical defects, intersex conditions, and genetically determined hormonal, neurologic, and vascular factors. The other category of constitutional factors include individual temperament like shyness, inhibition, excitation, impulsiveness, and personality traits like histrionic, obsessive-compulsive, and resilience of the individual.

The Developmental Factors of Sexual Dysfunctions

Psychological development for an individual continues throughout life. Sexually atypical adolescents may discover their homosexual orientation and in some extreme instances may be diagnosed as to having a gender identity disorder/conflict. In a few other individuals a sexual paraphilia such as voyeurism, exhibitionism, fetishism, sadism, masochism, or pedophilia may also develop [3]. Two types of developmental factors are thought to increase the likelihood of sexual dysfunction, event-based trauma (single episode), and process-based trauma (ongoing). An example of event-based trauma is rape. Children of parents who don't express warmth or affection can't establish healthy intimate relationship as an adult, and this is an example of process-based trauma [4]. Boys and girls at puberty receive sociosexual scripts from parents, society, and culture. Erotically rigid scripts provide a platform for the onset of sexual dysfunction later in adult life. Clinically, it is often reported that traumatic or humiliating sexual initiation and coitus may be associated with later sexual anxiety and/or aversion.

Child sexual abuse in girls is associated with vaginismus and/or orgasmic difficulties. Sexual abuse is considered a salient risk factor for later adult sexual dysfunction and an increased prevalence of high-risk sexual behavior/psychopathology [5].

Religious/cultural restrictions and/or expectations play a contributory role in the causation of sexual dysfunction. Medical illness, medical treatments, and surgical interventions specially in cancer predispose the men and women to sexual dysfunctions. Men frequently worry about penis size and women about body shape and weight. ED prevalence was much higher in men dissatisfied with their penis size than satisfied men, 77.2% versus 42.7% [6]. In women, body image issues can affect all domains of sexual function. Genital mutilation surgeries for carcinoma breast, carcinoma of testis, and carcinoma of penis can adversely affect sex in all domains of sexual function. An individual's vulnerability to sexual dysfunction later on is determined by the ratio of risk factors versus protective factors as well as their personal resilience [7]. When stress factors are greater than the individual's protective factors, then even resilient individuals can develop sexual dysfunction.

Precipitating Factors

It is difficult to determine which factor under which circumstance precipitates sexual dysfunction both within and between individuals. There is no clear-cut distinction between predisposing, precipitating, and maintaining factors. The same factor can precipitate and/or maintain a sexual dysfunction. Life-stage stressors like infertility, childbirth, child-rearing, divorce, death of the partner, partner's sexual inadequacy, extra marital relations of self or partner, and life situations like unemployment, loss of job, and financial troubles can also be precipitating factors.

The following play a major role in precipitating and maintaining sexual dysfunctions:

(a) Personality traits of the individual, (b) partner's problems, and (c) interpersonal relationships

(a) Personality Traits

Anger: Psychological responses during anger and during sexual activity are similar as pointed out by Kinsey. Some clinicians speculate that sexual dysfunction may be a means of expressing anger at partner.

Depression: In men with depression who are not on medication, 42% report a decrease in sexual drive, sexual fantasies, viewing sexually explicit material, and masturbation. About 26% are not sexually active [8]. In the men who are sexually active, 34% have less vigorous erections, 40% are unable to sustain erection, 12% had PE, and 23% reported delayed ejaculation. The relationship between depressive mood symptoms and sexual dysfunctions is bidirectional in nature and is further convoluted by the side effects of antidepressants. In Massachusetts Male Aging Study, moderate-to-severe erectile dysfunction was 1.82 times more in depressed men than in general population. Depression was also a strong predictor of arousal and orgasmic dysfunction in women.

Personality disorders like OCD, histrionic personality, and borderline personality: 50% of the individuals with OCD report sexual problems and over 60–73% are dissatisfied with their sexual lives [9]. Women with histrionic personality were associated with lower self-esteem, lower sexual assertiveness, greater erotophobic attitudes, and greater marital dissatisfaction. In contrast, women with borderline personality disorders showed higher sexual self-esteem, sexual assertiveness, and greater likelihood of extramarital affairs.

Anxiety: Anxiety is the central point of etiology and therapy of sexual dysfunction in both psychodynamic and behavior techniques. Anxiety is very commonly seen in individuals with sexual dysfunction. There is a strong correlation between sexual dysfunction and anxiety. This does not imply causality. Contrary to findings from clinical studies that explored the inhibition effect of anxiety on sex, laboratory studies indicate that anxiety either facilitates or does not affect sexual arousal in functional subjects. In sexually dysfunctional subjects, the response is mixed. Studies that explored the relationship between sympathetic activation and anxiety and/or sexual response have shown that anxiety is not universally disruptive to sexual functioning [10]. Anxiety in moderate levels in safe settings may catalyze sexual arousal, but at higher levels for longer duration may likely impair sexual functioning [10]. General anxiety, trait anxiety, sexual anxiety, and performance anxiety act differently in creating sexual dysfunction.

Sexual dysfunction in one of the partners can affect the sexual function of the other partner. 26% of the female partners of men with ED have inhibited sex: HSDD in 20%; arousal problem in 30%; orgasm difficulty in 24%; and/or urinary symptoms in 36%. Treatment of these men with ED with PDE-5 inhibitors resulted in significant reduction in all the female sexual dysfunctions. In partners of the women with sexual problems, 50% suffer with PE. Male partners of women with sexual pain disorders also report lower sexual satisfaction.

Maintaining Factors

Maintaining factors prolong or exacerbate the sexual dysfunction or may convert an episodic problem into a chronic problem. Performance anxiety, low confidence, and deteriorating interpersonal relationships can all contribute to causing a dysfunction on a long-term basis.

Performance anxiety: Performance anxiety is the fear of failure in the present sexual act based on the previous failures [11]. This perpetuates the sexual dysfunction in both men and women. The individual approaches sex with a failed mind or an anticipated fear of failing, resulting in no erection or loss of erection. The individual then loses confidence, and imagines the consequences of sexual failure leading to further deterioration and sexual avoidance. In partnered sex, mentally stepping outside of oneself and thus monitoring one's own sexual performance is called spectatoring. This distracts his/her attention from the pleasure of sexual activity. Spectatoring leads to sexual dysfunction in the long term.

A man or woman might have never achieved confidence to view themselves as sexual beings, and, they might have lost the confidence to perform good sexual function. In men with ED and PE, improving sexual confidence along with medical management gives good results. Success of medical treatment by itself increases the level of confidence in the man. But psychological intervention may be necessary to restore his/her confidence completely.

Relationship Issues and Sexual Dysfunction

There is a correlation between unsatisfactory or dysfunctional couple relations and sexual dysfunctions in individuals or couples. Which occurs first remains difficult to deduce. Sexual dysfunction can be a cause of relationship problem or can be an effect of poor interpersonal relationships [11]. In relationship problems and sexual dysfunctions whichever comes first, treating both together is the most effective form of intervention. If not done together, the problem that is not addressed may continue to influence the problem that is the focus of treatment.

Contextual Factors

Contextual factors include day-to-day nonsexual stressors and situations: not having privacy, working in different shifts, working in different cities, unemployment, financial loss, infertility, infertility treatments, child-rearing, and taking care of sick family members or partner. These contextual issues are usually short-lived, but may become chronic, leading to inability in having a satisfying sexual life or developing a sexual dysfunction.

Psychosexual Therapy and Techniques

Psychosexual therapy is a specialized form of psychological intervention that focuses on the sexual aspect of the human problems. The basic principles of general psychotherapeutic techniques are followed in sex therapy as well. The treatment modalities evolved over time from psychoanalytical approach to integrative biopsychosocial therapy.

Psychoanalytical and Psychodynamic Aspects of Sex Therapy

As per Freudian hypothesis—The child takes the parent of opposite sex as the object of his/her erotic wishes [12]. The child then moves away from his/her first and forbidden object of erotic wishes to develop mature adult sexuality. Today, the oedipal complex is used as a metaphor for the child's ability to separate individual from the parental unit. The conflict between libido and sexual impulse embedded in an unconscious Id, society and morality, and Super Ego and organized in the realistic part of the mind-Ego forms the basis of infant psyche and sexuality [13]. Failure to resolve the oedipal complex and incomplete infantile psychosexual development express as sexual dysfunctions. In adult relationships, there is always a conflict between desire of individuality and necessity of togetherness. This can create a conflict in which each partner gains from the other, maintaining its individuality. Early childhood anxieties and fears make this conflict destructive, a battleground necessitating sex therapy or which if unresolved may end in separation.

Psychodynamic therapy uses the clinical tools of transference and counter transference to access the internal world of the patient. Tolerance is a clinical term for projection. An individual transfers feelings and attitudes from a person or a situation in the past on to a person or situation in the present. For example, a child who had difficult experiences from an authoritarian father unconsciously transfers or projects these feelings on to the rest of the world, specially on to the persons in authority—a negative transference. If a child had a kind and supportive mother, it transfers these feelings on to everyone around—positive transference. The client's attitude towards the therapist will reflect the client's inner world. The client elicits feelings in friends, colleagues, and therapists and they respond to the client's feelings. These unconscious feelings the therapists and friends experience towards the client are called counter transference. The psychodynamic therapy helps clients to free themselves from unconsciously living out in the past experience—to live fully in the present. In psychodynamic therapy, the therapist helps the patient to review emotions and thoughts, and beliefs, along with early life experiences to gain insight into their present day problems and develop defensive mechanisms. Brief psychodynamic therapy may take up to 25 sessions, and long-term psychodynamic therapy may take 2 years.

Cognitive Aspects of Psychosexual Therapy

Throughout life, people develop certain beliefs about sexuality in general and their own sexuality, like a man should have erection on demand; orgasm is a must during sex; I am inadequate; and I am a failure if I don't satisfy a woman. When faced with a sexual situation, these automatic thoughts spring from the person's mind [14]. These automatic thoughts are different in sexually functional and sexually dysfunctional men. The client identifies the beliefs that are disturbing him. Using logic and evidence, the client and the therapist evaluate these beliefs. The therapist then guides the client to modify these distorted thoughts.

The first step in the cognitive therapy is identifying the automatic and involuntary thoughts that arise in the client's mind at successful and unsuccessful sexual encounters. The client can have myths, misleading ideas, maladaptive beliefs about sex, sexual responses, and sexual satisfaction [15]. Confronting the client with accurate information about the psychophysiology of sex is then done. The client is next asked to weigh the advantages and disadvantages of his sexual beliefs. Once the client identifies his distorted ideas and false beliefs, the therapist suggests or helps the client to identify alternative beliefs. A role-play technique is helpful wherein the client and the therapist enter into point–counterpoint dialogue, the client initially for his maladaptive belief and later against his maladaptive belief and for his new alternative belief. Then the client is given an opportunity to practice alternative beliefs. This is called cognitive restructuring.

Behavioral Aspects of Psychosexual Therapy

Behavior is learned and so can be unlearned via therapy. This is the basic principle of behavioral therapy. A behavior that elicits positive emotions is continued, repeated, and reinforced and a maladaptive behavior that elicits negative emotion is inhibited and discontinued. When sexual arousal is associated with negative feelings of guilt and fear, the result is a learned inhibition of sexual response. In practice, cognitive therapy is almost always combined with behavioral therapy. The CBT works based on the fact that cognition, emotions, and behaviors are interrelated and a change in one of these three dimensions will facilitate the change in the other two. In CBT, structured behavioral assignments are given to the individual or couple to be practiced in privacy. From a psychosexual context, therapies like sensate focus, systematic desensitization, stop and start technique, guided stimulation, and directed masturbation are popularly used in the treatment of male and female sexual dysfunctions.

Systemic Aspects of Psychosexual Therapy

Sexual relationship is an integral part of general relationship between a couple. So, nonsexual relationship can affect sexual functioning. In the sexual interaction of a couple, each partner brings a set of experiences from their family and society at large [16]. These embedded values influence the way they understand and respond to their partners. The basic concepts of sexual problems in a couple are as follows [17]:

1. A sexual problem of one partner always has an influence on the other. For example—the husband of a woman with vaginismus can develop ED.
2. Some sex problems are caused by the faulty relationship itself.
3. In every couple, there can be a difference in sex desire or in sexual arousal methods. When the couple can't find ways to cope up with this difference, sexual difficulties arise.
4. After a sexual dysfunction in one partner, the couple learns to live with the problem. They establish a new equilibrium in sexual relationship.

In couple therapy, the partners learn to talk to each other and the therapist facilitates the communication. The therapist won't formulate the goals. The therapist can then help the partners make an agreement, but he/she never imposes the contract. The fears of attraction, aversion, abandonment, and extramarital affairs in the couple are brought out by the couple's interaction. The therapist helps the partners to break the vicious cycle of sexual problems and relationship problems.

Mindfulness Aspects of Psychosexual Therapy

Awareness of physical sensation at the moment and acceptance of these sensations in a nonjudgmental attitude are the essence of mindfulness. Physical sensations are real. Without experiencing a sensation, we judge them as not right, or not good enough; this ultimately leads to negative emotions.

The thoughts are the product of the mind. Majority of these thoughts are useless, repetitive, ruminations, catastrophic thinking, and future projections which cause distress. Mindfulness is practiced in the Eastern hemisphere with roots in Buddhist meditation. Mindfulness is used or incorporated into various psychosocial interventions to treat psychological, medical, and psychosomatic disorders [18]. The therapeutic program uses mindful exercises like mindfulness of breath, mindful walking, eating, and meditation. In the mindfulness of breath, sitting comfortably over a chair or in a Buddha position, the client brings the attention to the sensation of touch of the body to the floor or chair, and then focuses the attention on the breath, and movements of the abdominal wall with each breath; they don't control breath. The mindfulness-based psychoeducation can be given in a group format, usually for female sexual dysfunctions like sexual desire, arousal, and orgasmic disorders.

The steps followed are [19]:

1. General mindfulness exercises for 10 min.
2. Body scan exercises for 20 min.
3. Focusing exercises for 20 min (during and after bath women are encouraged to observe and describe their body and repeat the statements like—It is my body and I appreciate … aspects of my body).
4. Self-observation exercise for 20 min (women are taught the anatomy of the genitals and they have to observe their genitals with a hand-held mirror and describe, and appreciate in a nonjudgmental way).
5. Self-observation and touch for 20 min (women are encouraged to touch their genitals along with observation and focus on the sensations).
6. The same principle can be applied to male sexual dysfunctions like ED, PE, and DE.

Integrative/Combined Biopsychosocial Model of Sex Therapy

The various perspectives of sexual problems are viewpoints of the problem and the problem may have multiple psychogenic factors. Understanding the problem in different perspectives is necessary [17]. Today's psychotherapy synthesizes the cognitive behavioral intervention, systems/couple interventions, and sometimes psychodynamic interventions also. The patient-centric goal of therapy is restoration of lasting and satisfying sexual function.

In addition, biological factors causing sexual dysfunctions like vascular and endocrinological diseases also may be in the same patient. The client may also be lacking psychosexual skills. So, they have to be taught the cognitive and/or behavioral aspect of lovemaking. The different dimensions of relationships like couples' expectations, autonomy, commitment, cooperation, conflicts, empathy, and emotional intimacy are also to be addressed in achieving this goal. Integrating biological, psychological, relationship, and skill training is the essence of integrative biopsychosocial model of sex therapy.

Sex Therapy

Sex therapy is a structured, short-term, intensive therapeutic intervention devised by Masters and Johnson [20]. The basic concepts of this therapy are the following:

1. In a sexual dysfunction, one partner may have a problem, but both are involved. So, the marital unit is the patient and marital relationship is to be treated.
2. The underlying deep-rooted psychopathology may be the reason for the sexual dysfunction, but it is the "here and now" events that cause and maintain the sexual problem. Sexual dysfunction is a symptom of a psychological disease. The symptom and the immediate causes of the symptom are treated, not the root cause. Unlike psychoanalytical therapy or marital therapy, sex therapy has a specific and limited goal, alleviating sexual dysfunctions, and the therapy ceases once the problem is resolved.
3. It is a couple therapy. Individual is not treated. Surrogate partner concept is discouraged.
4. The dual sex therapist team, one therapist male and the other female, one of them a physician, is adopted.
5. The couple stays for 2–3 weeks in the vicinity of the therapy area leaving family, work, finances, and worries at home. It is a romantic outing in a holiday resort.
6. In practice, the couple is interviewed separately and together, a round table discussion between the couple and the therapists is done and a treatment strategy is formulated. Broadly, the therapy has two parts, initial sensate focus exercises practiced by all couples. The latter half of the therapy is devoted to the specific sexual dysfunctions and hence the techniques are different for each sexual dysfunction. In sensate focus, the couple is instructed not to indulge in sexual intercourse, and not to view the sexual responses like erections in them or in their partner. Instead, focus on the sensations—"sensate focus." Nondemanding, nongenital, mutual pleasuring technique is taught to the couple and they practice the technique in the privacy of their homes regularly. Later genital pleasure is added. The couple is instructed to feel the pleasure of doing exercises in them and in their partner. When there is no demand for performance of sex, the performance anxiety is relieved. When the couple is comfortable, intercourse is introduced. They are instructed to focus on the pleasures of coital touch than the penetration act.

For ED, entry with woman on the top, containment of the male organ in her without thrusting, avoiding orgasm, nonorgasmic thrusting, and finally entry with man on the top, thrusting, and ejaculating are introduced in a sequential order. For PE, the start and stop and the squeeze technique; for DE, the guided stimulation technique; for vaginismus, systematic desensitization; and lastly for primary anorgasmia, directed masturbation are incorporated into the sex therapy sessions in the second half.

The classical sex therapy technique of Masters and Johnson is not followed by many now. The basic concept of sensate focus, nondemand pleasuring, is followed by all and individual variations are incorporated. Helen Kaplan's New Sex Therapy [21] incorporates all the behavioral and psychoanalytical techniques with the limited purpose of alleviating the sexual dysfunctions, not going deep into the root cause of psychopathology. Emergence of resistance during the course of treatment in the symptomatic patient or the client reveals the hidden cause of the sexual problem. Resolution of this resistance by confrontation or by psychoanalysis is the basic module of the New Sex Therapy.

Psychosexual Therapy for Specific Sexual Dysfunctions

Psychosexual Therapy for Erectile Dysfunction

The psychological factors that cause ED are analyzed in different ways by the different schools of thought. Psychoanalytical formulations believe that unresolved oedipal problems leading to unconscious castration anxiety, intrapsychic conflicts, and concomitant feelings of fear and guilt are the causations od ED. Learning theory believes that the oedipal conflicted child learns to fear sex and when he grows up, he, the unhappy husband learns to avoid sex; phobic ideas about woman genitals are also learnt. Cognitive theory is based on sexual myths and beliefs like erection should occur at will, sex is rigid penis, sex is strong thrusts only, women demand sex, wife is always to be satisfied, and simultaneous orgasm is a must; ideas of catastrophic consequences of erection failure are the causes of ED [22]. Ideas derived from past sexual experiences, manifesting in the current sexual experience and guiding future sexual behavior, are called sexual schema, e.g.: I can't have erection, I am incompetent, I am different, and I am not able to keep erection, which lead to automatic thoughts during sexual activity [22, 23]. As a result, he internally distracts from sexual cues which inhibit sexual arousal.

Immediate causal factors of erection failure: In a vulnerable man or a relationship, the factors operative "here and now" are performance anxiety, spectatoring, and lack of abandonment. Performance anxiety is a process that involves the interplay of cognitive, addictive, behavioral, and psychological responses [23]. At a sexual stimulus, negative automatic thoughts, anticipation of failure, and negative emotions lead to anxiety, sympathetic stimulation, and release of adrenaline leading to no erection or loss of erection. Spectatoring is a man focusing on him, his erection from a third person's perspective during sexual activity rather than focusing on his pleasurable sensation. He is a performer of sex and also a judge of his sex. A man abandons himself to his sexual feelings during sexual activity. Relieving the immediate causes of erection failure without addressing the deep-rooted psychopathy is the crux of sex therapy developed by Masters and Johnson [20]. The sex therapy for ED advocated and practiced by Masters and Johnson, modified by Helen Kaplan, is the most effective psychotherapeutic tool for treating ED.

Sex therapy for ED involves the following:

1. Sex education, and exploration of genital organs.
2. Couple is involved in communication.
3. Period of abstinence from ejaculation and coitus.
4. Nongenital pleasuring.
5. Nondemanding genital pleasuring.
6. Nondemanding stimulation of the penis by the partner.
7. Getting him tuned to lessening erections and regaining erection by stopping stimulation and restarting it.
8. Permission to be selfish—sex is to pleasure himself and not to please his partner.
9. Few days of strong erection with manual stimulation, entry of lubricated penis with woman on top.
10. Containment of the penis in the vagina without thrusts.
11. Thrusts by the woman in a teasing, nondemanding way without ejaculation.
12. Entry with the man on top without ejaculation and finally ejaculation.
13. Fantasizing about his wishes and extra-genital stimulation can also be incorporated.

In the treatment of nonorganic ED, the strategies adopted are:

1. Drug therapy alone
2. Psychotherapy alone
3. Psychotherapy with addition of oral medication
4. Psychotherapy with attention to the couple problems

Drug therapy alone: Reassurance, and use of PDE-5 inhibitors to get erections and successful coitus, relieves him of his immediate psychological issues. Daily dosing of PDE5 Inhibitor, and gradually tapering the dose is the practical way of treating. Psychotherapy alone is advocated when the couple is reluctant to use oral medication, when the man complains of low confidence despite having good intravaginal erectile function, when the partner also has untreated sexual dysfunction, when the couple has significant interpersonal problems, or when the couple has abandoned all sexual activity [24].

Oral medication can be added to sex therapy when the couple completed sensual and sexual touch and entered into a sexual excitation stage. Daily dosing of PDE5 inhibitor is preferred over on-demand dosing.

Psychotherapy for Premature Ejaculation

The basic criteria in all the definitions of PE are short intravaginal ejaculatory latency time, inability to control ejaculation, and concern and distress about the condition. There are two major categories of PE—lifelong PE and acquired PE and two additional categories—natural PE and premature like ejaculatory dysfunction.

Lifelong PE is when intravaginal ejaculatory latency time is of less than a minute, global, from first sexual encounter. Some may ejaculate before attempt at entry (ejaculation anteportas) and some may ejaculate at attempt at entry (ejaculation intraportas). Two to three percent of men have lifelong PE. There is genetic predisposition and may be of neurological origin [25].

Acquired PE on the other hand is PE developing after some years of normal ejaculatory latency and may be due to urological problems, ED, hypothyroidism, or psychological and relationship problems. Naturally variable PE is defined by rapid ejaculation that is inconsistent and irregular, diminished or poor control of ejaculation, and moderate IELT of 3–8 min. This is a normal variation of ejaculatory process. In subjective PE, the IELT is normal or may be more. There is a subjective perception of consistent or inconsistent early ejaculation and preoccupation with an imagined early ejaculation. This is the psychological misperception of ejaculation. The psychological factors causing PE are the following:

1. Psychoanalysts believe that premature ejaculators harbor intense, unconscious, sadistic feelings towards women. Rapid ejaculation soils the woman and deprives her of the pleasure.
2. PE is a psychosomatic disturbance, with the psychological conflict directed towards genitals [26].
3. Masters and Johnson proposed that PE is a learned behavior. Initial rapid sexual intercourse leads to habituation and performance anxiety sustains it [20].

All of these however are not evidence based. Anxiety, cognitive factors, and relationship factors are not causative factors but may be maintaining or exacerbating factors. Men with PE have lower frequency and lower satisfaction with intercourse, lower confidence in sex, lower self-esteem, and higher personal distress. Wives of man with PE also have lower sexual satisfaction and higher personal distress. Relationship dysfunction and marital discord ensue.

Management of PE

The central concept of psychosexual therapy for PE is to teach the man to identify the premonitory sensations that precede emission. Men with PE are usually unable to identify this sensation. In addition, these men cannot respond quickly to their premonitory symptoms to delay their ejaculation [27]. Behavioral techniques use this principle to treat PE.

The start-stop method developed by Semans involves stopping sexual stimulation or thrusts at impending emission; once the ejaculation urgency wanes, the man starts stimulation. Masters and Johnson modified this into stop-squeeze method. The man signals his partner as the ejaculatory wave builds. They stop sexual stimulation and the partner applies manual pressure to the glans penis until the urge is reduced. Slight reduction in erection is noticed and the sexual stimulation restarted. Initially, it is practiced at masturbation with three stop-squeeze pauses followed by ejaculation. Afterwards, the couple progresses to sex with woman-on-top position with two or three stop-squeeze pauses and finally shifts to man-on-top position.

A variant of stop-start technique is where the wife stimulates him manually. The man is advised to concentrate on the erotic sensations. When he feels premonitory orgasmic sensation, he signals his wife to stop stimulation. When the sensation subsides in a few seconds, stimulation is resumed. After 3–4 such pauses, he lets her to stimulate to ejaculation. Then the same is practiced with sex with woman on top and later man on top.

Sensate focus may be incorporated as preliminary to these techniques. Dysfunctional beliefs about ejaculation, man's sexual capacity, and woman's satisfaction have to be managed by cognitive therapy. When there is a communication problem or relationship problem, couple therapy is to be instituted. The success rate of Masters and Johnson or Helen Kaplan of more than 98% has never been replicated. Randomized controlled trials of psychotherapy for PE are few. A study compared (a) bibliotherapy without therapist contact, (b) bibliotherapy with minimal contact of the therapist, (c) sex therapy for couples, and (d) wait list control group. All these showed significant improvement in IELT [28]. However, long-term follow-up results of studies using sex therapy as monotherapy have revealed relapse rates of 60–75% after cessation of treatment [29].

Psychotherapy for Delayed Ejaculation

Marked delay in ejaculation or infrequent or absent ejaculation without the individual deliberately causing delay is called delayed ejaculation [30]. It can be lifelong or acquired, and generalized or situational. The causative factors may be neurogenic, endocrinological, iatrogenic, or psychogenic. Ninety percent of men with psychogenic DE can ejaculate at masturbation, but not after coital sex. The psychological reasons for DE are the following:

1. High frequency of masturbation.
2. Idiosyncratic masturbatory style not mimicking coital act like teasing the glans, tossing the penis, squeezing the penis, and rubbing against sheets; the speed, pressure, intensity, and spot of masturbation may be different [31].
3. Disparity between the reality of sex with their partner and their preferred sexual fantasy at masturbation is seen in these men with coital anejaculation. Psychodynamic formulations like fear of losing self, fear of losing semen, and fear of impregnation may be the causes of lifelong DE. Hostility and relationship difficulties may also be the causes.
4. Autosexual orientation—that is, men who prefer masturbation to coital sex can also be the reason for DE [32].

The modality of the psychotherapeutic treatment is based on the etiological factors for DE—sex education; genitally focused stimulation; masturbatory retraining; realignment of sexual fantasies or use of his own sexual fantasies at coital sex are the strategies adopted in the Kaplan model of sex therapy. Nongenital pleasing, nondemand genital play to increase sexual arousal → solitary masturbation to ejaculation → solitary masturbation in the presence of the wife → manual or oral stimulation by the wife → manual stimulation by the wife at the vaginal entrance, using vaginal fluid as lubricant → manual stimulation till impending orgasm and entry into the vagina → entry and ejaculation inside the vagina are the sequential steps. At coital sex, additional stimulation can be given by the wife's fingers to the base of the penis. No controlled studies are there to ascertain the efficacy of any of these techniques.

Psychotherapy of Sexual Interest/Arousal Disorder

Menopause and drug induced or surgeries over genital organs and pelvis are the medical causes of this disorder. Natural or surgical menopausal women with HSDD were treated with testosterone or tibolone with varying successes. Bupropion is of use in SSRIs-induced FSDD. Flibanserin is the only FDA-approved drug for HSDD.

Sexuality education, communication skills with the husband, and sex therapy of Masters and Johnson are used together. Moving from sensual pleasuring to sexual pleasuring leading to sexual activity is the essence of the treatment. Sensate focus alone and sensate focus with masturbation were compared in efficacy, with the latter giving better result [33]. Identifying the automatic thoughts that cause libido loss and behaviors that suppress desire, followed by CBT, is ideal. Mindfulness in daily nonsexual and sexual activities is proved to be of use in women with female sexual desire disorder (FSDD) following hysterectomy for cervical and endometrial cancer [34].

The combination of mindfulness exercises, cognitive therapy, and behavioral exercises like sensate focus achieved significant improvement in subjective arousal and marginal improvement in physiological sexual arousal.

Psychotherapy of Female Orgasmic Disorder

Anorgasmia can be lifelong or acquired and generalized or situational. Lifelong generalized anorgasmia is mostly due to guilt about sexuality, fear of losing self-control, not allowing "letting go" initially consciously and later unconsciously, and holding back sexual feelings which later become automatic. Acquired anorgasmia can be organic (menopausal, hormonal deprivation, drug induced) or can be a manifestation of dysfunctional relationship. Directed masturbation training is highly effective for lifelong and generalized anorgasmia [35].

The patient visually examines her body and genitals with the use of a mirror and charts of female genital organs. She then explores her body and genitals visually and by touch to locate sensitive areas that produce pleasure. The woman is instructed to manually stimulate these areas and concentrate on the feelings. The intensity and the duration of the stimulation are increased to achieve orgasm. Fantasy is liberally used. Topical lubricants, vibrators, and erotic videos are often added. Once the woman is able to achieve orgasm in solitude, the partner is included in the sessions to desensitize her to achieve orgasm in his presence. For acquired anorgasmia, addressing body image concerns, sex education, sexual skill training, sensate focus therapy, and couple therapy are employed singly or in combination.

Coital anorgasmia is situational wherein the woman is orgasmic at masturbation but not at coital sex. Fear of losing control and relationship issues may be the cause. Cognitive behavioral interventions and sensate focus exercises alone and with her partner give modest result in coital anorgasmia and significantly increase her marital and sexual satisfaction.

Coital alignment technique: Peno-clitoral contact is poor in missionary position of sex. Coital alignment technique is a variation of missionary position. Man enters in missionary position, and moves his body along the woman's body in cephalic direction by about two inches, so that the dorsal surface of the penis is now pressing against the clitoris. The woman approximates her legs or wraps her legs around his legs. During inward thrust, the male moves his pelvis downwards and caudally and upwards and cephalic in outward stroke. The penile-clitoral connection is maintained by the pressure and counterpressure simultaneously exerted by both the partners.

Psychotherapy of Female Sexual Pain Disorders

Dyspareunia is defined as persistent or recurrent pain with attempted or complete vaginal entry and/or vaginal sexual intercourse [30]. Vaginismus is persistent or recurrent difficulties to allow vaginal entry of a penis/finger/any object despite the woman's wish to do so [30]. In DSM-5, both these are grouped into single entity and termed genito-pelvic pain/penetration disorder [30]. The diagnostic criteria are persistent or recurrent difficulty, causing distress, lasting for at least 6 months at (1) vaginal penetration during intercourse, (2) marked vulvovaginal or pelvic pain during vaginal intercourse or penetration attempts, (3) marked fear or anxiety about vulvovaginal or pelvic pain in anticipation of, during, or as a result of vaginal penetration, and (4) marked tensing or tightening of the pelvic floor muscles during attempted vaginal penetration.

Vulvodynia on the other hand is a vulvar discomfort most often described as burning pain, occurring in the absence of relevant visible findings or a specific clinically identifiable neurologic disorder [36]. Vulvodynia can be generalized or localized, provoked or unprovoked, or mixed. Provoked vulvodynia is the commonest. Infections, antigens, inflammatory reactions, hormones, and genetic and psychological factors are implicated in the causation of vulvar pain. Tricyclic antidepressants, anticonvulsants, local application of lidocaine, capsaicin, corticosteroids, and botulinum toxin injection are the medical treatments given for alleviation of the symptoms. Vestibulectomy is done in intractable cases. Psychotherapy to target emotional, relational, cognitive, and behavioral aspects of sexual pain is used alone or together in the management of vulvodynia.

Pain-focused cognitive behavioral therapy: The CBT aims at assisting patients with conceptualizing their pain in terms of thoughts, feelings, and behavior, making them understand the interaction of these to each other, modifying these maladaptive behaviors, and building positive coping strategies like distraction relaxation [37].

Mindful-based cognitive therapy: Mindful based cognitive therapy help patients live in the moment, accept and tolerate pain as it is and this strategy is used for provoked vulvodynia. During the course of treatment, they identify the factors that increase or decrease the pain [38]. Sex therapy or couple therapy can be used to improve communication reducing feelings of guilt and shame and building positive sexual encounters.

Pelvic floor physiotherapy: The techniques used are biofeedback, electrical stimulation, and manual dilatation. Phallic shaped dilators in increasing shape and sizes are used in home practice. These techniques make the patient aware of the muscle tension, and help control the muscles, allow reducing the resting muscle tone, and lastly increase the flexibility of vaginal introitus, finally facilitating penetration. Psychotherapy and pelvic floor physiotherapy are used simultaneously as complementary to each other. Acupuncture and hypnosis are other emerging alternate treatment strategies.

Vaginismus: Contraction or spasm of the muscles around the vaginal introitus at attempted entry of a finger or penis is considered as the cause and hallmark of vaginismus. Now it is considered to be a phobic avoidance phenomenon. Anticipation of pain, fear of pain, and experience of pain also elicit pelvic muscle contraction. Attempts at penetration may elicit pain due to defensive increased muscle tone and confirm the anticipated pain. This negative perpetuation impairs genital and sexual responses and leads to dyspareunia and vaginismus. In conservative societies, where virginity is cherished, it may be defloration phobia than penetration phobia. Relief of vaginal spasm by progressive dilation of tightened vagina is the essential component in the treatment of vaginismus. However before this can be accomplished, the patient's phobic avoidance of vaginal entry is to be alleviated.

Failure to resolve penis envy in the phallic stage of development or her unconscious wish to castrate him as revenge to her own castration is the hypothesis proposed by psychoanalysts. Resolution of these conflicts by psychoanalytical techniques is a prolonged process and hence not used regularly. Behavioral therapy involves systematic desensitization in which in deeply relaxed states, she fantasizes the approach of the husband, later lying down on bed with him, later him approaching her with his erection, and finally attempting penetration. In contrast, another technique—flooding—can be used. The therapist might ask the patient to imagine that she is being "ripped apart" by her husband's penis [21]. Once she can tolerate this fantasy, she will be able to tolerate actual intercourse. In majority of the cases, the exhaustive desensitization techniques are not necessary and simple sex education and reassurance are enough.

Masters and Johnson's sensate focus can be initiated first [20]. The couple is instructed to visualize the genitals with a mirror and to identify the vaginal opening. In vivo vaginal dilatation can be done by the patient, husband, or the therapist. Patient's finger, husband's finger, or graded vaginal dilators can be used. The smallest dilator is inserted to a little depth beyond hymenal ring and kept there for some time till the uncomfortable feeling of insertion disappears. The patient or the husband can be instructed to move the finger back and forth in her vagina. Slow and gradual dilatation is done over some time until she is able to insert two fingers or a dilator of the size of erect penis. At first entry, the woman directs the lubricated penis into her. He then withdraws and later reenters and starts thrusting.

Conclusion

The importance of psychotherapy in treating sexual dysfunctions is to be emphasised to the practicing sexual medicine specialist. These therapies are safe and harmless and can also be used for a variety of disorders. When combined with medications, these therapies work better for alleviating the sexual dysfunction.

References

1. McCarthy B, Metz M. The 'Good-Enough Sex' model: a case illustration. Sex Relationship Ther. 2008;23:227–34.
2. Althof SE, Abdo CH, Dean J, Hackett G, McCabe M, McMahon CG, et al. International Society for Sexual Medicine's guidelines for the diagnosis and treatment of premature ejaculation. J Sex Med. 2010;7:2947–69.
3. Levine S, Risen C, Althof S. Essay on the diagnosis and nature of paraphilia. J Sex Marital Ther. 1990;16:89–102.
4. Levine S. Sexual life: a clinician's guide. New York: Plenum Press; 1992.
5. Freud S. Three essays on the theory of sexuality (1905). In: Strachey J, editor. The standard edition of the complete psychological works of Sigmund Freud. London: Hogarth Press; 1971. p. 135–243.
6. Shaeer O, Shaeer K. The global online sexuality survey (GOSS): ejaculatory function, penile anatomy, and contraceptive usage among Arabic-speaking internet users in the Middle East. J Sex Med. 2012;9(2):425–33.
7. Luthar S. The concept of resilience. Child Dev. 2000;71:534–62.
8. Bancroft J. Sexual arousal and response—the psychosomatic circle. In: Bancroft J, editor. Human sexuality and its problems. 3rd ed. Edinburg: Churchill Livingstone Elsevier; 2009.
9. Freund B, Steketee G. Sexual history, attitudes and functioning of obsessive-compulsive patients. J Sex Marital Ther. 1989;15:31–41.
10. Van Minnen A, Kampman M. The interaction between anxiety and sexual functioning: a controlled study of sexual functioning in women with anxiety disorders. Sex Relationship Ther. 2000;15:47–57.
11. Quinta Gomes AL, Nobre P. Personality traits and psychopathology on male sexual dysfunction: an empirical study. J Sex Med. 2011;8:461–9.
12. Freud S. Lecture four. In: Five lectures on psycho-analysis. The standard edition of the complete psychological works of Sigmund Freud. Vol. XI. 1910
13. Freud S. The ego and the id. In: The standard edition of the complete psychological works of Sigmund. Vol. XIX. 1923. p. 1–66.
14. Nobre P, Pinto-Gouveia J. Dysfunctional sexual beliefs as vulnerability factors to sexual dysfunction. J Sex Res. 2006;43(1):68–75.
15. Baker CD, de Silva P. The relationship between male sexual dysfunction and belief in Zilbergeld's myths: an empirical investigation. Sex Marital Ther. 1988;3:229–38.
16. Weiderman M. The state of theory in sex therapy. J Sex Res. 1998;35(1):88–99.
17. Barlow D. Causes of sexual dysfunction: the role of anxiety and cognitive interference. J Consult Clin Psychol. 1986;54(2):140–8.
18. Kabat-Zinn J. An outpatient program in behavioral medicine for chronic pain patients based on the practice of mindfulness meditation: theoretical considerations and preliminary results. Gen Hosp Psychiatry. 1982;4:33–47.

19. Brotto LA, Basson R, Luria M. A mindfulness-based group psychoeducational intervention targeting sexual arousal disorder in women. J Sex Med. 2008;5(7):164659.
20. Masters W, Johnson V, editors. Human sexual inadequacy. Boston: Little, Brown; 1970.
21. Kaplan HS, editor. The new sex therapy. New York: Brunner; 1974.editor
22. Zilbergeld B. The new male sexuality. New York: Batam Books; 1999.
23. Nobre P, Gouveia J. Erectile dysfunction: an empirical approach on Beck's cognitive theory. Sex Relationship Ther. 2000;15(4):351–66.
24. Santtila P, et al. Recreational use of erectile dysfunction medication may decrease confidence in ability to gain and hold erections in young males. Int J Impot Res. 2007;19(6):591–6.
25. Waldinger M, et al. An empirical operationalization study of DSM-IV diagnostic criteria for premature ejaculation. Int J Psychiatry Clin Pract. 1998;2:287293.
26. Schapiro B. Premature ejaculation, a review of 1130 cases. J Urol. 1943;50:3749.
27. Perelman MA. A new combination treatment for premature ejaculation: a sex therapist's perspective. J Sex Med. 2006;3(6):1004–12.
28. Berner M, Gunzler C. Efficacy of psychosocial interventions in men and women with sexual dysfunctions—a systematic review of controlled clinical trials: part 1-the efficacy of psychosocial interventions for male sexual dysfunction. J Sex Med. 2012;9(12):3089–107.
29. Hawton J. Treatment of sexual dysfunction by sex therapy and other approaches. Br J Psychiatry. 1995;167:307–14.
30. American Psychiatric Association. Diagnostic and statistical manual of mental disorders. 5th ed. Washington, DC: American Psychiatric Publishing; 2013.
31. Perelman MA. Idiosyncratic masturbation patterns: a key unexplored variable in the treatment of retarded ejaculation by the practicing urologist. J Urol. 2005;173:340.
32. Apfelbaum B. Retarded ejaculation: a much-misunderstood syndrome. In: Leiblum SR, Rosen RC, editors. Principles and practice of sex therapy: update for the 1990s. 2nd ed. New York: Guilford Press; 1989.
33. Hurlbert D. A comparative study using orgasm consistency training in the treatment of women reporting hypoactive sexual desire. J Sex Marital Ther. 1993;19:41–55.
34. Brotto L, Heiman J, Goff B, Greer B, Lentz G, Swisher E, et al. A psychoeducational intervention for sexual dysfunction in women with gynecologic cancer. Arch Sex Behav. 2008;37(2):317–29.
35. Meston CM, Hull E, Levin RJ, Sipski M. Women's orgasm. In: Lue TF, Basson R, Rosen R, Giuliano G, Khoury S, Montorsi F, editors. Sexual medicine: sexual dysfunctions in men and women. Paris: Health Publications; 2004. p. 783–850.
36. Goldstein A. Medical history, physical examination, and laboratory tests for the evaluation of dyspareunia. In: Goldstein A, Pukall CF, Goldstein I, editors. Female sexual pain disorders: evaluation and management. Oxford: Wiley-Blackwell; 2009. p. 14–20.
37. Landry T, Bergeron S, Dupuis M-J, Desrochers G. The treatment of provoked vestibulodynia: a critical review. Clin J Pain. 2008;24(2):155–71.
38. Brotto L, Basson R, Carlson M, Zhu C. Impact of an integrated mindfulness and cognitive behavioural treatment for provoked vestibulodynia (IMPROVED): a qualitative study. Sex Relationship Ther. 2013;28(1–2):3–19.

Micropenis

10

Karthik Gunasekaran and Shah Dupesh Khan

Introduction

One of the most commonly encountered problems in the practice of sexual medicine has been the serious concern men frequently have about penis size starting from puberty to adulthood. Men are extremely anxious about their penile length [1]. The penis is credited with the dual function of coitus and micturition. In biology, the ability to transfer sperms denotes maleness of an organism To a man, no matter what his socioeconomic status is, the size of the penis always matters [2].

Online content, visuals, peer pressure, and the belief that a bigger penis leads to better sexual satisfaction for the partner are lingering concerns that do not go away. Most of these men however, taken into consideration the great variation in size, turn out to be anatomically normal [3]. Across all cultures, the penis symbolizes masculinity, strength, and courage. History is abound with stories of men who have tried in desperation various techniques to increase penis size. It is said that the sadhus from India used weights suspended from the penis to stretch it much like a penile expander. These penises were not usable. They were simply stretched for the sake of size [4]. Some went to the extent of encouraging poisonous snakes to bite their penis like the Topinama of Brazil. Repeated bites would cause the penis to enlarge to a monstrous size [4].

The diagnosis of micropenis in clinical medicine is often a case of oversight. Micropenis is significantly different from small penis which is not clinically a true micropenis [3]. When misdiagnosed it can cause considerable anxiety to the patient

K. Gunasekaran, MS, FRCS (Glasgow), FECSM (✉) · S. D. Khan
The Metromale Clinic and Fertility Center,
No 1, Crescent Park Street, T-Nagar, Chennai, India

© Springer Nature Singapore Pte Ltd. 2019

K. Gunasekaran, S. D. Khan (eds.), *Sexual Medicine*,
https://doi.org/10.1007/978-981-13-1226-7_10

and the parents. It can lead to unnecessary examinations and tests. The term micropenis should not be confused or included under broader headings like small penis or inconspicuous penis. A diagnosis of micropenis is made by measuring stretched penile length. This concept was first introduced by Schonfeld and Beebe in 1942 [5, 6]. Based on this, the definition of micropenis was accepted as a stretched penile length 2.5 standard deviations less than the mean for age group without the presence of any other penile anomalies [5, 6]. It can occur on its own or as a part of a syndrome. In the United States, the reported incidence was 1.5 in 10,000 male births between the years 1997 and 2000 [7].

Pathophysiology of Micropenis

Growth of the penis is controlled by androgenic hormones. The gonadal ridge differentiates into testis during embryonic development and placental human chorionic gonadotrophin (HCG) production drives secretion of testosterone in the Leydig cells of the testis. Dihydrotestosterone that is derived from testosterone drives penile differentiation that is completed by the 12th week of intrauterine life [8]. A significant increase in penile size occurs between the 2nd and 3rd trimesters of intrauterine life due to elevated levels of androgens that are seen between the 8th and 24th weeks [9].

There is an increase of penile length of approximately 20 mm from weeks 16 to 38 [8]. Thus we can understand that a true micropenis could be one that results from abnormal or an imbalance in the hormonal milieu that occurs after 12 weeks of gestation [10, 11]. So, either there is an inadequate production of androgens for stimulation of penile growth or an inadequate response of the penis to stimulation.

Etiology

The etiology of micropenis can be classified into the following three broad categories.

Hypogonadotropic hypogonadism: This is also known as pituitary hypothalamic failure. Here the hormones from the hypothalamus and pituitary are not adequate for stimulation of the gonads. Conditions such as Kallmann syndrome and Prader-Willis syndrome are part of this entity and micropenis is associated with it [11].

Hypergonadotropic hypogonadism: This is a condition where there is a failure of the gonads also known as primary testicular failure. The condition may be associated with syndromes like Robinow syndrome and Poly-X syndromes like Klinefelter syndrome, gene translocations, and trisomies of chromosomes 8, 13, and 18 [11].

Idiopathic: For reasons unknown, here the hypothalamus-pituitary-testicular axis is essentially normal. Irrespective of the etiology the question that should run foremost in the physician's mind is whether the penis will respond sufficiently to hormonal stimulation for the infant to continue being raised as a boy or should gender reassignment be considered for him [12]. Table 10.1 summarizes all the possible causes of Micropenis.

Table 10.1 A brief overview of the various causes of micropenis

Causes of micropenis
Hypergonadotropic hypogonadism
Testicular anorchia
Klinefelter syndrome
Trisomy 21
Trisomies of chromosomes 8, 13, and 18
Noonan syndrome
LH and FSH end receptor defects
Hypogonadotropic hypogonadism
Kallmann syndrome
Isolated GnRH deficiency
Pituitary tumors
Lawrence-Moon syndrome
Bardet-Biedl syndrome
Prader-Willis syndrome
Defects in testosterone action
Partial androgen insensitivity syndrome
5-Alpha reductase deficiency
Growth hormone defects

Diagnostic Criteria

The key to treating a true micropenis lies in its early diagnosis as it allows for the different treatment modalities to be applied early. For an individual to be considered as having a micropenis, the phenotype should be male with a XY karyotype.

A small penis, foreskin, median raphe, and a normal location of the urethral meatus are required [13]. The length of the penile shaft along with the state of erection or nonerect can make the appearance of the micropenis to be either retracted or flaccid. Presence or absence of the corpora also aids in the appearance. The scrotal development may be one of underdevelopment or normal [14]. Usually the testicles are located in the scrotum, but testicular function is not guaranteed especially with certain syndromes. Volume may be below normal. Sometimes as part of a syndrome the normal descent of the testis may be affected. Features of feminization are usually absent.

How to measure penile length: Measurement of penile length is of utmost importance in a patient with suspected micropenis. If the stretched penile length of the penis is less than 2.5 SD (standard deviation of the mean) for the individual's age a diagnosis of micropenis is made [15]. Also a 46XY karyotype with normal internal and external genitalia supports the diagnosis. Penile length should be strictly measured in a fully stretched penis and not in a flaccid one. A scale or a ruler traditionally is used to measure length [11]. To begin with the suprapubic fat pad should be compressed and if there is a foreskin it should be retracted. The glans is then held between the thumb and forefinger and the penis is stretched. The penis length is then estimated in the dorsal aspect from the tip of the glans till the pubic rami.

An alternative method for estimating penis size will be with the help of syringe, where the needle end is cut and the piston is introduced in the opposite end (needle side). The flange aspect is then introduced over the penis that has to be measured; mild and gentle suction will then cause the penis to move up the syringe while simultaneously pressing down on the pubic fact gently. The penis size is then read by scale on the side of the syringe [15].

Differential Diagnosis

A number of conditions can mimic the diagnosis of a micropenis and it is of utmost importance that these conditions be diagnosed correctly so that there is no confusion. A web of skin under the penis, scar tissue which shrinks the penis by contracture, excess fat, insufficient or imperfect penile skin, and loose penile skin need to be differentiated from the diagnosis of a micropenis [16].

A buried penis occurs in obese children who are prepubertal. Here the main culprit is the suprapubic fat pad which covers and buries the penis [17]. Careful physical examination and correct measurement of penile length is key. The exact penile length can be estimated by applying gentle pressure on the fat tissue. A condition known as trapped penis results from fat pads in the suprapubic region that results from a lack of skin that should be available to cover the shaft [18]. This usually results following a circumcision or a trauma to the penis resulting in scarred prepubic skin. In this condition there is adhesion between the scrotal skin and the skin of the penis. Webbed penis is another differential diagnosis characterized by the penis that attaches by a skin tissue to the front of the scrotum [16]. Penile curvatures and penile agenesis are other conditions which need due consideration before confirming a diagnosis of micropenis [16, 17].

Investigating a Micropenis

Considering the many differential diagnoses, the diagnosis of micropenis can be quite challenging.

Laboratory investigation: A thorough endocrinology assessment helps determine the level of defect in the hypothalamic-pituitary axis. A concomitant evaluation of testicular function and central endocrine activity should be ideally done at the same time [19]. Serum estimates of FSH, LH, and total testosterone are usually adequate to assess adult testicular function. Elevated FSH and LH to twice the upper limit of normal reference range indicates hypergonadotropic hypogonadism, while extremely low FSH and LH and low testosterone indicates hypogonadotropic hypogonadism. In patients where bilateral undescended testis or anorchia is suspected, a HCG challenge test is done. A HCG challenge involves measuring testosterone response before and after administration of HCG. In this test, for children between 6 months and 14 years a dose of 1000–1500 i.m. can be given on an alternate day up to seven doses. The testosterone value is assessed before and after about 48 h of the last dose. Testosterone values rising beyond 200 ng/dL after a HCG test indicate the presence of a functional testis tissue [20, 21]. Determination of inhibin B and AMH levels, both which are produced by sertoli cells in the testis, gives us an idea of functioning testis tissue [21, 22]. A persistent mullerian duct syndrome is indicated by normal levels of inhibin B and low AMH [21, 22].

Imaging studies: Modalities such as ultrasound and MRI can be used for imaging. MRI imaging should be done for all children born with micropenis. MRI imaging helps assess the hypothalamus and pituitary. In children with craniofacial abnormalities assessment of the optic chiasm, corpus callosum, and fourth ventricle is done. In addition transverse brain images will best show the size of the olfactory sulci, which can be used to assess Kallmann syndrome as it is associated with anosmia [21].

Genetic testing: Genetic testing may be necessary to rule out syndromes that contribute to micropenis. Karyotype assessment using chromosomal analysis can be done for sex determination. Y fluorescence also helps in this matter [19].

Treatment

Goals of treatment: Goals of treating a man with micropenis should be realistic. The three key treatment objectives are (1) to provide the patient with a body image that will not lead to any embarrassment, (2) to engage in normal sexual intercourse, and (3) to help the patient achieve urination while standing normally. Achieving and/or reaching the target penile length for age is not a therapeutic goal.

An important aspect to keep in mind before we embark on treatment of micropenis is to understand what men and their female partners think about penis size as this may help dictate/decide management. An Internet survey of 52,000 heterosexual men and women was done to determine whether men with bigger penises had a more favorable body image compared to men who did not [2]. The study conducted by Lever et al. had one limitation in that it was based completely on patient's perspective of penis size and other physical attributes. The study revealed that men who considered themselves to have a large penis had a more positive image of their body and considered themselves more attractive than those men who did not. Women were found to be more satisfied with their partners' penis size than men with their own (84% vs. 55%). Studies in most cases have also found that most men complaining of a small penis in fact have a normal-sized penis [22].

Role of testosterone: The role of androgens is crucial in infancy for sex selection [23]. A trial administration of testosterone is done to assess the response either by intramuscular route or topical application. For a start 25 mg of either testosterone enanthate or cypionate is administered i.m. once in every 21 days for a 3-month period. Temporary rise of growth rate and a bone age advancement may be seen [24]. Guthrie et al. administered testosterone depot every 3 weeks for 3 months [24]. Main et al. suggested testosterone suppositories in boys with hypogonadotropic hypogonadism and noticed increase in penile length [25]. There has been no consensus method, duration, and dose of testosterone therapy for micropenis [20]. Moreover, it is a fact that none of these authors observed changes in testicular volume and AMH levels [26]. A good response is to expect a 100% increase in the penile length, although there is no global consensus on this. Sultan et al. consider a size increase of 3.5 cm to be adequate response to treatment. Some authors concur on repeating the applications within a short period [27].

Topical testosterone can be applied in infancy. Five percent testosterone cream was applied by Arisaka et al. in 50 infants and in children between the ages of 5 months and 8 years for 30 days [28]. Long-term dermal application of testosterone is found to promote skeletal as well as penile growth. Testosterone has positive effects on the growth of the penis during infancy. However, whether this growth continues into adolescence and even adulthood is not known [29]. During early adulthood a decrease in the number of androgen receptors is seen; thus application of testosterone early during development allows an upregulation of receptors. Hence treatment with testosterone before early adulthood is recommended [27].

Topical 5-alpha dihydrotestosterone (DHT) gel: Androgen insensitivity in prepubertal patients may benefit with the application of DHT gel to the periscrotal region. A thrice-daily application over a 5-week period showed an increase in penile length and acceleration in genital development [30]. It also worked in infants with 5-alpha reductase deficiency according to a study done by Bertelloni et al. [31]. Side effects were similar to testosterone; however minor skin irritations were seen [31]. This line of treatment can be tried in testosterone-resistant patients.

Luteinizing hormone (LH) and follicle-stimulating hormone (FSH): Recombinant LH and FSH have been tried during infancy and early childhood with varying success especially in patients diagnosed with hypogonadotropic hypogonadism. With the addition of testosterone to subcutaneous injections of 20 IU of LH and 21.3 IU of FSH for a 6-month time frame given twice a week, an increase in penile length from 1.6 to 2.4 cm was noted as well as a 170% increase in testicular volume [25, 32].

Surgical Management

When medical treatment fails to achieve desired penile length surgical options may be considered. Hinman reported as early as 1970s the first reconstructive surgery on the penis. Despite the evolution of various techniques for penile reconstruction, the radial artery forearm flap remains the most popular technique of all [33]. Implants have also been combined with reconstructive surgery with better cosmetic outcomes [34]. However, complications still remain high with surgery [35].

Conclusion

In conclusion, micropenis is a diagnosis which is to be made bearing in mind the right technique to correctly estimate and compare mean penile length. It can occur independently or as a part of a syndrome. Endocrinologic assessment is key in helping to establish the diagnosis. Early diagnosis and early treatment should be instituted for best results. Surgery is fraught with complications and should be carefully chosen and performed by the most experienced. Finally, evidence suggests that even with an untreated micropenis, majority of patients who grow up as male seem to have normal sexual function.

References

1. Van Seters AP, Slob AK. Mutually gratifying heterosexual relationship with micropenis of husband. J Sex Marital Ther. 1988;14(2):98–107.
2. Lever J, Frederick DA, Peplau LA. Does size matter? Men's and women's views on penis size across the lifespan. Psychol Men Masculinity. 2006;7(3):129.
3. Wylie KR, Eardley I. Penile size and the 'small penis syndrome'. BJU Int. 2007;99(6):1449–55.
4. Talalaj J. The strangest human sex, ceremonies and customs. Melbourne: Hill of Content Publishing Company Pty Ltd; 1994.
5. Schonfeld WA, Beebe GW. Normal growth and variation in the male genitalia from birth to maturity. J Urol. 1942;48(6):759–77.
6. Aaronson IA. Micropenis: medical and surgical implications. J Urol. 1994;152:4–14.
7. Nelson CP, Park JM, Wan J, Bloom DA, Dunn RL, Wei JT. The increasing incidence of congenital penile anomalies in the United States. J Urol. 2005;174(4):1573–6.
8. Johnson P, Maxwell D. Fetal penile length. Ultrasound Obstet Gynecol. 2000;15:308–10.
9. Zalel Y, Pinhas-Hamiel O, Lipitz S, Mashiach S, Achiron R. The development of the fetal penis-an in utero sonographic evaluation. Ultrasound Obstet Gynecol. 2001;17:129–31.
10. Evans BA, Williams DM, Hughes IA. Normal postnatal androgen production and action in isolated micropenis and isolated hypospadias. Arch Dis Child. 1991 66:1033–6.
11. Hatipoğlu N, Kurtoğlu S. Micropenis: etiology, diagnosis and treatment approaches. J Clin Res Pediatr Endocrinol. 2013;5(4):217.
12. Ludwig G. Micropenis and apparent micropenis—a diagnostic and therapeutic challenge. Andrologia. 1999;31(S1):27–30.
13. Tsang S. When size matters: a clinical review of pathological micropenis. J Pediatr Health Care. 2010;24(4):231–40.
14. Kayes O, Shabbir M, Ralph D, Minhas S. Therapeutic strategies for patients with micropenis or penile dysmorphic disorder. Nat Rev Urol. 2012;9(9):499.
15. Ozbey H, Temiz A, Salman T. A simple method for measuring penile length in newborns and infants. BJU Int. 1999;84:1093–4.
16. Bergeson PS, Hopkin RJ, Bailey RB, MCGill LC, Piatt JP. The inconspicuous penis. Pediatrics. 1993;92(6):794–9.
17. Wollin M, Duffy PG, Malone PS, Ransley PG. Buried penis. A novel approach. BJU Int. 1990;65(1):97–100.
18. Palmer JS, Elder JS, Palmer LS. The use of betamethasone to manage the trapped penis following neonatal circumcision. J Urol. 2005;174(4):1577–8.
19. Menon PS, Khatwa UA. The child with micropenis. Indian J Pediatr. 2000;67(6):455.
20. Sultan C, Paris F, Jeandel C, Lumbroso S, Galifer RB. Ambiguous genitalia in the newborn. Semin Reprod Med. 2002;20:181–8.
21. McEachern R, Houle AM, Garel L, Van Vliet G. Lost and found testes: the importance of the hCG stimulation test and other testicular markers to confirm a surgical declaration of anorchia. Horm Res Paediatr. 2004;62(3):124–8.
22. Shamloul R. Treatment of men complaining of short penis. Urology. 2005;65:1183–5.
23. Burstein S, Grumbach MM, Kaplan SL. Early determination of androgen-responsiveness is important in the management of microphallus. Lancet. 1979;2:983–36.
24. Guthrie RD, Smith DW, Graham CB. Testosterone treatment for micropenis during early childhood. J Pediatr. 1973;83:247–52.

25. Main KM, Schmidt IM, Skakkebaek NE. A possible role for reproductive hormones in newborn boys: progressive hypogonadism without the postnatal testosterone peak. J Clin Endocrinol Metab. 2000;85:4905–7.
26. Bin-Abbas B, Conte FA, Grumbach MM, Kaplan SL. Congenital hypogonadotropic hypogonadism and micropenis: effect of testosterone treatment on adult penile size why sex reversal is not indicated. J Pediatr. 1999;134:579–83.
27. Borsellino A, Spagnoli A, Vallasciani S, Martini L, Ferro F. Surgical approach to concealed penis: technical refinements and outcome. Urology. 2007;69:1195–8.
28. Arisaka O, Hoshi M, Kanazawa S, Nakajima D, Numata M, Nishikura K, Oyama M, Nitta A, Kuribayashi T, Kano K, Nakayama Y, Yamashiro Y. Systemic effects of transdermal testosterone for the treatment of microphallus in children. Pediatr Int. 2001;43:134–6.
29. Baskin LS, Sutherland RS, DiSandro MJ, Hayward SW, Lipschutz J, Cunha GR. The effect of testosterone on androgen receptors and human penile growth. J Urol. 1997;158:1113–8.
30. Bertelloni S, Scaramuzzo RT, Parrini D, Baldinotti F, Tumini S, Ghirri P. Early diagnosis of 5alpha-reductase deficiency in newborns. Sex Dev. 2007;1:147–51.
31. Kaya C, Bektic J, Radmayr C, Schwentner C, Bartsch G, Oswald J. The efficacy of dihydrotestosterone transdermal gel before primary hypospadias surgery: a prospective, controlled, randomized study. J Urol. 2008;179:684–8. Epub 2007 Dec 20
32. Han TS, Bouloux PM. What is the optimal therapy for young males with hypogonadotropic hypogonadism? Clin Endocrinol. 2010;72(6):731–7.
33. Hinman F Jr. Microphallus: characteristics and choice of treatment from a study of 20 cases. J Urol. 1972;107:499–505.
34. Babaei A, Safarinejad MR, Farrokhi F, Iran-Pour E. Penile reconstruction: evaluation of the most accepted techniques. Urol J. 2010;7:71–8.
35. Monstrey S, Hoebeke P, Selvaggi G, Ceulemans P, Van Landuyt K, Blondeel P, Hamdi M, Roche N, Weyers S, De Cuypere G. Penile reconstruction: is the radial forearm flap really the standard technique? Plast Reconstr Surg. 2009;124:510–8.

Sexual Paraphilia

11

Shah Dupesh Khan and Karthik Gunasekaran

Introduction

Human beings are inherently sexual in nature. An individual's sexual behaviour can have a profound impact on the person's sexuality regardless of how this behaviour occurs, be it masturbation in isolation or penetrative intercourse with a partner. Sex per say is not always done with an aim for procreation [1]. The individual's propensity for sex can be both procreative and non-procreative. The degree of inclination and the extent of engagement in the act though will depend on the individual's society, his/her culture, upbringing, religious beliefs/taboos, other people's expectation and opportunities [2]. What constitutes a normal sexual behaviour? There is no straightforward answer. What may be normal in one culture/society may be abnormal in another. The definition of 'normalcy' is driven by society and/or cultural values, and the extent of 'deviance' is also influenced by the same. Furthermore the 'degree of deviance' in some sexual behaviours can be quantified by comparing with already established norms, but this is not possible for all sex-related behaviours and conditions [3].

Most of the time the individual in question will never reveal his/her sex-related problem especially when the said sexual behaviour is considered highly deviant and illegal by his/her society [4]. This is more so with societies that encourage a medicalization of a particular sexual behaviour. Homosexuality, for example, is still considered a mental illness and the practice of the same is banned and a punishable offence in most Islamic societies/cultures [5]. This is despite the fact that homosexuality is

S. D. Khan (✉) · K. Gunasekaran, MS, FRCS (Glasgow), FECSM
The Metromale Clinic and Fertility Center,
No 1, Crescent Park Street, T-Nagar, Chennai, India

© Springer Nature Singapore Pte Ltd. 2019
K. Gunasekaran, S. D. Khan (eds.), *Sexual Medicine*,
https://doi.org/10.1007/978-981-13-1226-7_11

now well accepted in the West [6]. A person's end sexual behaviour to a certain extent is significantly influenced by both society/culture/religion and opportunity [7]. A boy studying in a boarding school may not have the opportunity for heterosexual contact and thus may engage in homosexual behaviour. This does not mean he is 'homosexually oriented'. He may still have a heterosexual preference and may engage in heterosexual contact later in adulthood. Thus the clinician should clearly differentiate and understand that sexual behaviour is different from sexual fantasy/preference and/or sexual identity.

Enculturation

Culture to a certain extent influences the degree of occurrences of sexual behaviour that is deviant. Enculturation is defined as what an individual imbibes while he/she grows up. Castillo suggested that enculturation involves learning a religion, and following a set pattern of behaviour and response which can shape neural networks. This state of enculturation is fluid in nature and depends on the time the individual spends with a particular culture and its values. The more time the individual spends, the greater the impact on his/her social responses [8]. Cultures can differ on the extent of masculinity/femininity. Some cultures favour both genders equally while some do not. Masculine cultures have more of a 'male' individual-led role and position of power- and finance-based reward system, while women have lesser opportunities in a masculine society [9]. As suggested by De bhugra and Hofstede, these cultures may have a greater incidence of paraphilias [9, 10]. Gender roles and gender expectations and its variation in different cultures could also influence the occurrence of particular paraphilia, since in the early days a woman's sexual need was mostly ignored. Women were mostly required just for procreation. This could probably explain as to why paraphilias occurred and/or still occur more commonly in men as compared to women across different cultures. There are other postulated reasons. In general men's frequency of sexual thoughts is significantly more and physical pleasure in sex is more important. For women the emotional connect derived from intercourse predominates as a motivational factor. The relationship between culture and paraphilias is highly dynamic since cultures and societies change rapidly with time [11].

It also seems probable that much of the early sex-related behaviour and deviance were shaped by religion and/or philosophy. Christianity and Islam both forbade sexual desire/arousal and sexual contact outside the context of wedlock [12]. Sexual activity was considered as a sacred duty but any and all forms of sexual desire/arousal were in general prohibited. This thought was well propagated by early religious scholars. Hinduism just like Islam and Christianity prohibited adultery and incest but was a sex-positive culture as seen in the drawings from the Kamasutra that describes almost all aspects of mateship [13]. This was a seminal shift as compared to the Greco-Roman society where gender preferences were more fluid rather than strict male-to-female intercourse. Sexual behaviour in the Greco-Roman society was more based on power dominance [14]. Regardless of gender, the man who penetrated was considered more superior, and the man/women who allowed penetration was considered feminine and inferior [14].

Individuals in different cultures learn from cultural stimuli, sexual scripts and/or habits that are acquired throughout their life from observation. They conform to a specific set of sex-related habits to avoid being called deviant. For example, in the Indian subcontinent, based on the practice of Ayurveda, the semen is considered to be extremely precious and derived from food and loss of semen by masturbation is well associated with fatigue and exhaustion. This condition called the *dhat* syndrome is exclusive to the Indian subpopulation [15]. Thus when dealing with a paraphilia, the clinician should always try to bear in mind the cultural context of the behaviour rather than simply branding the individual with complex and fancy medical terminologies. Most of the time, a behaviour that could be deviant in one society/culture may be normal in the other.

Paraphilia Is Different from Paraphilic Disorders

Paraphilias are poorly researched and poorly understood in the context of human sexual behaviour. We would like to loosely state that a paraphilic disorder as per the DSM-5 is defined as a 'persistent or recurrent urge, desire or fantasy that involves non human objects, non consenting individuals, and involves distress to oneself and/or partners'. The impairment should have also been present for at least 6 months before a conclusive diagnosis is made [16].

We state here loosely because paraphilias have a highly variable presentation [17]. As Moses clearly pointed out the definition of paraphilia is highly imprecise and can include a list of all sexual behaviour that is not considered normophilic by the current society [18]. The definition of paraphilias is in part driven by societal pressure and legal regulations. For example in the USA, over 20 states have a rule where sex offenders are allowed to be treated in a mental hospital after serving mandatory sentence; as a result the wordings used to define paraphilias have come under considerable scrutiny from lawmakers and forensic examiners. Making a DSM diagnosis is considered as a key evidence in most litigations that involve sex offence crimes. Thus any change in wordings that involve defining a paraphilia can have a significant impact on the sentencing of the individual as well as other legal consequences [19]. A parent for example may be allowed only limited visiting and/or custodian rights.

Sexual deviance is a very non-specific term. How deviant is deviant? This has not been rigorously quantified. The difference between normal and abnormal sexual behaviour is extremely fuzzy. The APA (American Psychiatry Association) ultimately came to a conclusion by vote that sexual deviant behaviour is mental disorders, and sadly this classification seems more authority based rather than evidence based. Why is homosexuality not classified as mental disorder then? The 7th print of the DSM-2 removed homosexuality and as Laws and Donohue have discussed most of the time moral judgement and society drive the definition of what is considered a deviant behaviour or classification of a disorder [20]. Wakefield also thoughtfully states that a disorder is diagnosed when there are symptoms of a dysfunction in an individual [21]. A conflict between an individual and social mores that leads to an act does not mean the individual is suffering. Consider the example of adultery; while most religions and societies condemn it, the individual in question has only acted out his desire, which still falls in the biological range of normalcy rather than deviant. Apart from the human species most other species are not largely monogamous.

The DSM-3 first utilized the term paraphilia to displace the word sexual deviance from the DSM-2. The term 'paraphilia' has since then been used till the DSM-4 manual [17]. In the DSM-5 manual a distinction has been made between paraphilia and paraphilic disorder which was non-existent until the DSM-4 [22]. The term *paraphilia* in now defined as the persistent or recurrent urge or intense pattern of atypical sexual arousal without any associated distress or clinically significant impairment. A *paraphilic disorder* on the other hand is an atypical sexual arousal that is associated with clinically significant distress. The DSM-5 also gives two criteria when a diagnosis has to be made. Criterion A defines the qualitative aspect of the particular paraphilia (that is, the presence of arousal on exposing one's genitals to strangers or arousal when being inflicted with pain during sex). Criterion B on the other hand describes the possible outcome from a paraphilia, i.e. the risk of harm or harm caused to oneself and others. Furthermore the disorder should have caused clinically significant distress for a period of 6 months [22].

A diagnosis of *paraphilic disorder* is only given when the atypical sexual interest meets criteria A and B. An ascertainment of *paraphilia* is made when only criterion A is met; this is to avoid the use of the term 'diagnosis' in an individual who only has an atypical interest that is not strictly pathological in nature [22]. While the intent of the change is to primarily reduce the general stigma associated with paraphilias, the outcome of this change will only result in more confusion in the legal context when judges and juries who are less well versed with the speciality take a decision. A relevant scenario would be making a decision of a child's custodian right when the parent is diagnosed with a paraphilia such as paedophilia.

In general, a paraphilia consists of altered sexual interest and arousal patterns that are different from the conventionally well-accepted erotic foreplay. It is difficult to objectively define paraphilia based on aetiology since a study focussed on aetiology cannot be done due to social, legal and ethical implications that involve study participants. Thereby a achieving a clear scientific diagnosis of paraphilia will not be possible in the near future. We are thus limited with only a descriptive diagnosis for all practical clinical purposes. Table 11.1 highlights the different types of paraphilic disorders.

Table 11.1 A brief overview of the various paraphilias

Paraphilic disorder	Defining criteria
Voyeuristic disorder	Intense arousal from looking at people undress or involved in sexual activity
Exhibitionistic disorder	Intense arousal from exposing one's genitals to strangers
Sexual sadism	Intense arousal obtained from inflicting pain both physical and psychological on another person
Frotteuristic disorder	Intense arousal from rubbing one's organ against a non-consenting person
Masochistic disorder	Intense arousal from being beaten, humiliated or made to suffer
Fetshistic disorder	Intense arousal from focus on non-genital body parts or use of non-living objects
Transvestic disorder	Arousal from cross-dressing
Paedophilia	Intense arousal, urge, fantasy that involves prepubescent child and/or children less than 13 years of age

Sexual Offending

Among a random sample of general population (n = 2450), approximately 11% of men and over 4% of women had reported at least one episode of being aroused when spying on other having sex [23]. Numerous studies have suggested that sexual paraphilias seem to have some association and/or seem to be a motivational factor in offending sexual behaviour. Studies also suggest that the paraphilia could be the motivating factor for recidivism of the criminal act [24]. The most common paraphilias that were found among sex offenders were paedophilia and sadism. How are different paraphilias distributed among a group of sex offenders? Can an offender have more than one specific paraphilia? The exact incidence is not well researched. Abel reports three paraphilias per child molester and two paraphilias for other sex offenders [24].

The discrepancies in the reported data could also arise from diagnostic discrepancies in accurately defining a paraphilia. More recent studies have also confirmed the presence of multiple paraphilias in a sex offender sample [25]. Offenders with more than one paraphilia were also found to have more victims and were found to engage in incestuous behaviour compared to offenders without paraphilias [26].

While psychopathy has been well associated with sexual offending, the relationship between sexual paraphilia and psychopathy is still not clear. A handful of studies have suggested that self-reported psychopathy along with sexually deviant behaviour is a high risk for an individual to act out his fantasy [27–29]. Psychopaths who were sexual murderers and child molesters were also found to have sexual paraphilias like sadism and/or voyeurism. They were also at a higher risk to recidivate and frequently had multiple victims [30].

More recent studies have explored the association between sexual fantasies and paraphilias. Due to public concern, most studies have focussed on sexual fantasies of child offenders while paying little importance to other offender subtypes. Child molesters frequently have sexually deviant fantasies about children [31]. However sexually deviant fantasies are not exclusive to sex offenders as a population and non-offenders also engage in sexually deviant fantasy [32]. More clarity and research are required into relationship between deviant sexual fantasy, paraphilias and sex offending.

Treatment Strategies in Paraphilias

Surgical treatment by way of castration was done in the early 1980s and 1990s. While considered effective, the method is not foolproof and even post-castration the paedophilic offender can still engage in sexual intercourse. Chemical castration involves the use of anti-androgens and is more expensive due to the ongoing nature of the treatment [33]. Both surgical and chemical castration are not first-line and/or recommended treatment strategies in the management of paraphilic disorders.

Psychotherapy, especially cognitive behavioural therapy (CBT), is frequently used to treat different types of paraphilias. The results have been found to be extremely variable and part reason for the failure of these therapies is because the individual in question should first accept he has a problem and feel guilt before embarking on therapy. Recidivism is particularly high with these therapies [34]. Masturbation conditioning and aversion therapies have not been found to be effective.

Neurotransmitters play an important role in mediating sexual arousal. Animal studies have suggested that serotoninergic neurotransmission helps in reducing sexual arousal [35]. The effect of selective serotonin neurouptake inhibitor (SSRI) like fluoxetine in treating paraphilic disorders in daily doses ranging from 20 to 80 mg/day has been evaluated in small open-label studies and individual case reports [36, 37]. Most of these studies reported a mild-to-moderate decrease in the total sexual outlet, fantasies, desire intensity and deviant thoughts along with behaviour. In another study naltrexone was administered to 21 male sex offenders in the adolescent age group in an open-label manner; approximately 71% of study participants reported benefits after daily dosing of 1600 mg/day after 8 weeks of therapy. Reported benefits included reduced frequency of masturbation from 2/day to 2/week, and a general reduction in both sexual arousal and fantasies [38].

Studies have indicated that dopamine neurotransmission is well associated with increased sexual arousal. Neuroleptics have been explored in the treatment of paedophilia as they block dopamine neurotransmission. Small open-label crossover studies however found very weak treatment effects from small significant effect on sexual thought frequency; moreover these medications were also associated with extra pyramidal symptoms [39].

GnRH agonists have been explored in the treatment of paedophilia. GnRH agonist reduces the pituitary gonadotropes' responsiveness to endogenously produced

FSH and LH. Initially there will be flare and increased production of FSH and LH followed by a reduction in production as agonist use continues. In most trials that involve GnRH agonists leuprolide and triptorelin have been commonly used in doses varying from 3.75 to 7.5 mg IM/SC on a monthly basis. Here again, open-label studies with a small number of participants found that leuprolide given IM on a monthly basis for a period ranging from 1 to 3 years significantly helped reduce paedophilic sexual thoughts/urges/desire and masturbatory frequency. Testosterone levels also fell to castration levels along with accompanying erectile dysfunction. Bone demineralization along with hot flashes was reported as a side effect. Relapse after stopping the medication however was consistently reported across different studies [40].

Anti-androgens and progestational drugs like cyproterone acetate (dose range 50 –200 mg/day) have been used to treat paraphilias. Small randomized crossover trials have found some benefit compared to placebo in terms of reduced sexual outlet scores, spontaneous daytime erection and/or orgasm during masturbation in sex offenders [41]. No major adverse events were noted. Total testosterone values also modestly fell in this group. In another study on 300 paraphilic men who received cyproterone acetate 50–200 mg/day along with IM 300 mg between a minimum of 2 months and an 8-year period, over 80% of study participants reported adequate inhibition of sexual desire [42].

A major hurdle in the pharmacotherapy of sexual paraphilia is that all current pharmacotherapeutic modalities have limited scientific evidence to support their use. However most studies conducted so far have a high degree of sample biases and are not randomized as well. Sample biases occur since most studies have explored the efficacy of different drugs on specific populations like sex offenders from prisons. This may not be strictly representative of the actual paraphilic study population. Furthermore, the main paraphilia in focus in most studies seems to be paedophilia and not other paraphilias. Guay and Garcia have both independently published excellent reviews on the various pharmacotherapies available for paraphilias [41, 43]. However crucial points have been missed. As rightly pointed out in an excellent commentary by Balon [17], what is the primary guiding principle for a treatment? Is it the distress felt by the patient? Is it the number of victims or any other diagnostic factor listed in the DSM? Most importantly what about patients who do not feel distressed by their paraphilia? Should we treat them? Should the treatment be for life? Who pays for it?

Conclusion

Sexual paraphilias are deceivingly complex. We do not know anything about the actual aetiology of paraphilias nor do we know anything about how and when to treat these disorders. Paraphilia and its management are an unchartered territory of problems filled with complex ethical/medical and/or legal issues. While the updated DSM-5 guidelines seem a subtle improvement in categorizing paraphilias as compared to previous editions, much more scientific work remains to be done in this enigmatic spectrum of atypical sexual arousal patterns called paraphilias.

References

1. Bhugra D, de Silva P. Uniforms: fact, fashion, fantasy or fetish. Sex Marital Ther. 1996;11:393–406.
2. Berridge KC, Kringlebach ML. Affective neuroscience of pleasure: reward in humans and animals. Psychopharmacology. 2008;199:457–48.
3. Baumeister RF. Gender and erotic plasticity: sociocultural influences on the sex drive. Sex Relationship Ther. 2004;19(2):133–9.
4. Baxter DJ, Marshall WL, Barbaree HE, Davidson PR, Malcolm PB. Deviant sexual behavior: differentiating sex offenders by criminal and personal history, psychometric measures, and sexual response. Crim Justice Behav. 1984;11(4):477–501.
5. Kligerman N. Homosexuality in Islam: a difficult paradox. Macalester Islam J. 2007;2(3):8.
6. Loftus J. America's liberalization in attitudes toward homosexuality, 1973 to 1998. Am Sociol Rev. 2001;66:762–82.
7. Odimegwu C. Influence of religion on adolescent sexual attitudes and behaviour among Nigerian university students: affiliation or commitment? Afr J Reprod Health. 2005;9:125–40.
8. Castillo RJ. Culture, trance, and the mind-brain. Anthropol Conscious. 1995;6(1):17–34.
9. Ayonrinde O, Bhugra D. Paraphilias and culture. In: Troublesome disguises: managing challenging disorders in psychiatry. 2014. p. 199.
10. Hofstede G. Culture's consequences: comparing values, behaviors, institutions and organizations across nations. Thousand Oaks, CA: Sage; 2003.
11. Bhugra D, Popelyuk D, McMullen I. Paraphilias across cultures: contexts and controversies. J Sex Res. 2010;47(2–3):242–56.
12. Adamczyk A, Hayes BE. Religion and sexual behaviors: understanding the influence of Islamic cultures and religious affiliation for explaining sex outside of marriage. Am Sociol Rev. 2012;77(5):723–46.
13. Doniger W. The "Kamasutra": it isn't all about sex. Kenyon Rev. 2003;25(1):18–37.
14. Ibrahim I. From ancient Greco-Roman culture the contemporary LGBTQ community: the transfer of sex and power dynamics. Denison J Religion. 2016;15(1):4.
15. Sumathipala A, Siribaddana SH, Bhugra D. Culture-bound syndromes: the story of dhat syndrome. Br J Psychiatry. 2004;184(3):200–9.
16. First MB, Frances A. Issues for DSM-V: unintended consequences of small changes: the case of paraphilias.
17. Balon R. Controversies in the diagnosis and treatment of paraphilias. J Sex Marital Ther. 2013;39(1):7–20.
18. Moser C. Yet another paraphilia definition fails. Arch Sex Behav. 2011;40(3):483–5.
19. Woodworth M, Freimuth T, Hutton EL, Carpenter T, Agar AD, Logan M. High-risk sexual offenders: an examination of sexual fantasy, sexual paraphilia, psychopathy, and offence characteristics. Int J Law Psychiatry. 2013;36(2):144–56.
20. Laws DR, O'Donohue WT, editors. Sexual deviance: theory, assessment, and treatment. New York: Guilford Press; 2008.
21. Wakefield JC. DSM-5 proposed diagnostic criteria for sexual paraphilias: tensions between diagnostic validity and forensic utility. Int J Law Psychiatry. 2011;34(3):195–209.
22. American Psychiatric Association. Diagnostic and statistical manual of mental disorders (DSM-5®). Arlington, VA: American Psychiatric Publishing; 2013.
23. Långström NI, Zucker KJ. Transvestic fetishism in the general population. J Sex Marital Ther. 2005;31(2):87–95.
24. Abel GG, Becker JV, Cunningham-Rathner J, Mittelman M, Rouleau JL. Multiple paraphilic diagnoses among sex offenders. J Am Acad Psychiatry Law Online. 1988;16(2):153–68.
25. Smallbone SW, Wortley RK. Criminal diversity and paraphilic interests among adult males convicted of sexual offenses against children. Int J Offender Ther Comp Criminol. 2004;48(2):175–88.

26. Lebegue B. Paraphilias in US pornography titles: "pornography made me do it" (Ted Bundy). Bull Am Acad Psychiatry Law. 1991;19:43–8.
27. Porter S, Demetrioff S, Ten Brinke L. Sexual psychopath: current understanding and future challenges. In: Schlank A, editor. The sexual predator, vol. 4. Kingston, NJ: Civic Research Institute; 2010. p. 13-1–13-12.
28. Porter S, Woodworth M, Earle J, Drugge J, Boer D. Characteristics of sexual homicides committed by psychopathic and nonpsychopathic offenders. Law Hum Behav. 2003;27(5):459.
29. Porter S, Fairweather D, Drugge J, Herve H, Birt A, Boer DP. Profiles of psychopathy in incarcerated sexual offenders. Crim Justice Behav. 2000;27(2):216–33.
30. Rice ME, Quinsey VL, Harris GT. Sexual recidivism among child molesters released from a maximum security psychiatric institution. J Consult Clin Psychol. 1991;59(3):381
31. Maniglio R. The role of deviant sexual fantasy in the etiopathogenesis of sexual homicide: a systematic review. Aggress Violent Behav. 2010;15(4):294–302.
32. Gray NS, Watt A, Hassan S, Macculloch MJ. Behavioral indicators of sadistic sexual murder predict the presence of sadistic sexual fantasy in a normative sample. J Interpers Violence. 2003;18(9):1018–34.
33. Fitzgerald EA. Chemical castration: MPA treatment of the sexual offender. Am J Crim Law. 1990;18:1.
34. Thibaut F, Barra FD, Gordon H, Cosyns P, Bradford JM. WFSBP task force on sexual disorders. The World Federation of Societies of Biological Psychiatry (WFSBP) guidelines for the biological treatment of paraphilias. World J Biol Psychiatry. 2010;11(4):604–55.
35. Bancroft J. The endocrinology of sexual arousal. J Endocrinol. 2005;186(3):411–27.
36. Stein DJ, Hollander E, Anthony DT, Schneier FR, Fallon BA, Liebowitz MR, Klein DF. Serotonergic medications for sexual obsessions, sexual addictions, and paraphilias. J Clin Psychiatry. 1992;53:267–71.
37. Kafka MP. Successful antidepressant treatment of nonparaphilic sexual addictions and paraphilias in men. J Clin Psychiatry. 1991;52:60–5.
38. Ryback RS. Naltrexone in the treatment of adolescent sexual offenders. J Clin Psychiatry. 2004;65:982–6.
39. Kobayashi T. Effect of haloperidol on a patient with hypersexuality following frontal lobe injury. Psychogeriatrics. 2004;4(2):49–52.
40. Briken P, Hill A, Berner W. Pharmacotherapy of paraphilias with long-acting agonists of luteinizing hormone-releasing hormone: a systematic review. J Clin Psychiatry. 2003;64:890–7.
41. Guay DR. Drug treatment of paraphilic and nonparaphilic sexual disorders. Clin Ther. 2009;31(1):1–31.
42. Laschet U, Laschet L. Antiandrogens in the treatment of sexual deviations of men. In: Proceedings of the Fourth International Congress on Hormonal Steroids, Mexico City. 1976. p. 821–826.
43. Garcia FD, Thibaut F. Current concepts in the pharmacotherapy of paraphilias. Drugs. 2011;71(6):771–90.

Sexual Health in the Aging Couple

12

Prashanth Baspure

Introduction

Human advancement has allowed people to live longer and healthier lives the world over—and the numbers say it all. 2006 recorded almost 500 million people over the age of 65 worldwide, and this number is expected to double by 2030 [1]. This means that seniors will comprise one out of eight people on earth. In addition, developing countries will see a rapid jump in their senior population by 2030, with some estimates as high as 140% increase.

While these numbers are encouraging from a social, medical, and economic standpoint, they also bring forth monumental challenges. An aging population strains existing support models such as social and pension systems, affecting everything from economic growth and trade to disease patterns and migration. It challenges the fundamental assumptions of growing older.

Other important issues representing the aging population pertain to sexuality and various determinates [2], which are often neglected. In fact, even the World Health Organization (WHO) acknowledges that reproduction and sexuality are fundamental components to the health and well-being of human beings [2]. Sexual health is defined by the WHO as a state of mental, physical, as well as social well-being. It requires a positive and dignified approach to matters such as sexuality, relationships, as well as safe and pleasurable sexual experiences. Sexual health is determined based on complex interactions between various domains such as the sexual desire, frequency of intercourse, orgasm and/or ejaculation, erectile function, early-morning erections, and overall satisfaction with an individual's general health as well as sex life. These domains are defined by the fitness levels of the individual as well as their partner [2].

P. Baspure
Passion Fruit Relationship & Sexual Wellness, Bangalore, Karnataka, India

© Springer Nature Singapore Pte Ltd. 2019

K. Gunasekaran, S. D. Khan (eds.), *Sexual Medicine*,
https://doi.org/10.1007/978-981-13-1226-7_12

A clear understanding of sexuality becomes increasingly important as beliefs surrounding aging, gender, sexuality, and personal happiness continue to transform as individuals live longer and healthier. Owing to this, the interest in studying and characterizing modifications in the relationship between sexual health and aging has increased significantly.

Changes in the Sexual Response Cycle

As defined by Masters and Johnson [3], all stages of an individual's sexual response cycle are influenced by age and its associated factors. In addition, there is no conclusive scientific evidence to prove that sexual dysfunction is inevitable with increasing age of both men and women, who are otherwise physiologically and psychologically healthy.

Sexual response cycle in aging men: With increasing age, men tend to experience age-related changes in the excitement stage of the sexual cycle such as a steady decline in β-adrenergic receptors as well as cholinergic receptors. This consequently leads to an increased activity in α-adrenergic receptors, and in turn interferes with relaxation of the corporal smooth muscles that is necessary to initiate and maintain erectile response [4]. Furthermore, an increase in the connective tissue deposits can decrease distending capacity of the penis. These factors further lead to decreased elasticity in the corpora cavernosa, making it difficult to achieve and maintain normal erections [4].

Common physiological changes in aging men include:

- Atrophic changes in the sexual organs
- Decreased testosterone levels
- Delay in achieving erection
- Poor erection function and quality
- Failure to sustain erection
- Reduced desire due to reduced hormone levels

As compared to young men who can achieve erection in a couple of seconds, older men may require several minutes to do the same [4]. Hence, partners might have to help in actively facilitating an erectile response through intense stimulation before intromission. With aging, penile sensitivity and rigidity also decline gradually [4]. Penile erection may be satisfactory for intromission but couples may need to supplement intercourse with other forms of stimulation (manual or oral) or experiment with different coital positions to sustain arousal and mood.

The plateau stage is prolonged with age, whereas the duration of orgasm declines. Further, the duration of the refractory period is also significantly increased. With respect to the postorgasmic refractory period, older men may require several days to recover when compared to younger men. This is fundamentally because with increasing age, the restoration of ionic neurotransmitters requires a longer time [4].

Sexual response cycle in aging women: The female sexual response cycle sees similar changes as with men. The onset of lubrication in the vagina takes a couple of seconds in younger women versus a few minutes in older menopausal women. The quantity may also be reduced [4]. This vaginal dryness is usually caused by a decreased vasocongestion and lubrication in the vagina, leading to painful coitus. As with men, the plateau phase of the sexual response cycle is delayed in older women. However, orgasmic response in women is not particularly affected by age, as several women report multiorgasmic capabilities [4].

Some of the most common physiological changes in aging women include:

- Declining secretion of estrogen after menopause
- Decrease in vaginal lubrication
- Shrinking of cervix and uterus
- Decreased elasticity in breast tissue
- Decreased breast dimensions
- Atrophy in the vaginal canal
- Decrease in length and width of the vagina

Psychological Impact on Men and Women

Apart from physiological changes, another prevailing factor that should be considered in the equation is ageism—where social beliefs and attitudes deem sexual behavior in seniors to be inappropriate or even abnormal. Older people also find it difficult to come to terms with their declining attractiveness, physical attributes, and sexual potency. As a result, their sexual health is affected by negative attitudes towards sexuality, as well as social constraints caused by disturbed relationships, physical infirmities, economic worries, and psychological problems [5].

A study conducted in Finland [6]to gauge the attitudes of sexuality and satisfaction of these needs concurs with the statements above. Fifty residents in a nursing home were interviewed to gain a better understanding of basic human needs, particularly sexual, as well as need satisfaction in seniors. More than half the participants did not consider it appropriate for older people to enjoy an active sex life [6]. Twenty-five percent felt that addressing sexual needs and desires was shameful or sinful [6]. Less than 25% of the participants were willing to speak to the nursing home staff regarding sexual matters [6].

Sexual Behavior in the Aging

Epidemiological studies: comparisons between men and women: The Masters and Johnson report [3], supplemented by multiple other studies, suggests that older men and women remain sexually active throughout their lives. They did not find an upper age limit for healthy sexual function. However, some evidence shows that with increasing age the frequency of sexual activity diminishes.

Between 2001 and 2002, the Global Study of Sexual Attitudes and Behaviors (GSSAB) interviewed 27,000 participants across 29 countries. This group included men and women between the ages of 40 and 80 years. Twenty-one percent of women and almost half of men aged between 70 and 80 years reported having intercourse in the past year of the interview [7]. Within the age group of 40–49 years, this number included 93% of men and 88% of women [7]. An interesting find in the study indicated that 17% and 23% of men and women, respectively, said that "elderly people did not want sex" [7]. However, 68% of men and 60% of women were also in favor of seniors seeking treatment to enjoy sexual pleasure [7].

Similarly, the National Social Life, Health, and Aging Project (NSHAP) worked with 3005 men and women aged between 57 and 85 across the USA. This national probability sample reported that while men were more likely to remain sexually active than women across all ages, they did not discuss their problems with doctors. The study also found that the most common sexual dysfunctions in men included erectile dysfunction, lack of interest, and inability to climax [8]. The prevalence of these conditions increased with age, with the exception of premature ejaculation (PE)—a condition that affected 28% of all men and was more common in younger age groups [8]. On the other hand, common sexual problems among women included low sex drive, inadequate vaginal lubrication, and inability to climax [8].

A case-control analysis by Syme et al. revealed that 62.4% of subjects between 63 and 67 years had sex once a month or less frequently, to once or more a day. In general, men were found to be more sexually active than women. However, there have been fewer differences in the sexual behaviors of men and women in more recent studies in comparison to those in the past.

Studies specific to men: Helgason et al. studied sexual functions in 319 randomly selected Swedish men ranging from the ages of 50 to 80 years. Seventy-one percent of the group were sexually active with many men reporting adequate erections during sexual intercourse [9]. However, the rate of poor maintenance was equally high, adding up to 72% [9].

A population-based study conducted in Krimpen assessed 1688 Dutch men to study the prevalence of ED. Three percent of men ranging from 50 to 54 years were diagnosed with ED, a number that rose to 26% in men between 70 and 78 years [10]. A related Health in Men Study indicated that while 49% of the participants reported ED, only 3.2% claimed to have unpleasurable sex.

Studies specific to women: Validated scales are not frequently used in women-centric studies, limiting the accuracy with which sexual function and dysfunction can be measured [11]. Further, factors such as limited age ranges, low rate of response, as well as restrictive inclusion criteria affected the limit of generalizability of these studies. Similar to men, evidence indicated that sexual functions of women decreased with age, beginning from the late 20s to late 30s [11]. In particular, desire as well as frequency of orgasm and sexual intercourse declined sharply with advancing age.

It is also important to note that studies that utilized a broader and more inclusive definition of sexual activity (i.e., including not just sexual intercourse but any activity that involves sexual arousal) showed that despite the negative correlation between sexual activity and age, senior women remained sexually active [11].

Determinates of Sexual Behavior Modification with Aging

Sexual performance is impaired with aging owing to the interference of vascular, endocrine, and neurological functions. That's not all; other relational and psychological factors such as the partner's age and sexual function, length of the relationship, and their emotional response to the partner also play an important role in the process. In a study on 2187 men, relational, intrapsychic, and organic factors could independently predict impaired erections [2].

Comorbidities in Men

Cardiovascular diseases: Studies suggest that CV and ED-related diseases should be considered as different manifestations of underlying vascular pathology. In fact, ED should be treated as the first sign of forthcoming coronary artery disease (CAD). It also serves as an efficient predictor of silent CAD in diabetics independent of ED severity and glycometabolic control.

Obesity: Major epidemiological investigations such as PROCAM, NHANES, and Framingham have proved that obesity is an independent factor that increases mortality in men, caused largely due to coronary atherosclerosis and other cardiovascular diseases. The chances of developing ED are 2.5 times higher in obese men than those of healthy and normal weight.

Diabetes mellitus: Some studies indicate that men over the age of 66 years with type 2 diabetes have a 49% chance of developing ED. Some common complications associated with diabetes mellitus include retrograde ejaculation as well as anejaculation.

Comorbidities in Women

Cardiovascular diseases: An observational study conducted by the Women's Health Initiative depicted that dissatisfaction with sexual activity at baseline had a 44% higher risk of developing peripheral artery disease [12]. The longitudinal data also showed similar risks of developing myocardial infarction, coronary vascularization, or stroke even after controlling for smoking status [12].

Obesity: One hundred and six obese women with a median BMI of 44.5, who also underwent bariatric surgery, were analyzed under a prospective cohort study. Postsurgery, these women showed significant improvement in sexual activity across most reproductive hormones of sexual interest as well as psychosocial status [13]. This shows that obesity in itself is predictive of poor sexual function along with increasing age.

Relational Components

Couples of all ages face similar causes of sexual dissatisfaction, ranging from commitment issues, problems with communication and intimacy, and marital conflicts to an imbalance in relationships, boredom, and a mismatch in sexual desire [4].

In elderly couples, these factors are sometimes amplified by resentment and anger built over the years, even decades of the relationship. In addition, feelings of resignation and entrapment contribute further to sexual dissatisfaction, particularly if leaving the relationship is no longer an option.

Intrapsychic Components

The intrapsychic components that contribute towards sexual dissatisfaction in younger men are largely associated with problems in the work environment. However in older men, these components comprise psychosocial stresses such as loss of job, death of a partner, deteriorating support systems, worsening of social status, and other family problems related to health or finance [14]. These radical life changes may affect sexual performance and increase the likelihood of developing anxiety and/or depression, especially in older men. In addition, depressive symptoms and drugs used for other comorbid medical conditions may impair multiple aspects of sexual function in men such as erection, sexual desire, as well as ejaculatory reflex. Repetitive experiences of such failure can compound the issue and amplify performance anxiety, and personal vulnerability and distress [14].

Sexual Satisfaction and Aging

Much of the scientific literature evaluated and focussed on the various pathophysiological processes in aging that can affect sexual function and activity. There are limited studies on other emotional and psychological factors. In addition to physical benefits, sexual satisfaction can enhance the overall well-being of an individual and strengthen intimate relationships and marriages [15]. Sexual satisfaction is the result of these factors interacting on different levels—individual, relationship, and culture [15]. Physical changes as well as illnesses associated with aging can reduce physiological response and sexual desire. However, it is also important to emphasize and understand how sexual satisfaction is influenced by individual cultural norms embedded in individuals [15].

Conclusion

Aging is in general associated with a reduced frequency of sexual activity. While epidemiological evidence suggests that sexuality remains an important issue for aging men and women, cultural influences and stereotypes in our communities make it difficult for doctors and aged patients to communicate honestly. Some doctors still view sexual dysfunction as a natural biological aspect of aging instead of a medical issue. As a result, older patients hesitate to discuss sexuality and sexual health with their primary care physicians.

This lack of open discussion leads to sexual issues not being addressed, further resulting in social withdrawal, depression, and even delayed diagnosis of underlying conditions. These misconceptions and negative attitudes can only be addressed with proper education and encouragement from healthcare professionals on age-related changes to sexuality, as well as advice on meaningful sexual relations.

References

1. Kinsella K, Gist Y. Older workers, retirement, and pensions: a comparative International Chartbook. Washington, DC: U.S. Census Bureau and U.S. National Institute on Aging, and U.S. Census Bureau International Data Base; 1995.
2. Corona G, Rastrelli G, Maseroli E, Forti G, Maggi M. Sexual function of the ageing male. Best Pract Res Clin Endocrinol Metab. 2013;27:581–601.
3. Masters MH, Johnson V. Human sexual response. Boston: Little Brown & Co; 1966.
4. Meston CM. Aging and sexuality. West J Med. 1997;167(4):285–90.
5. Phanjoo AL. Sexual dysfunction in old age. Adv Psychiatr Treat. 2000;6(4):270–7. https://doi.org/10.1192/apt.6.4.270.
6. Paunonen M, Häggman-Laitila A. Sexuality and the satisfaction of sexual needs. Scand J Caring Sci. 1990;4(4):163–8.
7. Laumann EO, Paik A, Glasser DB, Kang JH, Wang T, Levinson B, Moreira E, Nicolosi A, Gingell C. Sexual behavior and sexual dysfunctions after the age 40: the global study of sexual attitudes and behaviors. Urology. 2004;64:991–7.
8. Suzman R. The National Social Life, Health, and Aging Project: an introduction. J Gerontol B Psychol Sci Soc Sci. 2009;64B(Suppl 1):i5–i11.
9. Helgason A, Adolfsson J, Dickman P, Arver S, Fredrikson M, Göthberg M, Steineck G. Sexual desire, erection, orgasm and ejaculatory functions and their importance to elderly Swedish men: a population-based study. Age Ageing. 1996;25:285–91.
10. Blanker MH, Bohnen AM, Groeneveld FP, Bernsen RM, Prins A, Thomas S, Bosch JL. Correlates for erectile and ejaculatory dysfunction in older Dutch men: a community-based study. J Am Geriatr Soc. 2001;49(4):436–42.
11. Hayes R, Dennerstein L. The impact of aging on sexual function and sexual dysfunction in women: a review of population-based studies. J Sex Med. 2005;2(3):317–30.
12. McCall-Hosenfeld JS, Freund KM, Legault C, Jaramillo SA, Cochrane BB, Manson JE, Wenger NK, Eaton CB, McNeeley SG, Rodriguez BL, Bonds D. Sexual satisfaction and cardiovascular disease: the Women's Health Initiative. Am J Med. 2008;121(4):295–301.
13. Sarwer DB, Spitzer JC, Wadden TA, Mitchell JE, Lancaster K, Courcoulas A, Gourash W, Rosen RC, Christian NJ. Changes in sexual functioning and sex hormone levels in women following bariatric surgery. JAMA Surg. 2014;149(1):26–33.
14. Reynolds CF 3rd, Kupfer DJ. Depression and aging: a look to the future. Psychiatr Serv. 1999;50(9):1167–72.
15. Carpenter L, Nathanson C, Kim YJ. Physical women, emotional men: gender and sexual satisfaction in midlife. Arch Sex Behav. 2007;38:87–107. https://doi.org/10.1007/s10508-007-9215-y.

MIX
Papier aus verantwortungsvollen Quellen
Paper from responsible sources
FSC® C105338

If you have any concerns about our products,
you can contact us on
ProductSafety@springernature.com

In case Publisher is established outside the EU,
the EU authorized representative is:
Springer Nature Customer Service Center GmbH
Europaplatz 3, 69115 Heidelberg, Germany

Printed by Libri Plureos GmbH
in Hamburg, Germany

SpringerBriefs in Applied Sciences and Technology

AF665686

SpringerBriefs present concise summaries of cutting-edge research and practical applications across a wide spectrum of fields. Featuring compact volumes of 50 to 125 pages, the series covers a range of content from professional to academic.

Typical publications can be:

- A timely report of state-of-the art methods
- An introduction to or a manual for the application of mathematical or computer techniques
- A bridge between new research results, as published in journal articles
- A snapshot of a hot or emerging topic
- An in-depth case study
- A presentation of core concepts that students must understand in order to make independent contributions

SpringerBriefs are characterized by fast, global electronic dissemination, standard publishing contracts, standardized manuscript preparation and formatting guidelines, and expedited production schedules.

On the one hand, **SpringerBriefs in Applied Sciences and Technology** are devoted to the publication of fundamentals and applications within the different classical engineering disciplines as well as in interdisciplinary fields that recently emerged between these areas. On the other hand, as the boundary separating fundamental research and applied technology is more and more dissolving, this series is particularly open to trans-disciplinary topics between fundamental science and engineering.

Indexed by EI-Compendex, SCOPUS and Springerlink.

Dingyi Pan · Zhaosheng Yu · Nhan Phan-Thien

Langevin Analysis of Microstructured Fluids

A Perspective of Microstructured Fluids

Springer

Dingyi Pan
Department of Engineering Mechanics
Zhejiang University
Hangzhou, Zhejiang, China

Zhaosheng Yu
Department of Engineering Mechanics
Zhejiang University
Hangzhou, Zhejiang, China

Nhan Phan-Thien
Department of Mechanical Engineering
National University of Singapore
Singapore, Singapore

ISSN 2191-530X ISSN 2191-5318 (electronic)
SpringerBriefs in Applied Sciences and Technology
ISBN 978-981-95-2317-7 ISBN 978-981-95-2318-4 (eBook)
https://doi.org/10.1007/978-981-95-2318-4

© The Editor(s) (if applicable) and The Author(s), under exclusive license to Springer Nature Singapore Pte Ltd. 2026

This work is subject to copyright. All rights are solely and exclusively licensed by the Publisher, whether the whole or part of the material is concerned, specifically the rights of reprinting, reuse of illustrations, recitation, broadcasting, reproduction on microfilms or in any other physical way, and transmission or information storage and retrieval, electronic adaptation, computer software, or by similar or dissimilar methodology now known or hereafter developed.
The use of general descriptive names, registered names, trademarks, service marks, etc. in this publication does not imply, even in the absence of a specific statement, that such names are exempt from the relevant protective laws and regulations and therefore free for general use.
The publisher, the authors and the editors are safe to assume that the advice and information in this book are believed to be true and accurate at the date of publication. Neither the publisher nor the authors or the editors give a warranty, expressed or implied, with respect to the material contained herein or for any errors or omissions that may have been made. The publisher remains neutral with regard to jurisdictional claims in published maps and institutional affiliations.

This Springer imprint is published by the registered company Springer Nature Singapore Pte Ltd.
The registered company address is: 152 Beach Road, #21-01/04 Gateway East, Singapore 189721, Singapore

If disposing of this product, please recycle the paper.

Dedicated to Kim Thoa, Ena (Jian-wei) and Xiao Xin (Jian-xin), whose unwavering support helps us to see further ahead

Preface

This Lecture Note is an outgrowth of an eight-week short course on *Modeling of Microstructured Fluids*, delivered in the spring of 2025 at Zhejiang University. The topics covered were modeling techniques for complex structured fluids, including polymer solutions and suspensions, mainly in the dilute regime, where exact and rigorous results can be obtained.

Research students often find it challenging to gather relevant information on these topics from multiple sources—monographs and published papers—especially when attempting to apply the concepts in their own research. This Lecture Note aims to address this challenge: it brings together basic but essential tools needed to understand and model complex structured fluids; it does not emphasize the latest developments in the literature, nor does it claim to be comprehensive.

The Lecture Note begins with Chap. 1 summarizing basic results in Cartesian tensors. Chapter 2 covers, in sufficient detail, the kinematics of motion and the equations of balance. Chapter 3 offers a mechanical (rather than mathematical) perspective on the Langevin equations. In this, the equipartition of energy principle and the fluctuation-dissipation theorem are discussed, relating the strength of the Brownian forces to the mobility of the Langevin system, and leading to the Fokker–Planck Kolmogorov Smoluchowski diffusion equation. Chapters 4 and 5 apply the concepts from Chap. 3 to the modeling of dilute polymer solutions and rigid rod systems. Finally, Chap. 6 offers some simple ideas on suspensions in highconcentration regimes.

It was decided that the level pitched in the lectures is that of first-year graduate students with a basic knowledge in calculus and differential equations. The length and scope of the Lecture Note reflects the focus and depth of this short course. The Note comes with a set of assignments at varying levels of difficulty; solving them is a part of the education process and is highly recommended. In addition, PowerPoint files for the course are available to assist instructors in delivering the course.

We are grateful to the Graduate School of Zhejiang University for supporting NP-T during this short course, which enabled the writing of this Lecture Note.

Hangzhou, China — Dingyi Pan
Hangzhou, China — Zhaosheng Yu
Singapore, Singapore — Nhan Phan-Thien
April 2025

Contents

Chapter 1
Basic of Tensors and Fields

A Short Summary of Tensor Analysis

1.1 Notation of Scalars, Vectors and Tensors

Physical quantities encountered in physics of fluids are either scalars, vectors, or tensors. These quantities are distinguished by the following generic notation.

Scalars (zero-order tensors) are typical denoted by lightface italic (e.g., s denotes a scalar), they are independent of coordinate directions. Common scalars are time, temperature, pressure, volume, and density.

Vectors (first-order tensors) are typical denoted by boldface (e.g., $\mathbf{u}$ denotes a vector), they have both a magnitude and a direction. In the Cartesian frame of reference, $\mathcal{F} = \{O; \mathbf{e}_1, \mathbf{e}_2, \mathbf{e}_3\}$, which consists of an origin O, a clock, and an orthonormal basis $\{\mathbf{e}_1, \mathbf{e}_2, \mathbf{e}_3\}$, a vector $\mathbf{u}$ (Fig. 1.1) are given by

$$\mathbf{u} = \mathbf{e}_1 \cdot u_1 + \mathbf{e}_2 \cdot u_2 + \mathbf{e}_3 \cdot u_3. \tag{1.1}$$

Common vectors are displacement, velocity, acceleration, force, torque.

Second-order tensors (or two-tensors, we deal mostly with second-order tensors) are denoted by boldface (e.g., $\mathbf{F}$ denotes a tensor). They have a scalar for each pair of coordinate directions, and therefore they are a set of 3×3 scalars referred to a frame of reference. Common second-order tensors are stress, displacement gradient, velocity gradient. If there is a set of $3 \times 3 \times 3$ scalars referred to a frame of reference, then it becomes a third-order tensor, such as alternating tensors.

For simplicity, indices, such as i, j, or k on the values 1, 2, or 3, are employed for notation of vectors and tensors. One may write the vector

$$\mathbf{u} = \sum_{i=1}^{3} u_i \mathbf{e}_i = u_i \mathbf{e}_i. \tag{1.2}$$

Here we have employed the *summation convention*.

© The Author(s), under exclusive license to Springer Nature Singapore Pte Ltd. 2025

D. Pan et al., *Langevin Analysis of Microstructured Fluids*,
SpringerBriefs in Applied Sciences and Technology,
https://doi.org/10.1007/978-981-95-2318-4_1

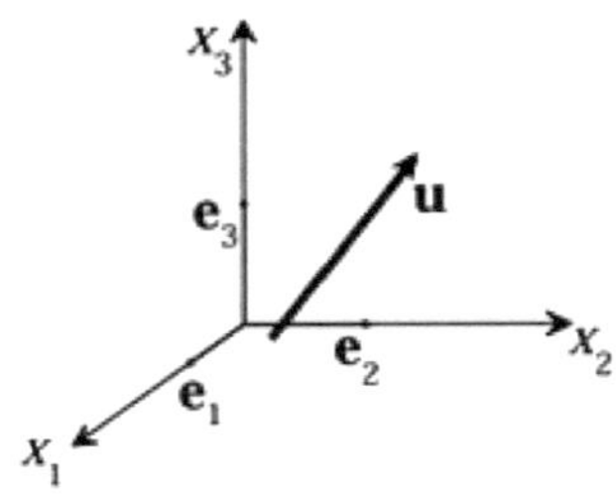

Fig. 1.1 Cartesian frame of reference (only right-handed frame of reference is considered), where $(\mathbf{e}_1 \times \mathbf{e}_2) \cdot \mathbf{e}_3 = 1$

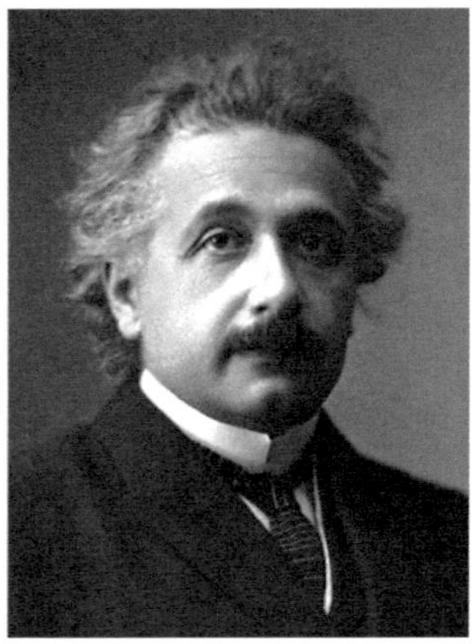

Fig. 1.2 Albert Einstein (1879–1955) got the Nobel Prize in Physics in 1921 for his explanation in photoelectricity. He derived the effective viscosity of a dilute suspension of neutrally buoyant spheres, $\eta = \eta_s(1 + \frac{5}{2}\phi)$, η_s: the solvent viscosity, ϕ: the sphere volume fraction. (Official 1921 Nobel Prize in Physics photograph possibly by Herman Mishkin (1871–1948), public domain photograph.)

Remark 1.1 (*Summation convention*) Whenever there are repeated subscripts, a summation is implied over the range of the subscripts, from (1, 2, 3). For example,

$$A_{ij} B_{jk} = \sum_{j=1}^{3} A_{ij} B_{jk}. \tag{1.3}$$

This short-hand notation is due to Einstein (Fig. 1.2), who argued that physical laws must not depend on coordinate systems, and therefore must be expressed in tensorial format. This is the essence of the *Principle of Frame Indifference*.

Both boldface (vector or *dyadic*) and indicial (tensor) notations are used throughout this text. One may write

$$\mathbf{W} = W_{ij}\mathbf{e}_i\mathbf{e}_j. \tag{1.4}$$

This is the basis for the *dyadic* notation, the $\mathbf{e}_i\mathbf{e}_j$ play the role of the basis "vectors" for the tensor $\mathbf{W}$.

1.2 Frame Rotation

Consider the two frames of references, $\mathcal{F} = \{O; \mathbf{e}_1, \mathbf{e}_2, \mathbf{e}_3\}$ and $\mathcal{F}' = \left\{O; \mathbf{e}'_1, \mathbf{e}'_2\ \mathbf{e}'_3\right\}$, as shown in Fig. 1.3, one obtained from the other by a rotation. First, on the orthonormal basis

$$\mathbf{e}_i \cdot \mathbf{e}_j = \delta_{ij}, \quad \mathbf{e}'_i \cdot \mathbf{e}'_j = \delta_{ij}.$$

where δ_{ij} is the *Kronecker delta*.

Remark 1.2 (*Kronecker delta & alternating tensor*) The *Kronecker delta* is defined as

$$\delta_{ij} = \begin{cases} 1, & i = j, \\ 0, & i \neq j. \end{cases} \tag{1.5}$$

The *Kronecker delta* is a second-order tensor. In fact it is invariant in any coordinate system, and therefore is an *isotropic* tensor of second order. δ_{ij} are said to be the components of the second-order unit tensor $\mathbf{I}$. δ_{ij} is sometimes called the *substitution tensor*, since the operation $\delta_{ij}u_j = u_i$ replaces the subscript j by i.

The *alternating tensor* is defined as

$$\varepsilon_{ijk} = \begin{cases} +1\ , \text{ if } (i, j, k) \text{ is an even permutation of } (1, 2, 3) \\ -1\ , \text{ if } (i, j, k) \text{ is an odd permutation of } (1, 2, 3) \\ \ \ 0\ , \text{ otherwise.} \end{cases} \tag{1.6}$$

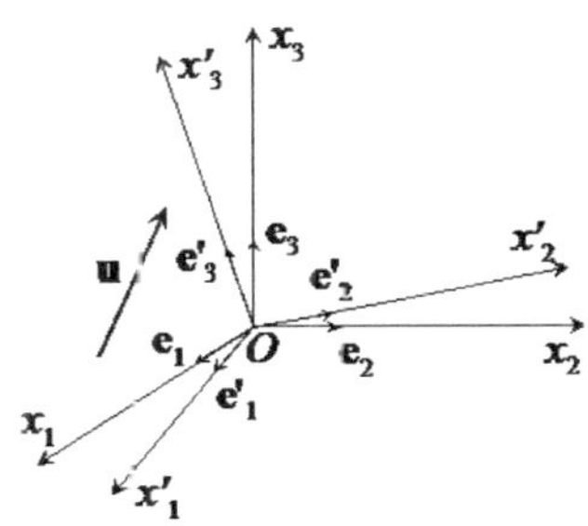

Fig. 1.3 Two frames of reference sharing a common origin

Then, define the cosine of the angle between $\left(\mathbf{e}_i, \mathbf{e}'_j\right)$ as

$$A_{ij} = \mathbf{e}'_i \cdot \mathbf{e}_j.$$

Thus A_{ij} can be regarded as the components of $\mathbf{e}'_i$ in $\mathcal{F}$, or the components of $\mathbf{e}_j$ in $\mathcal{F}'$. We write

$$\mathbf{e}'_p = A_{pi}\mathbf{e}_i \quad \therefore \quad A_{pi}A_{qi} = \delta_{pq}.$$

Similarly

$$\mathbf{e}_i = A_{pi}\mathbf{e}'_p \quad \therefore \quad A_{pi}A_{pj} = \delta_{ij}.$$

We now consider a vector $\mathbf{u}$, expressed in either frame $\mathcal{F}$ or $\mathcal{F}'$,

$$\mathbf{u} = u_i\mathbf{e}_i = u'_j\mathbf{e}'_j.$$

Thus, a vector can be formally defined as any quantity whose components change similarly to the components of the position vector under a frame rotation. Taking scalar product with either base vector,

$$\begin{aligned} u'_i &= \mathbf{e}'_i \cdot \mathbf{e}_j u_j = A_{ij}u_j, \\ u_j &= \mathbf{e}_j \cdot \mathbf{e}'_i u'_i = A_{ij}u'_i. \end{aligned}$$

In matrix notation,

$$[\mathbf{A}] = \begin{bmatrix} A_{11} & A_{12} & A_{13} \\ A_{21} & A_{22} & A_{23} \\ A_{31} & A_{32} & A_{33} \end{bmatrix}, \quad [\mathbf{u}] = \begin{bmatrix} u_1 \\ u_2 \\ u_3 \end{bmatrix}, \quad \left[\mathbf{u}'\right] = \begin{bmatrix} u'_1 \\ u'_2 \\ u'_3 \end{bmatrix},$$

we have

$$\begin{aligned} \left[\mathbf{u}'\right] &= [\mathbf{A}] \cdot [\mathbf{u}], \quad & [\mathbf{u}] &= [\mathbf{A}]^T \cdot \left[\mathbf{u}'\right], \\ u'_i &= A_{ij}u_j, & u_j &= A_{ij}u'_i. \end{aligned} \tag{1.7}$$

The matrix A is called a rotation—in fact a proper orthogonal matrix ($det\mathbf{A} = +1$).

Remark 1.3 (*Orthogonal matrix*) A matrix is said to be an *orthogonal matrix* if its inverse is also its transpose; furthermore, if its determinant is +1, then it is a *proper orthogonal matrix*.

For a second-order tensor, $\mathbf{W} = [W_{ij}]$, it can be transformed to another set under a frame rotation according to

$$W'_{ij} = A_{im}A_{jn}W_{mn}. \tag{1.8}$$

In matrix notation, we write

$$\left[\mathbf{W}'\right] = [\mathbf{A}]\,[\mathbf{W}]\,[\mathbf{A}]^T \ \text{ or } \mathbf{W}' = \mathbf{AWA}^T \ \text{ or } W'_{ij} = A_{ik}W_{kl}A_{jl}.$$

In the direct notation, we denote a tensor by a bold face letter (without the square brackets). This direct notation is intimately connected to the concept of a linear operator, e.g., Gurtin [2].

Similary, an entity, $\mathbf{W}$ with components $[W_{i_1 i_2 \ldots i_n}]$ (n indices). is a n-order tensor if its components transform under a frame rotation according to

$$W'_{i_1 i_2 \ldots i_n} = A_{i_1 j_1} A_{i_2 j_2} \cdots A_{i_n j_n} W_{j_1 j_2 \ldots j_n}. \tag{1.9}$$

1.3 Tensor Operations

1.3.1 Inner Products

The set of all vectors forms a vector space $\mathcal{U}$ under addition and multiplication. In this space, the usual scalar product can be shown to be an inner product. With the norm induced by this inner product,

$$|\mathbf{u}|^2 = \mathbf{u} \cdot \mathbf{u},$$

$\mathcal{U}$ is a normed vector space. We also refer to a vector $\mathbf{u}$ by its components, u_i.

1.3.2 Outer Products

Consider now two tensors of first order, u_i and v_i. The product $u_i v_j$ represents the outer product of $\mathbf{u}$ and $\mathbf{v}$, and written as (the subscripts are assigned from left to right by convention),

$$[\mathbf{uv}] = \begin{bmatrix} u_1v_1 & u_1v_2 & u_1v_3 \\ u_2v_1 & u_2v_2 & u_2v_3 \\ u_3v_1 & u_3v_2 & u_3v_3 \end{bmatrix}.$$

In a frame rotation, from $\mathcal{F}$ to $\mathcal{F}'$, the components of this change according to

$$u'_i v'_j = A_{im} A_{jn} u_m v_n.$$

Usually, a higher-order (higher than 2) tensor is formed by taking outer products of tensors of lower orders.

1.3.3 Transpose

The components of the transpose of a tensor **W** are obtained by swapping the indices:

$$[\mathbf{W}]_{ij} = W_{ij}, \quad [\mathbf{W}]^T_{ij} = W_{ji}.$$

A tensor **S** is *symmetric* if it is unaltered by the transpose operation,

$$\mathbf{S} = \mathbf{S}^T, \qquad S_{ij} = S_{ji}.$$

It is *anti-symmetric* (or *skew*) if

$$\mathbf{S} = -\mathbf{S}^T, \quad S_{ij} = -S_{ji}.$$

An anti-symmetric tensor must have zero diagonal terms (when $i = j$).

1.3.4 Decomposition

Any second-order tensor can be decomposed into symmetric and anti-symmetric parts:

$$\mathbf{W} = \frac{1}{2}\left(\mathbf{W} + \mathbf{W}^T\right) + \frac{1}{2}\left(\mathbf{W} - \mathbf{W}^T\right). \tag{1.10}$$

Returning to (1.8), if we interchange i and j, we get

$$W'_{ji} = A_{jm}A_{in}W_{mn} = A_{jn}A_{im}W_{nm}.$$

The second equality arises because m and n are dummy indices, mere labels in the summation. The left side of this expression is recognized as the components of the transpose of **W**. The equation asserts that the components of the transpose of **W** are also transformed according to (1.8). Thus, if **W** is a two-tensor, then its transpose is also a two-tensor, and the Cartesian decomposition (1.10) splits an arbitrary two-tensor into a symmetric and an anti-symmetric tensor (of second order).

1.3.5 Contraction

Given a two-tensor W_{ij}, the operation

$$W_{ii} = \sum_{i=1}^{3} W_{ii} = W_{11} + W_{22} + W_{33}$$

is called a contraction. It produces a scalar. The invariance of this scalar under a frame rotation is seen by noting that

$$W'_{ii} = A_{ik}A_{il}W_{kl} = \delta_{kl}W_{kl} = W_{kk}.$$

This scalar is also called the trace of $\mathbf{W}$, written as

$$\mathrm{tr}\mathbf{W} = W_{ii}. \tag{1.11}$$

If the trace of $\mathbf{W}$ is zero, then $\mathbf{W}$ is said to be traceless. In general, given an n-order tensor, contracting any two subscripts produces a tensor of $(n-2)$ order.

1.3.6 On Products of Two Second-Order Tensors

Given two second-order tensors, $\mathbf{U}$ and $\mathbf{V}$,

$$\mathbf{U} = U_{ij}\mathbf{e}_i\mathbf{e}_j, \quad \mathbf{V} = V_{ij}\mathbf{e}_i\mathbf{e}_j,$$

one can form different products from them, which are listed as following.

The *tensor product*, $\mathbf{U}\otimes\mathbf{V}$, produces a fourth-order tensor, with component $U_{ij}V_{kl}$,

$$\mathbf{U}\otimes\mathbf{V} = U_{ij}V_{kl}\mathbf{e}_i\mathbf{e}_j\mathbf{e}_k\mathbf{e}_l. \tag{1.12}$$

The *single dot product*, $\mathbf{U}\cdot\mathbf{V}$, produces a second-order tensor (sometimes written without the dot), and the dot is the contraction operator,

$$\begin{aligned}\mathbf{U}\cdot\mathbf{V} = \mathbf{U}\mathbf{V} &= \left(U_{ij}\mathbf{e}_i\mathbf{e}_j\right)\cdot\left(V_{kl}\mathbf{e}_k\mathbf{e}_l\right)\\ &= U_{ij}\mathbf{e}_i\delta_{jk}V_{kl}\mathbf{e}_l = U_{ij}V_{jl}\mathbf{e}_i\mathbf{e}_l,\end{aligned} \tag{1.13}$$

with components $U_{ik}V_{kl}$, just like multiplying two matrices U_{ik} and V_{kj}.

The *double dot (or scalar, or inner) product*, $\mathbf{U}:\mathbf{V}$, produces a scalar,

$$\begin{aligned}\mathbf{U}:\mathbf{V} &= \left(U_{ij}\mathbf{e}_i\mathbf{e}_j\right):\left(V_{kl}\mathbf{e}_k\mathbf{e}_l\right) = \left(U_{ij}\mathbf{e}_i\right)\delta_{jk}\cdot\left(V_{kl}\mathbf{e}_l\right)\\ &= U_{ij}V_{kl}\delta_{jk}\delta_{il} = U_{ij}V_{ji}.\end{aligned} \tag{1.14}$$

The dot operates on a pair of base vectors until we run out of dots. The end result is a scalar (remember our summation convention). It can be shown that the scalar product is in fact an inner product. Subsequently, the *norm* of a two-tensor is defined from the inner product in the usual manner,

$$\|\mathbf{U}\|^2 = \mathbf{U}^T:\mathbf{U} = U_{ij}U_{ij} = \mathrm{tr}\left(\mathbf{U}^T\mathbf{U}\right). \tag{1.15}$$

The space of all linear vector functions therefore forms a normed vector space.

In addition, a tensor $\mathbf{U}$ is *invertible* if there exists a tensor, $\mathbf{U}^{-1}$, called the inverse of $\mathbf{U}$, such that

$$\mathbf{U}\mathbf{U}^{-1} = \mathbf{U}^{-1}\mathbf{U} = \mathbf{I}. \tag{1.16}$$

Finally, one can also define the vector *cross product* between two second-order tensors, and indeed any combination of dot and cross vector products.

1.3.7 Invariants

From a second-order tensor $\mathbf{S}$, there are three independent scalar invariants that can be formed, by taking the trace of $\mathbf{S}$, $\mathbf{S}^2$ and $\mathbf{S}^3$,

$$I = \text{tr}\mathbf{S} = S_{ii}, \quad II = \text{tr}\mathbf{S}^2 = S_{ij}S_{ji}, \quad III = \text{tr}\mathbf{S}^3 = S_{ij}S_{jk}S_{ki}.$$

However, it is customary to use the following invariants

$$I_1 = I, \ \ I_2 = \frac{1}{2}\left(I^2 - II\right), \ \ I_3 = \frac{1}{6}\left(I^3 - 3I\ II + 2III\right) = \det \mathbf{S}.$$

It is also possible to form ten invariants between two tensors [2].

1.3.8 Eigenvalue and Eigenvector

A scalar ω is an *eigenvalue* of a two-tensor $\mathbf{S}$ if there exists a non-zero vector $\mathbf{e}$, called the *eigenvector*, satisfying

$$\mathbf{S}\mathbf{e} = \omega\mathbf{e}. \tag{1.17}$$

The characteristic space for $\mathbf{S}$ corresponding to the eigenvalue ω consists of all vectors in the eigenspace, $\{\mathbf{v} : \ \mathbf{S}\mathbf{v} = \omega\mathbf{v}\}$. If the dimension of this space is n, then ω is said to have geometric multiplicity of n. The *spectrum* of $\mathbf{S}$ is the ordered list $\{\omega_1, \omega_2, \ldots\}$ of all the eigenvalues of S.

Remark 1.4 (*Positive definite tensor*) A tensor $\mathbf{S}$ is said to be *positive definite* if it satisfies

$$\mathbf{S} : \mathbf{v}\mathbf{v} > 0, \qquad \forall \mathbf{v} \neq \mathbf{0}. \tag{1.18}$$

It can be proved that the eigenvalues of a positive definite tensor are strictly positive.

1.3.9 Polar Decomposition Theorem

For any given tensor $\mathbf{F}$, there exist positive definite tensors $\mathbf{U}$ and $\mathbf{V}$, and a rotation tensor $\mathbf{R}$, such that

$$\mathbf{F} = \mathbf{RU} = \mathbf{VR}. \tag{1.19}$$

Each of these representations is unique, and

$$\mathbf{U} = \left(\mathbf{F}^T\mathbf{F}\right)^{1/2}, \quad \mathbf{V} = \left(\mathbf{F}\mathbf{F}^T\right)^{1/2}. \tag{1.20}$$

The first representation ($\mathbf{RU}$) is called the right, and the second ($\mathbf{VR}$) is called the left polar decomposition.

1.3.10 Cayley–Hamilton Theorem

The most important theorem is the Cayley–Hamilton theorem: Every tensor $\mathbf{S}$ satisfies its own characteristic equation

$$\mathbf{S}^3 - I_1\mathbf{S}^2 + I_2\mathbf{S} - I_3\mathbf{I} = \mathbf{0}, \tag{1.21}$$

where $I_1 = \mathrm{tr}\mathbf{S}$, $I_2 = \frac{1}{2}\left((\mathrm{tr}\mathbf{S})^2 - \mathrm{tr}\mathbf{S}^2\right)$, and $I_3 = \det\mathbf{S}$ are the three scalar invariants for $\mathbf{S}$, and $\mathbf{I}$ is the unit tensor in three dimensions.

1.4 Fields and Integral Theorems

1.4.1 Field

A function of the position vector $\mathbf{x}$ is called a *field*. We have scalar fields, e.g., the temperature field $T(\mathbf{x})$, vector fields, e.g., the velocity field $\mathbf{u}(\mathbf{x})$, or tensor fields, e.g., the stress field $\mathbf{S}(\mathbf{x})$. Conservation laws and equations of balance in continuum mechanics as discussed in next chapter involve derivatives of different fields, and it is absolutely essential to know how to calculate the gradients of fields in different coordinate systems. It is also convenient to employ the dyadic notation at this point.

1.4.2 Gradient Operator

Derivatives with respect to position vectors are called *gradients*, and the gradient operator is defined as

$$\nabla = \mathbf{e}_j \frac{\partial}{\partial x_j} = \mathbf{e}_1 \frac{\partial}{\partial x_1} + \mathbf{e}_2 \frac{\partial}{\partial x_2} + \mathbf{e}_3 \frac{\partial}{\partial x_3}. \tag{1.22}$$

This operator can be treated as a vector, operating on its arguments. By itself, it has no meaning; it must operate on a scalar, a vector, or a tensor.

For example, the gradient of a scalar is

$$\nabla \varphi = \mathbf{e}_j \frac{\partial \varphi}{\partial x_j} = \mathbf{e}_1 \frac{\partial \varphi}{\partial x_1} + \mathbf{e}_2 \frac{\partial \varphi}{\partial x_2} + \mathbf{e}_3 \frac{\partial \varphi}{\partial x_3}. \tag{1.23}$$

The gradient of a vector can be likewise calculated

$$\nabla \mathbf{u} = \left(\mathbf{e}_i \frac{\partial}{\partial x_i} \right) \left(u_j \mathbf{e}_j \right) = \mathbf{e}_i \mathbf{e}_j \frac{\partial u_j}{\partial x_i}. \tag{1.24}$$

Remark 1.5 (*Velocity gradient*) If $\mathbf{u}$ is the velocity field, then $\nabla \mathbf{u}$ is the gradient of the velocity. So

$$(\nabla \mathbf{u})_{ij} = \nabla_i u_j = \frac{\partial u_j}{\partial x_i}.$$

Mostly, the term velocity gradient is taken to mean the two-tensor $\mathbf{L} = (\nabla \mathbf{u})^T$ with components

$$L_{ij} = \frac{\partial u_i}{\partial x_j}. \tag{1.25}$$

The velocity gradient tensor can be decomposed into a symmetric part $\mathbf{D}$, called the strain rate tensor, and an anti-symmetric part $\mathbf{W}$, called the vorticity tensor:

$$\mathbf{D} = \frac{1}{2} \left(\nabla \mathbf{u} + \nabla \mathbf{u}^T \right), \quad \mathbf{W} = \frac{1}{2} \left(\nabla \mathbf{u}^T - \nabla \mathbf{u} \right). \tag{1.26}$$

1.4.3 Divergent Operator

The divergence of a vector is a scalar, and it is defined by

$$\nabla \cdot \mathbf{u} = \left(\mathbf{e}_i \frac{\partial}{\partial x_i} \right) \cdot \left(u_j \mathbf{e}_j \right) = \mathbf{e}_i \cdot \mathbf{e}_j \frac{\partial u_j}{\partial x_i} = \delta_{ij} \frac{\partial u_j}{\partial x_i}$$

$$\nabla \cdot \mathbf{u} = \frac{\partial u_i}{\partial x_i} = \frac{\partial u_1}{\partial x_1} + \frac{\partial u_2}{\partial x_2} + \frac{\partial u_3}{\partial x_3}. \tag{1.27}$$

The divergence of a vector is also an invariant, being the trace of a tensor.

The divergence of a tensor is a vector field defined by

$$\nabla \cdot \mathbf{S} = \left(\mathbf{e}_k \frac{\partial}{\partial x_k} \right) \cdot \left(S_{ij} \mathbf{e}_i \mathbf{e}_j \right) = \mathbf{e}_j \frac{\partial S_{ij}}{\partial x_i}. \tag{1.28}$$

1.4.4 Curl of a Vector

The curl of a vector is a vector, and it is defined by

$$\begin{aligned} \nabla \times \mathbf{u} &= \left(\mathbf{e}_i \frac{\partial}{\partial x_i} \right) \times \left(u_j \mathbf{e}_j \right) = \mathbf{e}_i \times \mathbf{e}_j \frac{\partial u_j}{\partial x_i} = \varepsilon_{kij} \mathbf{e}_k \frac{\partial u_j}{\partial x_i} \\ &= \mathbf{e}_1 \left(\frac{\partial u_3}{\partial x_2} - \frac{\partial u_2}{\partial x_3} \right) + \mathbf{e}_2 \left(\frac{\partial u_1}{\partial x_3} - \frac{\partial u_3}{\partial x_1} \right) + \mathbf{e}_3 \left(\frac{\partial u_2}{\partial x_1} - \frac{\partial u_1}{\partial x_2} \right). \end{aligned} \tag{1.29}$$

The curl of a vector is sometimes denoted by the operator rot, rot $\mathbf{u} \equiv \nabla \times \mathbf{u}$.

1.4.5 Gauss Divergence Theorem

Various volume integrals can be converted to surface integrals by the following theorems, due to Gauss (Fig. 1.4):

$$\int_V \nabla \varphi dV = \int_S \varphi \mathbf{n} dS, \tag{1.30}$$

$$\int_V \nabla \cdot \mathbf{u} dV = \int_S \mathbf{n} \cdot \mathbf{u} dS, \tag{1.31}$$

$$\int_V \nabla \cdot \mathbf{S} dV = \int_S \mathbf{n} \cdot \mathbf{S} dS. \tag{1.32}$$

The proofs may be found in Kellogg [3]. In these, V is a bounded regular region, with bounding surface S and outward unit vector $\mathbf{n}$. φ, $\mathbf{u}$, and $\mathbf{S}$ are differentiable scalar, vector, and tensor fields with continuous gradients.

1.4.6 Stokes Curl Theorem

Various surfaces integrals can be converted into contour integrals using the following theorems, known as Stokes' Curl theorems:

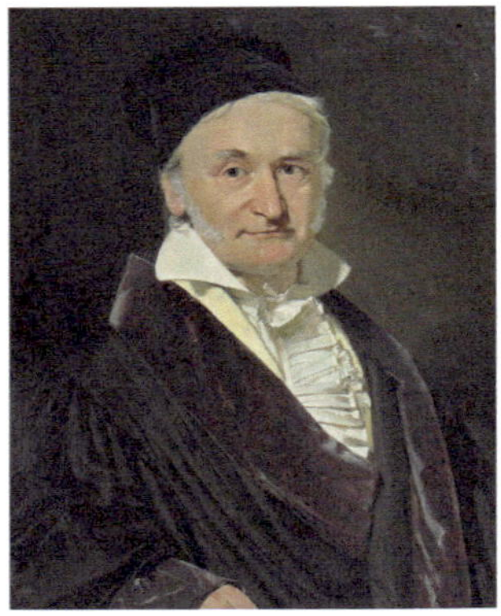

Fig. 1.4 Carl Friedrich Gauss (1777–1855) was a Professor of Mathematics at the University of Göttingen. He made several contributions to Number Theory, Geodesy, Statistics, Geometry, Physics. His motto was "few, but ripe" (*Pauca, Sed Matura*). He did not publish several important papers because they did not satisfy these requirements. (Painting by Christian Albrecht Jensen (1792–1870), public domain work of art.)

$$\int_S \mathbf{n} \cdot (\nabla \times \mathbf{u})\, dS = \oint_C \mathbf{t} \cdot \mathbf{u} dC, \tag{1.33}$$

$$\int_S \mathbf{n} \cdot (\nabla \times \mathbf{S})\, dS = \oint_C \mathbf{t} \cdot \mathbf{S} dC. \tag{1.34}$$

In these, $\mathbf{t}$ is a tangential unit vector along the contour C. The direction of integration is determined by the right-hand rule: thumb pointing in the direction of $\mathbf{n}$, fingers curling in the direction of C.

1.4.7 Leibniz Formula

If φ is a field (a scalar, a vector, or a tensor) define on a region $V(t)$, which is changing in time, with bounding surface $S(t)$, also changing in time with velocity $\mathbf{u}_S$, then we have the Leibniz (Fig. 1.5) formula,

$$\frac{d}{dt}\int_V \varphi dV = \int_V \frac{\partial \varphi}{\partial t} dV + \int_S \varphi \mathbf{u}_S \cdot \mathbf{n} dS. \tag{1.35}$$

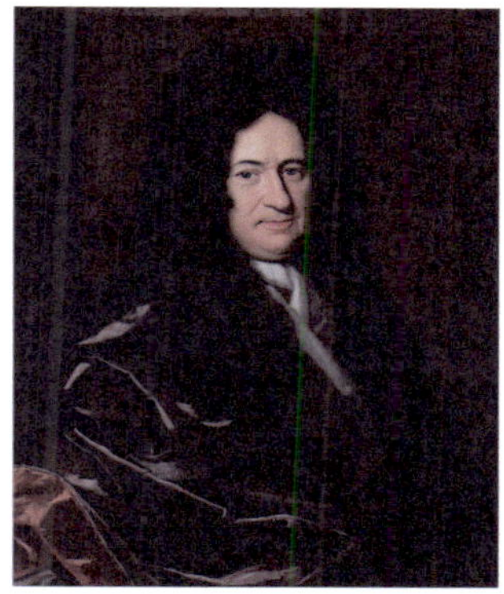

Fig. 1.5 Gottfried W. Leibniz (1646–1716) was a German philosopher and mathematician, who independently with Newton, laid the foundation for integral and differential calculus in 1675. (Painting by Christoph Bernhard Francke (1665–1729), public domain work of art.)

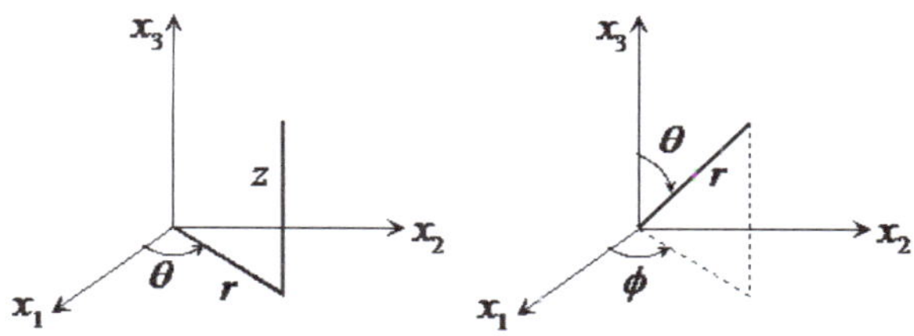

Fig. 1.6 Cylindrical and spherical frame of references

1.4.8 Non-Cartesian Frames

All the above definitions for gradient and divergence of a tensor remain valid in a non-Cartesian frame, provided that the derivative operation is also applied to the basis vectors as well. We illustrate this process in two important frames, cylindrical and spherical coordinate systems as shown in Fig. 1.6. Refer to Bird et al. [4] for others.

In a cylindrical coordinate system (Fig. 1.6, left), points are located by giving them values to $\{r, \theta, z\}$, which are related to $\{x = x_1, y = x_2, z = x_3\}$ by

$$\begin{aligned} x = r\cos\theta, \quad y = r\sin\theta, \quad z = z \\ r = \sqrt{x^2 + y^2}, \quad \theta = \tan^{-1}\left(\tfrac{y}{x}\right), \quad z = z \end{aligned}.$$

The basis vectors in this frame are related to the Cartesian ones by

$$\begin{aligned} \mathbf{e}_r = \cos\theta\mathbf{e}_x + \sin\theta\mathbf{e}_y, \qquad \mathbf{e}_x = \cos\theta\mathbf{e}_r - \sin\theta\mathbf{e}_\theta \\ \mathbf{e}_\theta = -\sin\theta\mathbf{e}_x + \cos\theta\mathbf{e}_y, \quad \mathbf{e}_y = \sin\theta\mathbf{e}_r + \cos\theta\mathbf{e}_\theta \end{aligned}.$$

In a spherical coordinate system (Fig. 1.6, right), points are located by giving them values to $\{r, \theta, \phi\}$, which are related to $\{x = x_1, y = x_2, z = x_3\}$ by

$$x = r\sin\theta\cos\phi, \quad y = r\sin\theta\sin\phi, \quad z = r\cos\theta,$$
$$r = \sqrt{x^2 + y^2 + z^2}, \quad \theta = \tan^{-1}\left(\frac{\sqrt{x^2 + y^2}}{z}\right), \quad \phi = \tan^{-1}\left(\frac{y}{x}\right).$$

The basis vectors are related by

$$\begin{aligned}
\mathbf{e}_r &= \mathbf{e}_1 \sin\theta\cos\phi + \mathbf{e}_2 \sin\theta\sin\phi + \mathbf{e}_3 \cos\theta,\\
\mathbf{e}_\theta &= \mathbf{e}_1 \cos\theta\cos\phi + \mathbf{e}_2 \cos\theta\sin\phi - \mathbf{e}_3 \sin\theta,\\
\mathbf{e}_\phi &= -\mathbf{e}_1 \sin\phi + \mathbf{e}_2 \cos\phi,
\end{aligned}$$

and

$$\begin{aligned}
\mathbf{e}_1 &= \mathbf{e}_r \sin\theta\cos\phi + \mathbf{e}_\theta \cos\theta\cos\phi - \mathbf{e}_\phi \sin\phi,\\
\mathbf{e}_2 &= \mathbf{e}_r \sin\theta\sin\phi + \mathbf{e}_\theta \cos\theta\sin\phi + \mathbf{e}_\phi \cos\phi,\\
\mathbf{e}_3 &= \mathbf{e}_r \cos\theta - \mathbf{e}_\theta \sin\theta.
\end{aligned}$$

Problems

Problem 1.1 The components of vectors **u**, **v**, and **w** are given by u_i, v_i, w_i. Verify that

$$\begin{aligned}
\mathbf{u}\cdot\mathbf{v} &= u_i v_i,\\
\mathbf{u}\times\mathbf{v} &= \varepsilon_{ijk}\mathbf{e}_i u_j v_k,\\
(\mathbf{u}\times\mathbf{v})\cdot\mathbf{w} &= \varepsilon_{ijk} u_i v_j w_k,\\
(\mathbf{u}\times\mathbf{v})\cdot\mathbf{w} &= \mathbf{u}\cdot(\mathbf{v}\times\mathbf{w}),\\
(\mathbf{u}\times\mathbf{v})\times\mathbf{w} &= (\mathbf{u}\cdot\mathbf{w})\,\mathbf{v} - (\mathbf{v}\cdot\mathbf{w})\,\mathbf{u},\\
(\mathbf{u}\times\mathbf{v})^2 &= u^2 v^2 - (\mathbf{u}\cdot\mathbf{v})^2,
\end{aligned}$$

where $u^2 = |\mathbf{u}|^2$ and $v^2 = |\mathbf{v}|^2$.

Problem 1.2 Let **A** be a 3×3 matrix with entries A_{ij},

$$[\mathbf{A}] = \begin{bmatrix} A_{11} & A_{12} & A_{13}\\ A_{21} & A_{22} & A_{23}\\ A_{31} & A_{32} & A_{33} \end{bmatrix}.$$

Verify that

$$\det[\mathbf{A}] = \varepsilon_{ijk}A_{1i}A_{2j}A_{3k} = \varepsilon_{ijk}A_{i1}A_{j2}A_{k3},$$
$$\varepsilon_{lmn}\det[\mathbf{A}] = \varepsilon_{ijk}A_{il}A_{jm}A_{kn} = \varepsilon_{ijk}A_{li}A_{mj}A_{nk},$$
$$\det[\mathbf{A}] = \frac{1}{6}\varepsilon_{ijk}\varepsilon_{lmn}A_{il}A_{jm}A_{kn}.$$

Problem 1.3 Verify that

$$\varepsilon_{ijk}\varepsilon_{imn} = \delta_{jm}\delta_{kn} - \delta_{jn}\delta_{km}.$$

Given that two 3×3 matrices of components

$$[\mathbf{A}] = \begin{bmatrix} A_{11} & A_{12} & A_{13} \\ A_{21} & A_{22} & A_{23} \\ A_{31} & A_{32} & A_{33} \end{bmatrix}, \quad [\mathbf{B}] = \begin{bmatrix} B_{11} & B_{12} & B_{13} \\ B_{21} & B_{22} & B_{23} \\ B_{31} & B_{32} & B_{33} \end{bmatrix}$$

verify that if $[\mathbf{C}] = [\mathbf{A}] \cdot [\mathbf{B}]$, then the components of $\mathbf{C}$ are $C_{ij} = A_{ik}B_{kj}$. Thus if $[\mathbf{D}] = [\mathbf{A}]^T[\mathbf{B}]$, then $D_{ij} = A_{ki}B_{kj}$.

Problem 1.4 Show that, if $\left[A_{ij}\right]$ is a frame rotation matrix,

$$\det\left[A_{ij}\right] = \left(\mathbf{e}'_1 \times \mathbf{e}'_2\right) \cdot \mathbf{e}'_3 = 1.$$
$$[\mathbf{A}]^T[\mathbf{A}] = [\mathbf{A}][\mathbf{A}]^T = [\mathbf{I}], \quad [\mathbf{A}]^{-1} = [\mathbf{A}]^T, \quad \det[\mathbf{A}] = 1.$$

Problem 1.5 Verify that

$$\varepsilon_{ijk}u_i v_j w_k = \det\begin{bmatrix} u_1 & u_2 & u_3 \\ v_1 & v_2 & v_3 \\ w_1 & w_2 & w_3 \end{bmatrix}.$$

Consider a second-order tensor W_{ij} and a vector $u_i = \varepsilon_{ijk}W_{jk}$. Show that if $\mathbf{W}$ is symmetric, $\mathbf{u}$ is zero, and if $\mathbf{W}$ is anti-symmetric the components of $\mathbf{u}$ are twice those of $\mathbf{W}$ in magnitude. This vector is said to be the axial vector of $\mathbf{W}$.
Hence, show that the axial vector associated with the vorticity tensor of (1.26) is $-\nabla \times \mathbf{u}$.

Problem 1.6 If $\mathbf{D}$, $\mathbf{S}$ and $\mathbf{W}$ are second-order tensors, $\mathbf{D}$ symmetric and $\mathbf{W}$ anti-symmetric, show that

$$\mathbf{D} : \mathbf{S} = \mathbf{D} : \mathbf{S}^T = \mathbf{D} : \tfrac{1}{2}\left(\mathbf{S} + \mathbf{S}^T\right),$$
$$\mathbf{W} : \mathbf{S} = -\mathbf{W} : \mathbf{S}^T = \mathbf{W} : \tfrac{1}{2}\left(\mathbf{W} - \mathbf{W}^T\right),$$
$$\mathbf{D} : \mathbf{W} = 0.$$

Further, show that

$$\begin{aligned}&\text{if } \mathbf{T} : \mathbf{S} = 0 \quad \forall \mathbf{S} \text{ then } \mathbf{T} = 0,\\&\text{if } \mathbf{T} : \mathbf{S} = 0 \quad \forall \text{ symmetric } \mathbf{S} \text{ then } \mathbf{T} \text{ is anti-symmetric},\\&\text{if } \mathbf{T} : \mathbf{S} = 0 \quad \forall \text{ anti-symmetric} \mathbf{S} \text{ then } \mathbf{T} \text{ is symmetric}.\end{aligned}$$

Problem 1.7 Show that $\mathbf{Q}$ is orthogonal if and only if $\mathbf{H} = \mathbf{Q} - \mathbf{I}$ satisfies

$$\mathbf{H} + \mathbf{H}^T + \mathbf{H}\mathbf{H}^T = 0, \quad \mathbf{H}\mathbf{H}^T = \mathbf{H}^T\mathbf{H}.$$

Problem 1.8 Show that, if $\mathbf{S}$ is a second-order tensor, then $I = \text{tr } \mathbf{S}$, $II = \text{tr } \mathbf{S}^2$, $III = \det \mathbf{S}$ are indeed invariants. In addition, show that

$$\det (\mathbf{S} - \omega \mathbf{I}) = -\omega^3 + I_1 \omega^2 - I_2 \omega + I_3.$$

If ω is an eigenvalue of $\mathbf{S}$ then $\det (\mathbf{S} - \omega \mathbf{I}) = 0$. This is said to be the characteristic equation for $\mathbf{S}$.

Problem 1.9 Apply the result above to find the square root of the Cauchy–Green tensor in a two-dimensional shear deformation

$$[\mathbf{C}] = \begin{bmatrix} 1 + \gamma^2 & \gamma \\ \gamma & 1 \end{bmatrix}.$$

Investigate the corresponding formula for the square root of a symmetric positive definite tensor $\mathbf{S}$ in three dimensions.

Problem 1.10 Write down all the components of the strain rate tensor and the vorticity tensor in a Cartesian frame.

Problem 1.11 Given that $\mathbf{r} = x_i \mathbf{e}_i$ is the position vector, $\mathbf{a}$ is a constant vector, and $f(r)$ is a function of $r = |\mathbf{r}|$, show that

$$\nabla \cdot \mathbf{r} = 3, \quad \nabla \times \mathbf{r} = \mathbf{0}, \quad \nabla (\mathbf{a} \cdot \mathbf{r}) = \mathbf{a}, \quad \nabla f = \frac{1}{r}\frac{df}{dr}\mathbf{r}.$$

Problem 1.12 Show that the divergence of a second-order tensor $\mathbf{S}$ in cylindrical coordinates is given by

$$\begin{aligned}\nabla \cdot \mathbf{S} = \mathbf{e}_r &\left(\frac{\partial S_{rr}}{\partial r} + \frac{S_{rr} - S_{\theta\theta}}{r} + \frac{1}{r}\frac{\partial S_{\theta r}}{\partial \theta} + \frac{\partial S_{zr}}{\partial z} \right) \\ + \mathbf{e}_\theta &\left(\frac{\partial S_{r\theta}}{\partial r} + \frac{2 S_{r\theta}}{r} + \frac{1}{r}\frac{\partial S_{\theta\theta}}{\partial \theta} + \frac{\partial S_{z\theta}}{\partial z} + \frac{S_{\theta r} - S_{r\theta}}{r} \right) \\ + \mathbf{e}_z &\left(\frac{\partial S_{rz}}{\partial r} + \frac{S_{rz}}{r} + \frac{1}{r}\frac{\partial S_{\theta z}}{\partial \theta} + \frac{\partial S_{zz}}{\partial z} \right).\end{aligned} \tag{1.36}$$

Problem 1.13 Show that, in cylindrical coordinates, the Laplacian of a vector **u** is given by

$$\begin{aligned}\nabla^2\mathbf{u} = \mathbf{e}_r &\left[\frac{\partial}{\partial r}\left(\frac{1}{r}\frac{\partial}{\partial r}(ru_r)\right) + \frac{1}{r^2}\frac{\partial^2 u_r}{\partial \theta^2} + \frac{\partial^2 u_r}{\partial z^2} - \frac{2}{r^2}\frac{\partial u_\theta}{\partial \theta}\right] \\ + \mathbf{e}_\theta &\left[\frac{\partial}{\partial r}\left(\frac{1}{r}\frac{\partial}{\partial r}(ru_\theta)\right) + \frac{1}{r^2}\frac{\partial^2 u_\theta}{\partial \theta^2} + \frac{\partial^2 u_\theta}{\partial z^2} + \frac{2}{r^2}\frac{\partial u_r}{\partial \theta}\right] \\ + \mathbf{e}_z &\left[\frac{1}{r}\frac{\partial}{\partial r}\left(r\frac{\partial u_z}{\partial r}\right) + \frac{1}{r^2}\frac{\partial^2 u_z}{\partial \theta^2} + \frac{\partial^2 u_z}{\partial z^2}\right].\end{aligned} \tag{1.37}$$

Problem 1.14 Show that, in cylindrical coordinates,

$$\begin{aligned}\mathbf{u}\cdot\nabla\mathbf{u} = \mathbf{e}_r &\left[u_r\frac{\partial u_r}{\partial r} + \frac{u_\theta}{r}\frac{\partial u_r}{\partial \theta} + u_z\frac{\partial u_r}{\partial z} - \frac{u_\theta u_\theta}{r}\right] \\ + \mathbf{e}_\theta &\left[u_r\frac{\partial u_\theta}{\partial r} + \frac{u_\theta}{r}\frac{\partial u_\theta}{\partial \theta} + u_z\frac{\partial u_\theta}{\partial z} + \frac{u_\theta u_r}{r}\right] \\ + \mathbf{e}_z &\left[u_r\frac{\partial u_z}{\partial r} + \frac{u_\theta}{r}\frac{\partial u_z}{\partial \theta} + u_z\frac{\partial u_z}{\partial z}\right].\end{aligned} \tag{1.38}$$

Problem 1.15 The stress tensor in a material satisfies $\nabla\cdot\mathbf{S} = \mathbf{0}$. Show that the volume-average stress in a region V occupied by the material is

$$\langle\mathbf{S}\rangle = \frac{1}{2V}\int_S (\mathbf{xt} + \mathbf{tx})\, dS, \tag{1.39}$$

where $\mathbf{t} = \mathbf{n}\cdot\mathbf{S}$ is the surface traction. The quantity on the left side of (1.39) is called the *stresslet* [5].

Problem 1.16 Calculate the following integrals on the surface of the unit sphere

$$\langle\mathbf{nn}\rangle = \frac{1}{S}\int_S \mathbf{nn}dS \tag{1.40}$$

$$\langle\mathbf{nnnn}\rangle = \frac{1}{S}\int_S \mathbf{nnnn}dS. \tag{1.41}$$

These are the averages of various moments of a uniformly distributed unit vector on a sphere surface.

References

1. N. Phan-Thien, N. Mai-Duy, *Understanding Viscoelasticity: An Introduction to Rheology*, 3rd edn. (Springer International Publishing AG, Berlin, 2017)
2. M.E. Gurtin, *An Introduction to Continuum Mechanics* (Academic Press, New York, 1981)
3. O.D. Kellogg, *Foundations of Potential Theory* (Dover, New York, 1954)
4. R.B. Bird, R.C. Armstrong, O. Hassager, Dynamics of Polymeric Liquids. Vol. 1: Fluid Mechanics, 2nd edn. Wiley, New York (1987)
5. G.K. Batchelor, The stress system in a suspension of force-free particles. J. Fluid Mech. **41**, 545–570 (1970)

Chapter 2
Kinematics and Conservation Laws

A Short Summary of Continuum Mechanics

2.1 Kinematics

2.1.1 Velocity and Acceleration Fields

Considering a continuous body $\mathcal{B}$ in three-dimensional space $\mathbb{E}_3$, we refer to the configuration at time $t = 0$, $\mathcal{B}_R$, as the *reference configuration*. The particle position is denoted by $\mathbf{X}$ in the reference configuration. Its current position is denoted by $\mathbf{x}$ which is a function of time after it traces out a path in $\mathbb{E}_3$. A motion is defined to be a twice-differentiable and invertible map

$$\mathbf{x} = \mathbf{M}(\mathbf{X}, t), \quad \mathbf{X} = \mathbf{M}^{-1}(\mathbf{x}, t), \tag{2.1}$$

where t is the time and $\mathbf{X} = \mathbf{M}(\mathbf{X}, 0)$ by definition. This is also called the *Lagrangian description* of the motion (after Lagrange, Fig. 2.1). Collectively $\mathbf{M}(\mathbf{X}, t)$, $\mathbf{X} \in \mathcal{B}_R$ gives us the spatial description of the motion, called the *current configuration*.

The velocity and the acceleration fields can be respectively defined as

$$\hat{\mathbf{u}} = \frac{\partial}{\partial t}\mathbf{M}(\mathbf{X}, t), \tag{2.2}$$

and

$$\hat{\mathbf{a}} = \frac{\partial^2}{\partial t^2}\mathbf{M}(\mathbf{X}, t). \tag{2.3}$$

It is customary to refer to velocity and acceleration fields as functions of the current position, the so-called *Eulerian description* (after Euler, Fig. 2.2). This is accomplished using (2.1).

Denoting $\mathbf{u} = \mathbf{u}(\mathbf{x}, t)$ as the Eulerian velocity field, we find that the Eulerian acceleration field is given by

© The Author(s), under exclusive license to Springer Nature Singapore Pte Ltd. 2026
D. Pan et al., *Langevin Analysis of Microstructured Fluids*,
SpringerBriefs in Applied Sciences and Technology,
https://doi.org/10.1007/978-981-95-2318-4_2

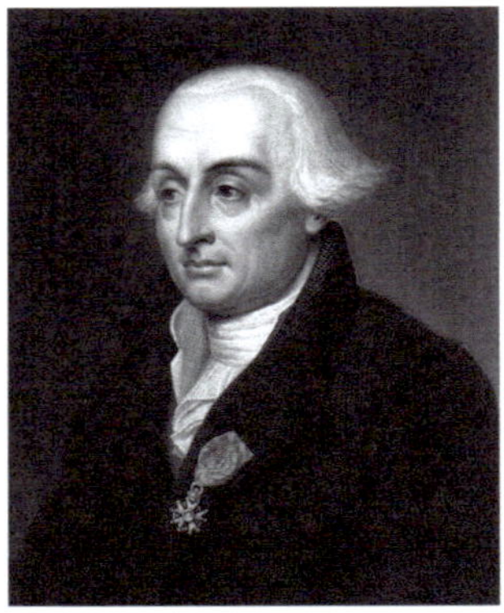

Fig. 2.1 Joseph-Louis Lagrange (1736–1813) was a Italian/French mathematician, who made important contributions to analytic mechanics, calculus of variations, and number theory. His book *Mécanique Analytique* was an approved publication by a committee with members including Laplace and Legendre in 1788. (Portrait of unknown author, public domain work of art.)

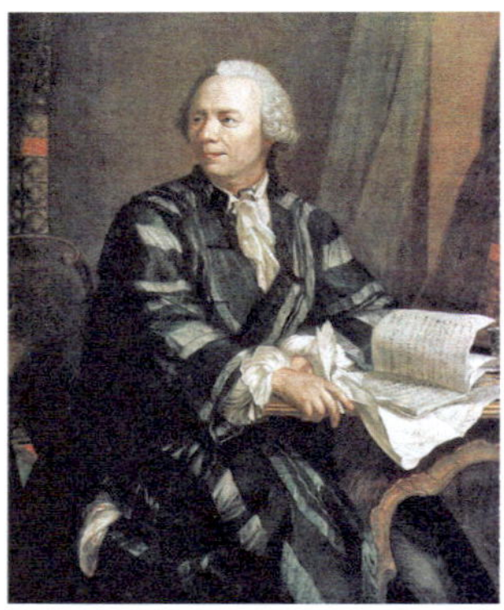

Fig. 2.2 Leonhard Euler (1707–1783) was one of the greatest mathematicians of the eighteenth century. He occupied Daniel Bernoulli's chair of mathematics at St. Petersburg. He perfected the integral calculus, worked in analytic geometry, theory of lunar motion, introduced Euler's identity and many other mathematical symbols that we are familiar with, π, $f()$, $\sum$. He published more than 856 articles and books. (Painting by Jakob Emanuel Handmann (1718–1781), public domain work of art.)

$$
\begin{aligned}
\mathbf{a} = \left.\frac{\partial}{\partial t}\mathbf{u}\left(\mathbf{x}, t\right)\right|_{\mathbf{X}} &= \frac{\partial \mathbf{u}}{\partial t} + \frac{\partial \mathbf{u}}{\partial \mathbf{x}} \cdot \left.\frac{\partial \mathbf{x}}{\partial t}\right|_{\mathbf{X}} \\
&= \frac{\partial \mathbf{u}}{\partial t} + \mathbf{u} \cdot \nabla \mathbf{u} = \frac{\partial \mathbf{u}}{\partial t} + \mathbf{L} \cdot \mathbf{u},
\end{aligned}
\tag{2.4}
$$

where we have introduced the velocity gradient tensor (note the transpose operation in its definition). An Eulerian velocity is called steady if it does not depend on time.

Remark 2.1 (*Material derivative*) The derivative on $\mathbf{u}$ as implied in (2.4) is called the *material derivative*, or *total time derivative*, or *simply time derivative* (if there is no confusion),

$$\frac{d}{dt}(\cdot) = \frac{\partial}{\partial t}(\cdot) + \mathbf{u} \cdot \nabla(\cdot). \tag{2.5}$$

2.2 Deformation Gradient and Strain Tensors

2.2.1 *Deformation Gradient*

The gradient of $\mathbf{x}$ with respect to $\mathbf{X}$ is called the *deformation gradient*,

$$\mathbf{F} = \left(\frac{\partial \mathbf{x}}{\partial \mathbf{X}}\right)^T. \tag{2.6}$$

The initial value of $\mathbf{F}$ (at time $t = 0$) is the identity tensor, $\mathbf{F}(0) = \mathbf{I}$. The mass in a region V is

$$\int_V \rho d\mathbf{x} = \int_{V_0} \rho \,|J|\, d\mathbf{X},$$

where $J = \det \mathbf{F}$ and V_0 is the region occupied by the reference configuration. Thus, we demand that $\det \mathbf{F} > 0$, so that the mapping is not degenerate. For an incompressible fluid, the kinematic constraint is of course $\det \mathbf{F} = 1$.

2.2.2 *Cauchy–Green Strain Tensor*

The concept of strain is introduced by comparing the length of a fluid element at the current time to that in the reference configuration. We have from the definition of the deformation gradient,

$$d\mathbf{x} = \mathbf{F} d\mathbf{X}.$$

Here $d\mathbf{X}$ is a fluid element at point $\mathbf{X}$, which at time t is mapped to $d\mathbf{x}$ at point $\mathbf{x}$. Its current length is

$$dx^2 = d\mathbf{x} \cdot d\mathbf{x} = F_{ij} dX_j F_{ik} dX_k = d\mathbf{X}\mathbf{F}^T \cdot \mathbf{F} d\mathbf{X} = \mathbf{F}^T \mathbf{F} : d\mathbf{X} d\mathbf{X}$$

The tensor

$$\mathbf{C} = \mathbf{F}^T \mathbf{F}, \tag{2.7}$$

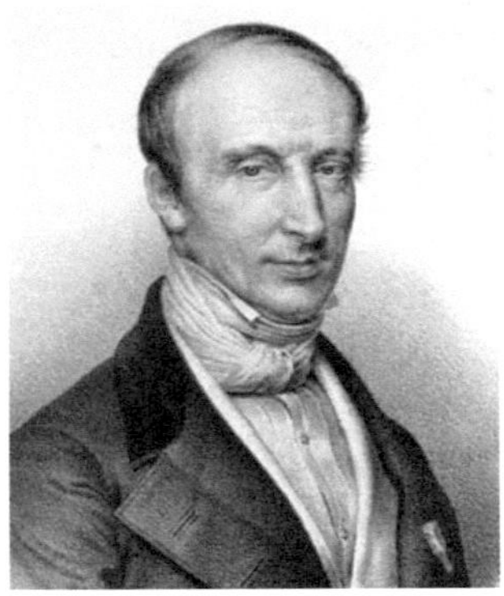

Fig. 2.3 Augustin-Louis Cauchy (1789–1857) was a prolific French mathematician. He contributed more than 16 fundamental concepts and theorems, and published more than 800 papers. His name is one of the 72 inscribed on the Eiffel tower. (Lithograph by Gregoire et Deneux, public domain work of art.)

is therefore a measure of the strain the fluid experiences. It is called the *right Cauchy–Green* tensor (for a portray of Cauchy, see Fig. 2.3). The *left Cauchy–Green* tensor is defined as

$$\mathbf{B} = \mathbf{F}\mathbf{F}^T. \tag{2.8}$$

It is also known as the Finger tensor.

2.2.3 Relative Strain Tensors

The reference configuration enjoys no particular mathematical status, although it may have a physical significance (e.g., the stress-free state). Suppose the particle $\mathbf{X}$ at time τ occupies the position $\boldsymbol{\xi}$, then the relative deformation gradient is defined as

$$\mathbf{F}_t(\tau) = \left(\frac{\partial \boldsymbol{\xi}}{\partial \mathbf{x}}\right)^T. \tag{2.9}$$

Correspondingly, the right and left relative Cauchy–Green tensor are given by

$$\mathbf{C}_t(\tau) = \mathbf{F}_t(\tau)^T \mathbf{F}_t(\tau), \quad \mathbf{B}_t(\tau) = \mathbf{F}_t(\tau)\mathbf{F}_t(\tau)^T, \tag{2.10}$$

respectively. Because of the chain rule, the relative deformation gradient satisfies

$$\mathbf{F}_t(\tau) = \left(\frac{\partial \boldsymbol{\xi}}{\partial \mathbf{x}}\right)^T = \left(\frac{\partial \mathbf{X}}{\partial \mathbf{x}} \cdot \frac{\partial \boldsymbol{\xi}}{\partial \mathbf{X}}\right)^T = \left(\frac{\partial \boldsymbol{\xi}}{\partial \mathbf{X}}\right)^T \cdot \left(\frac{\partial \mathbf{X}}{\partial \mathbf{x}}\right)^T$$
$$= \mathbf{F}(\tau)\,\mathbf{F}(t)^{-1}. \tag{2.11}$$

2.3 Rivlin–Ericksen Tensors

Suppose the relative Cauchy–Green tensor has been determined. The n-th *Rivlin–Ericksen tensor* (Fig. 2.4) is defined as

$$\mathbf{A}_n(t) = \frac{d^n}{d\tau^n}\mathbf{C}_t(\tau)\bigg|_{\tau=t}, \quad n = 1, 2, \ldots \tag{2.12}$$

Since $\mathbf{C}_t(\tau)|_{\tau=t} = \mathbf{I}$ (because $\mathbf{F}_t(t) = \mathbf{I}$), we may define

$$\mathbf{A}_0 = \mathbf{I}, \tag{2.13}$$

and extend the definition (2.12) to $n = 0, 1, \ldots$ In effect, the Rivlin–Ericksen tensors are defined as the coefficients of the following Taylor series about t:

$$\mathbf{C}_t(\tau) = \sum_{n=0} \frac{(\tau - t)^n}{n!}\mathbf{A}_n(t). \tag{2.14}$$

Rivlin–Ericksen tensors can be determined directly from the velocity field without having to find the strain tensor. For example, the first Rivlin–Ericksen tensor is twice the strain rate tensor:

$$\mathbf{A}_1(t) = \frac{d}{d\tau}\mathbf{C}_t(\tau)\bigg|_{\tau=t} = \mathbf{L}(t) + \mathbf{L}(t)^T = 2\mathbf{D}(t). \tag{2.15}$$

Detailed derivation is given in Phan-Thien and Mai-Duy [1].

Alternatively, if we consider the length square of a fluid element in the current time, we have

$$dx(t)^2 = d\mathbf{x} \cdot d\mathbf{x} = \mathbf{F}^T\mathbf{F} : d\mathbf{X}d\mathbf{X} = \mathbf{C}(t) : d\mathbf{X}d\mathbf{X}, \tag{2.16}$$

and similarly,

$$d\xi(\tau)^2 = \mathbf{C}(\tau) : d\mathbf{X}d\mathbf{X}. \tag{2.17}$$

Then, if we combine (2.10) and (2.11), and use the definition of right Cauchy–Green tensor (2.7), we have

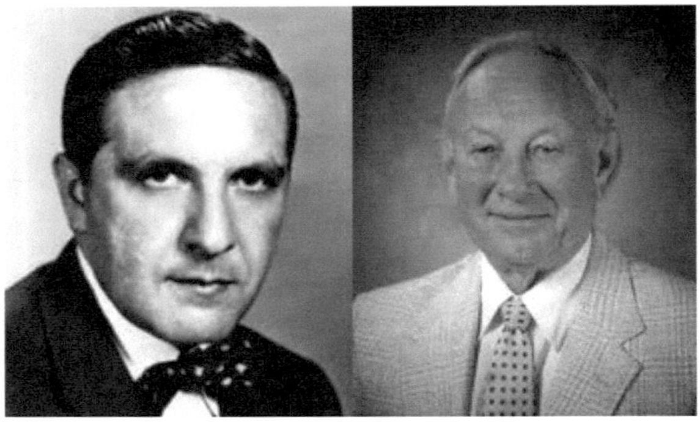

Fig. 2.4 Rivlin–Ericksen tensors were named after Ronald Samuel Rivlin (1915–2005), a British-American physicist, mathematician, rheologist, with significant contributions to Rheology and rubber elasticity (left photo. Copyright holder: The Franklin Institute, courtesy of AIP Emilio Segrè Visual Archives), and Jerald LaVerne Ericksen (1924–2021), an American mathematician with major contributions in Continuum Mechanics, especially *anisotropic liquids* (right photo, provided in Sluckin and Calderer [6])

$$\frac{d^n}{d\tau^n}\mathbf{C}_t(\tau) = \mathbf{F}(t)^{-T}\frac{d^n}{d\tau^n}\mathbf{C}(\tau)\,\mathbf{F}(t)^{-1}.$$

Thus

$$\mathbf{F}(t)^T\left[\frac{d^n}{d\tau^n}\mathbf{C}_t(\tau)\right]\mathbf{F}(t) = \frac{d^n}{d\tau^n}\mathbf{C}(\tau).$$

Taking the scalar product of this with $d\mathbf{X}d\mathbf{X}$ and $\tau = t$, and recall (2.17) and the definition of Rivlin–Ericksen tensors (2.12), we obtain

$$\mathbf{A}_n : d\mathbf{x}d\mathbf{x} = \left.\frac{d^n}{d\tau^n}d\xi(\tau)^2\right|_{\tau=t},$$

which relates the Rivlin–Ericksen tensors to the high-order stretching rate of a fluid element. Further, a recursive relation can be derived (referring to [1]), leading to the recursive formula due to Rivlin and Ericksen [7]

$$\mathbf{A}_{n+1} = \frac{d}{dt}\mathbf{A}_n + \mathbf{A}_n\mathbf{L} + \mathbf{L}^T\mathbf{A}_n, \quad \mathbf{A}_0 = \mathbf{I}, \quad n = 1, 2, \ldots \tag{2.18}$$

2.4 Conservation Laws

In this section, we are briefing the equations of balance which are mathematical statements of the conservation of mass, linear and angular momentum, and energy. We first introduce the Reynolds transport theorem (for a portray of Reynolds, see Fig. 2.5) which is useful in formulating the equations of balance.

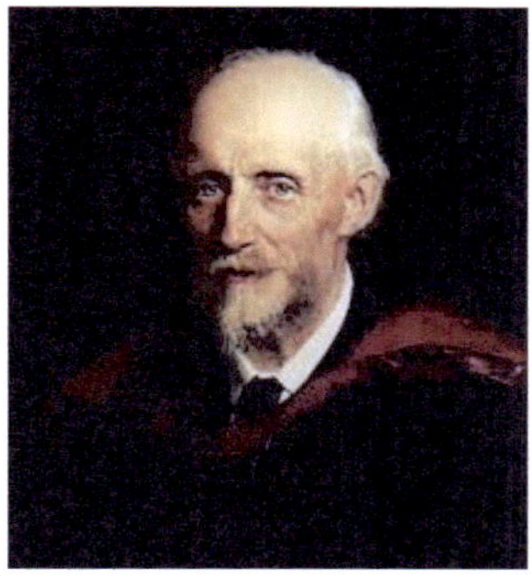

Fig. 2.5 Osborne Reynolds (1842–1912) introduced the lubrication theory and formulated the concept of turbulence flow. He was the first in the UK university system to hold the title *Professor of Engineering* at Owens College (now University of Manchester). The Reynolds number and stresses are named after him. (Painting by John Collier (1850–1934), public domain work of art.)

2.4.1 Reynolds Transport Theorem

Let $\Phi(\mathbf{x}, t)$ be a field (scalar, vector or tensor) defined over a region V occupied by the body $\mathcal{B}$ at time t. Reynolds transport theorem states that

$$\frac{d}{dt}\int_V \Phi dV = \int_V \left(\frac{d\Phi}{dt} + \Phi\nabla\cdot\mathbf{u}\right) dV = \int_V \left(\frac{\partial\Phi}{\partial t} + \nabla\cdot(\Phi\mathbf{u})\right) dV \qquad (2.19)$$

where $\mathbf{u}$ is the velocity field, and d/dt is the material derivative (2.5). This is Theorem 1 of Reynolds transport theorem and it is proved by expressing the volume integral in the reference configuration Phan-Thien and Mai-Duy [1].

The following form allows a physical interpretation of the theorem: the first term on the right represents the rate of creation of the quantity Φ, and the second term, the flux of Φ into the volume V through its bounding surface.

$$\frac{d}{dt}\int_V \Phi d\mathbf{x} = \int_V \frac{\partial\Phi}{\partial t} dV + \int_S (\Phi\mathbf{u})\cdot\mathbf{n} dS. \qquad (2.20)$$

We can also prove another theorem, given below

$$\frac{d}{dt}\int_V \rho\Phi dV = \int_V \rho\frac{d\Phi}{dt} dV, \qquad (2.21)$$

where $\rho(\mathbf{x}, t)$ is the density field at time t and this theorem can be proved by incorporating with balance equations which will be introduced in next subsection.

2.4.2 Conservation of Mass

Conservation of mass is expressed as the mass in the volume V is constant at all times, and also from Reynolds transport theorem (2.19), we have

$$\frac{d}{dt}\int_V \rho dV = \int_V \left(\frac{\partial \rho}{\partial t} + \nabla \cdot (\rho \mathbf{u})\right) dV = 0.$$

Since the volume V is arbitrary, a necessary and sufficient condition for the conservation of mass is

$$\frac{\partial \rho}{\partial t} + \nabla \cdot (\rho \mathbf{u}) = \frac{d\rho}{dt} + \rho \nabla \cdot \mathbf{u} = 0. \tag{2.22}$$

Remark 2.2 (*Incompressible fluid*) For an *incompressible* material, the density of fluid particles does not change, and the conservation of mass demands that

$$\nabla \cdot \mathbf{u} = \frac{\partial u_i}{\partial x_i} = \mathrm{tr}\mathbf{L} = \mathrm{tr}\mathbf{D} = \frac{1}{2}\mathrm{tr}\mathbf{A}_1 = 0. \tag{2.23}$$

Liquids are almost incompressible. Gases are compressible, while for low flow speeds (for Mach numbers < 0.3) the density changes in the flow are small and (2.23) is an excellent approximation.

2.4.3 Conservation of Momentum

Conservation of momentum is basically derived from Newton's second law, therefore, the forces acting on the body are considered, which include surface forces $\mathbf{t}$ (tractions), and body forces $\mathbf{b}$ (those that act at a distance).

2.4.3.1 Conservation of Linear Momentum

Newton's second law (a postulate), as applied to a volume V occupied by the body, requires that

$$\frac{d}{dt}\int_V \rho \mathbf{u} dV = \int_S \mathbf{t} dS + \int_V \rho \mathbf{b} dV. \tag{2.24}$$

Here S is the bounding surface of V. The first term on the right hand of (2.24) represents the surface force acting on V due to the body outside V, and the second term is the net body force on V. This is also called the balance equations of linear momentum.

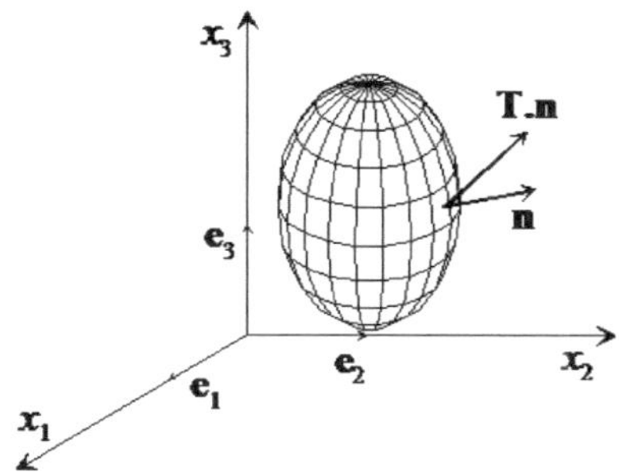

Fig. 2.6 Defining the stress tensor

Before we deal with the first term on the right hand of (2.24), we first define the so-called *Cauchy stress tensor* (**T** in Fig. 2.6) which has following properties

$$\mathbf{t}\,(\mathbf{x}, t; \mathbf{n}) = \mathbf{T}\,(\mathbf{x}, t) \cdot \mathbf{n}. \tag{2.25}$$

Regarding the balance of linear momentum (2.24) and using the definition of the stress tensor (2.25) and also corollary (2.21), we have

$$\int_V \rho \frac{d\mathbf{u}}{dt} dV = \int_S \mathbf{T} \cdot \mathbf{n} dS + \int_V \rho \mathbf{b} dV. \tag{2.26}$$

The surface integral on the right hand of the preceding equation can be converted into a volume integral to obtain

$$\int_V \rho \frac{d\mathbf{u}}{dt} dV = \int_V \nabla \mathbf{T}^T dV + \int_V \rho \mathbf{b} dV.$$

Since the integrand is continuous on an arbitrary V, the conservation of linear momentum becomes

$$\rho \frac{d\mathbf{u}}{dt} = \nabla \mathbf{T}^T + \rho \mathbf{b}. \tag{2.27}$$

When the fluid is Newtonian, the resulting Eq. (2.27) is Navier–Stokes equation, named after Claude-Louis Navier (1785–1836) and Georges Gabriel Stokes (1819–1903), Fig. 2.7.

2.4.3.2 Conservation of Angular Momentum

The balance of angular momentum (a postulate) without considering body couple can likewise be written as

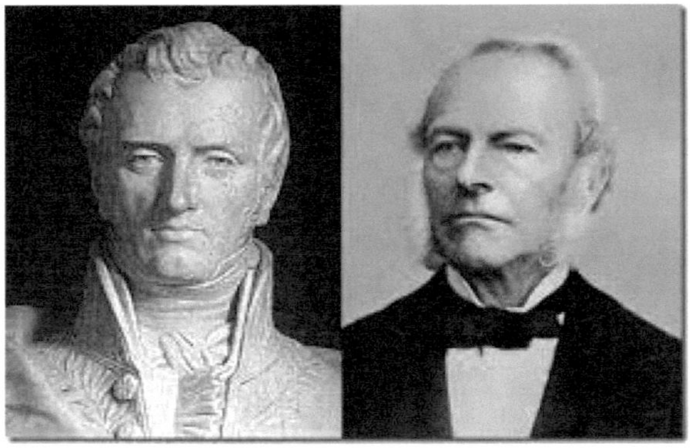

Fig. 2.7 The Navier–Stokes equations were named after Claude-Louis Navier (1785–1836), a French engineer and physicist (left photo, lacking author information, public domain work of art), and George Gabriel Stokes (1819–1903), an Irish mathematician and physicist (right public domian photograph by Fradelle & Young). The development of the equations took several years, from 1822 (Navier) to 1850 (Stokes)

$$\frac{d}{dt}\int_V \mathbf{x}\times\rho\mathbf{u}dV = \int_V \mathbf{x}\times\rho\frac{d\mathbf{u}}{dt}dV = \int_S \mathbf{x}\times\mathbf{t}dS + \int_V \mathbf{x}\times\rho\mathbf{b}dV. \tag{2.28}$$

Again, corollary (2.21) is used on the first equation of (2.28). Note that the term involving $d\mathbf{x}/dt = \mathbf{u}$ does not contribute to the left hand side of this because of the definition of the cross product.

Examining the first term on the right of the second equation of (2.28) and also employing Cauchy stress tensor,

$$\begin{aligned}\int_S \varepsilon_{ijk}x_j t_k dS = \int_S \varepsilon_{ijk}x_j T_{kl}n_l dS &= \int_V \frac{\partial}{\partial x_l}\left(\varepsilon_{ijk}x_j T_{kl}\right)dV \\ &= \int_V \left(\varepsilon_{ijk}\delta_{jl}T_{kl} + \varepsilon_{ijk}x_j\frac{\partial T_{kl}}{\partial x_l}\right)dV \\ &= \int_V \left(t_i^A + \varepsilon_{ijk}x_j\frac{\partial T_{kl}}{\partial x_l}\right)dV,\end{aligned}$$

where the "axial vector" is defined as $t_i^A = \varepsilon_{ijk}T_{kj}$. When these results are substituted back into (2.28),

$$\int_V \mathbf{x}\times\rho\frac{d\mathbf{u}}{dt}dV = \int_V \left(\mathbf{t}^A + \mathbf{x}\times\nabla\cdot\mathbf{T}^T\right)dV + \int_V \mathbf{x}\times\rho\mathbf{b}dV,$$

and therefore,

$$\int_V \mathbf{t}^A dV = \int_V \mathbf{x}\times\left[\rho\frac{d\mathbf{u}}{dt} - \nabla\cdot\mathbf{T}^T - \rho\mathbf{b}\right]dV.$$

From the conservation of linear momentum, and the continuity of the integrands in the arbitrary volume V, it follows that

$$\mathbf{t}^A = \mathbf{0} \quad \therefore \quad \varepsilon_{ijk} T_{kj} = 0 \quad \therefore \quad \mathbf{T} = \mathbf{T}^T \text{ or } \mathbf{T} \text{ is symmetric.} \tag{2.29}$$

A necessary and sufficient condition for the balance of angular momentum, in the absence of body couples, is that the stress be symmetric. In deriving (2.29), both the conservation of mass and linear momentum are needed.

2.4.4 Conservation of Energy

For the conservation of energy, we first define the kinetic energy K, and internal energy E as

$$K = \int_V \frac{1}{2} \rho u^2 dV, \quad E = \int_V \rho \varepsilon dV, \tag{2.30}$$

where ε is the specific internal energy per unit mass. If we define $\mathbf{q}$ to be the flux of energy out of S per unit area, and r the amount of energy created per unit mass, and meanwhile consider the rate of work done on the body by surface and body forces, then the mathematical statement for the first law of thermodynamics can be expressed as

$$\begin{aligned} \frac{d}{dt} \int_V \left(\frac{1}{2} \rho u^2 + \rho \varepsilon \right) dV = & \int_S (\mathbf{t} \cdot \mathbf{u} - \mathbf{q} \cdot \mathbf{n})\, dS \\ & + \int_V (\rho r + \rho \mathbf{b} \cdot \mathbf{u})\, dV. \end{aligned} \tag{2.31}$$

Using Reynolds transport theorem (2.21) for the left of (2.31), and convert the surface integral on the right of (2.31) into volume integral, (2.31) becomes

$$\begin{aligned} \int_V \rho (\mathbf{u} \cdot \mathbf{a} + \dot{\varepsilon})\, dV = & \int_V \left(\mathbf{u} \cdot \nabla \mathbf{T}^T + \mathbf{T} : \mathbf{L} - \nabla \cdot \mathbf{q} \right) dV \\ & + \int_V (\rho r + \rho \mathbf{b} \cdot \mathbf{u})\, dV. \end{aligned}$$

Here, the term $\mathbf{a}$ is

$$\mathbf{a} = \frac{d\mathbf{u}}{dt} = \frac{\partial \mathbf{u}}{\partial t} + \mathbf{u} \cdot \nabla \mathbf{u}$$

is recognized as the acceleration field. Because of the conservation of linear momentum, and the continuity of the integrands in the arbitrary volume V, the conservation of energy is reduced to

$$\rho \dot{\varepsilon} = \mathbf{T} : \mathbf{D} - \nabla \cdot \mathbf{q} + \rho r. \tag{2.32}$$

In deriving this, all the three balance equations for mass, linear momentum, and angular momentum are required. The term $\mathbf{T} : \mathbf{D}$ represents the rate of work done by the stress, or the "stress power". It is seen that

$$\mathbf{T} : \mathbf{D} = -P\text{tr}\mathbf{D} + \mathbf{S} : \mathbf{D}.$$

The rate of work done by the pressure for an incompressible fluid is zero, because $\text{tr}\mathbf{D} = 0$.

Problems

Problem 2.1 Using $\mathbf{F}\mathbf{F}^{-1} = \mathbf{I}$ for a deformation gradient $\mathbf{F}$, show that

$$\frac{d}{dt}\mathbf{F}^{-1} = -\mathbf{F}^{-1}\mathbf{L}, \quad \mathbf{F}^{-1}(0) = \mathbf{I}.$$

Problem 2.2 For a simple shear flow, where the velocity field takes the form

$$u = \dot{\gamma} y, \quad v = 0, \quad w = 0, \tag{2.33}$$

show that the velocity gradient and its exponent are given by

$$[\mathbf{L}] = \begin{bmatrix} 0 & \dot{\gamma} & 0 \\ 0 & 0 & 0 \\ 0 & 0 & 0 \end{bmatrix}, \quad \exp(\mathbf{L}) = \mathbf{I} + \mathbf{L}. \tag{2.34}$$

Show that the path lines are given by

$$\boldsymbol{\xi}(\tau) = \mathbf{x} + (\tau - t)\,\mathbf{L}\mathbf{x} \tag{2.35}$$

so that a fluid element dX can only be stretched linearly in time at most.

Problem 2.3 Repeat the same exercise for an elongational flow, where

$$u = ax, \quad v = by, \quad w = cz, \quad a + b + c = 0. \tag{2.36}$$

In this case, show that

$$[\mathbf{L}] = \begin{bmatrix} a & 0 & 0 \\ 0 & b & 0 \\ 0 & 0 & c \end{bmatrix}, \quad \left[e^{\mathbf{L}}\right] = \begin{bmatrix} e^a & 0 & 0 \\ 0 & e^b & 0 \\ 0 & 0 & e^c \end{bmatrix}. \tag{2.37}$$

Show that the path lines are given by

$$[\boldsymbol{\xi}(\tau)] = \begin{bmatrix} \xi \\ \psi \\ \zeta \end{bmatrix} = \begin{bmatrix} e^{a(\tau-t)} & 0 & 0 \\ 0 & e^{b(\tau-t)} & 0 \\ 0 & 0 & e^{c(\tau-t)} \end{bmatrix} \begin{bmatrix} x \\ y \\ z \end{bmatrix}. \tag{2.38}$$

Conclude that exponential flow can stretch the fluid element exponentially fast.

Problem 2.4 Consider a super-imposed oscillatory shear flow:

$$u = \dot{\gamma}_m y, \quad v = 0, \quad w = \omega \gamma_a y \cos \omega t.$$

Show that the path lines are

$$\begin{aligned} \xi(\tau) &= x + \dot{\gamma}_m (\tau - t) y, \\ \psi(\tau) &= y, \\ \zeta(\tau) &= z + \gamma_0 y (\sin \omega \tau - \sin \omega t). \end{aligned} \tag{2.39}$$

Problem 2.5 Calculate the Rivlin–Ericksen tensors for the elongational flow (2.36).

Problem 2.6 Calculate the Rivlin–Ericksen tensors for the unsteady flow (2.39).

Problem 2.7 Write down, in component forms the conservation of mass and linear momentum equations, assuming the fluid is incompressible, in Cartesian, cylindrical, and spherical coordinate systems.

References

1. N. Phan-Thien, N. Mai-Duy, *Understanding Viscoelasticity: An Introduction to Rheology*, 3rd edn. (Springer International Publishing AG, Berlin, 2017)
2. R.B. Bird, R.C. Armstrong, O. Hassager, *Dynamics of Polymeric Liquids. Vol. 1: Fluid Mechanics*, 2nd edn. (Wiley, New York, 1987)
3. R.I. Tanner, *Engineering Rheology*, revised edition edn. (Oxford University Press, Oxford, 1992)
4. R. Huilgol, N. Phan-Thien, *Fluid Mechanics of Viscoelasticity: General Principles, Constitutive Modelling, Analytical and Numerical Techniques* (Elsevier, Amsterdam, 1997)
5. F.A. Morrison, *Understanding Rheology: Topic in Chemical Engineering* (Oxford Unversity Press, Oxford, 2001)
6. T. Sluckin, M.C. Calderer, Jerry Ericksen (1924–2021). Liq. Cryst. **50**(2), 191–194 (2023). https://doi.org/10.1080/02678292.2023.2211814
7. R.S. Rivlin, J.L. Ericksen, Stress deformation relations for isotropic materials. J. Rat. Mecahnics Anal. **4**, 323–425 (1955)

Chapter 3
Langevin Dynamics

A Basic Understanding of Langevin Dynamics

Brownian forces were named after the botanist Robert Brown (Fig. 3.1), for his observations on the erratic motion of pollen in water, detailed in his seminal 1828 paper [1], followed by some further clarifications in his second 1829 paper [2], in response to remarks on his previous 1828 paper. A summary of Brown's contributions was detailed in Cohen [3, 4]. Brown's observations laid the foundation for the prediction of the existence of molecules by Einstein [5] (Fig. 1.2), which was confirmed by Perrin [6] (Fig. 3.2). The stage was ripe for Paul Langevin (1872–1946) (Fig. 3.3), who, three years after Einstein's molecule paper [5] and 80 years after Brown's observations [1], published his first paper [7] on a class of continuously random motions now known as the *Langevin dynamics*. The book by Graham [8] provided a great deal more information on Brownian motion, microhydrodynamics and complex fluids, and should be consulted in parallel to this Lecture Note. Some historical notes on the development of Langevin equations leading to Fokker–Planck, Smoluchowski diffusion equation are available in the book by Tanner and Walters [9].

Langevin is our main theme here, and a few words about his life may be appropriate. Langevin was a contemporary of Einstein; he was a post-doctoral student of Pierre Curie (1859–1906). Pierre shared the 1903 Nobel Prize in Physics with his wife, Marie Curie née Maria Sklodowska (1867–1934), and another physicist Antoine Henry Becquerel (1852–1908), for their pioneer work on radioactivity, a term of Maria coined. Maria was the first woman to win a Nobel Prize, and indeed she was the only person to win two Nobel Prizes in two disciplines (Physics and Chemistry). After Pierre Curie died in a car accident, Langevin started to develop a romantic relationship with Marie Curie. The relationship became public and they both became targets for the French newspapers, so much that Langevin fought a duel with a newspaper editor to defend Marie Curie's honor (the duel did not amount to anything of note, except to provide more fuel for the press). As fate would have it, Marie Curie's granddaughter, Helene Joliot-Curie, married Langevin's grandson, Michel Langevin [10].

© The Author(s), under exclusive license to Springer Nature Singapore Pte Ltd. 2026

D. Pan et al., *Langevin Analysis of Microstructured Fluids*,
SpringerBriefs in Applied Sciences and Technology,
https://doi.org/10.1007/978-981-95-2318-4_3

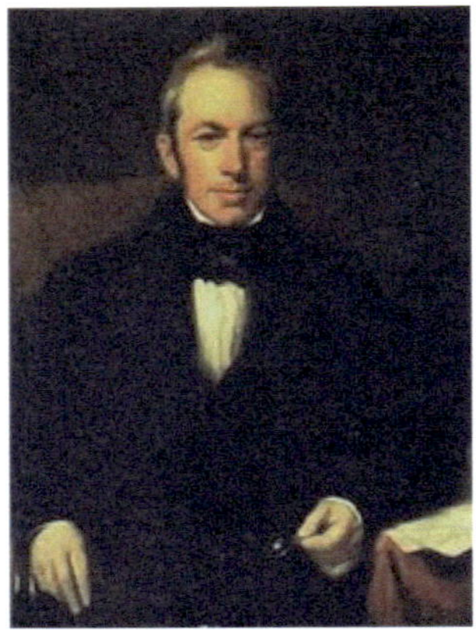

Fig. 3.1 Robert Brown (1773–1858) was a well-known English botanist. He traveled to Australia on the *Investigator* as an appointed *Naturalist*, collecting some 3400 specimens. His observations on the erratic motion of pollen in water under the microscope paved the way for the prediction and confirmation of *Brownian motion*, indirectly validated the molecular hypothesis. (Public domain painting from Henry William Pickersgill (1782–1875))

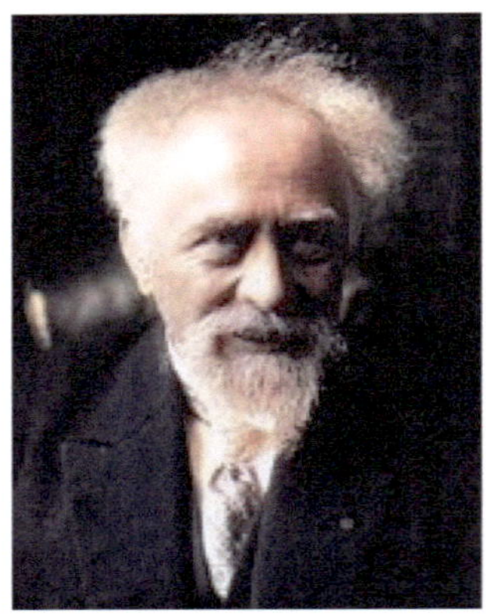

Fig. 3.2 Jean Perrin (1870–1942) confirmed the existence of molecules, and calculated the number of molecules per molar mass; he gave the name *Avogadro number* (an Italian physicist and chemist) to this. The work gained him the 1926 Nobel prize in Physics. (Public domain photograph in 1926)

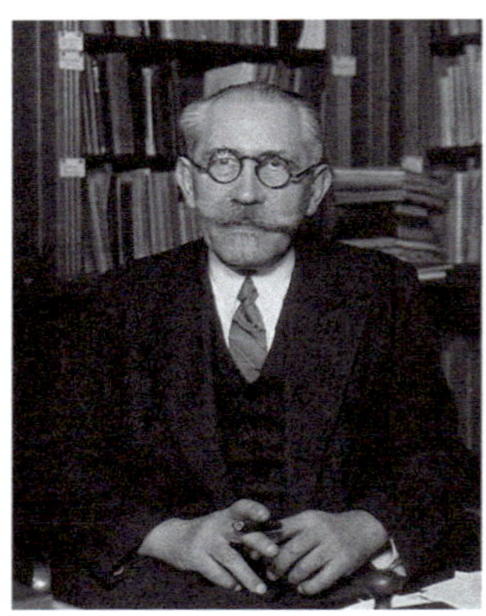

Fig. 3.3 Paul Langevin (1872–1946) was a doctoral student of Pierre Curie. He devised a mechanics description of Brownian motion which, in his words, "infinitely more simple" than Einstein's method. (Photograph by Henri Manuel (1874–1947), source: Wellcome Collection)

3.1 General Remarks on Microstructured Fluids

We talk about a *suspension* when there are two widely separated length scales, the length scale of a typical particle in the suspension, a, and the length scale of the flow apparatus $L, a \ll L$. We have a suspension when there are many particles in a volume L^3; otherwise we simply have a flow of a few discrete particles. Figure 3.4 illustrates a shear flow of a suspension. Examples of suspensions are, not exclusively, polymer chains in a viscous solvent (usually called a polymer solution), suspensions of magnetic particles, suspensions of active particles capable of self-propulsion (e.g., flagella), suspensions of fibers, rod-like or disc-like particles.

We collectively call these suspensions *microstructured fluids*; their microstructure comes about because of the interactions between their constituent components (suspended particles); these interactions may be intrinsically caused by their motions, or by flow-induced. In addition, the complications from the suspending liquid (solvent) cannot be overstated. When the solvent is viscoelastic, as often the case, some of the viscoelastic properties of the solvent, if not all, may be inherited, or amplified by the suspension. Choosing a relevant constitutive relation for the solvent can be a formidable task by itself (see, for example, Huilgol and Phan-Thien [11], Bird et al. [12], Tanner [13] for some popular constitutive equations). Almost any relevant constitutive equation for the solvent (except Newtonian) is non-linear, possibly with a time-dependent response (fading memory), and solving a boundary-value problem with this, given a suspended particle, is truly a formidable task, even numerically. When the solvent is Newtonian, we speak of *Newtonian suspension*, and when it is viscoelastic, *viscoelastic suspension*. Furthermore, the flow may be in different regimes: low Reynolds number, laminar or turbulent flow. Only in the low Reynolds number Newtonian flow, or Stokes flow, or slow flow regime, and additionally only for simple shape particles (rigid, viscous, or gaseous), that there are significant advances: excellent summaries of available solutions for flows past simple particles exist, see, Happel and Brenner [14], Kim and Karrila [15].

Our learning objective: to model technologically interesting suspensions

To make progress, explore and understand the physics behind these suspensions, we must make some assumptions, as stated below.

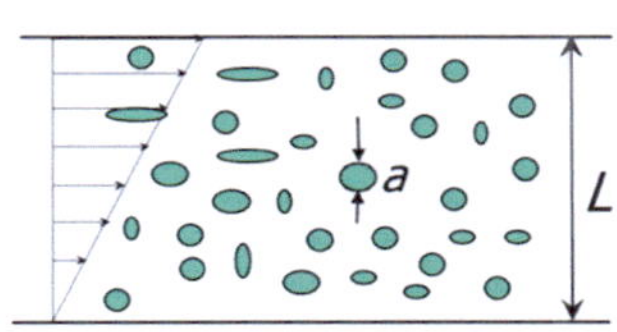

Fig. 3.4 The existence of two widely separate length scales, $a \ll L$, and the sheer number of suspended particles turn a flow over some discrete particles into a suspension

---

Remark 3.1 (*Newtonian solvent*)
We assume that the solvent is a Newtonian incompressible fluid in slow viscous flow on the microscale; that is, only Newtonian suspension is considered in the zero Reynolds number (based on particle size a) limit.

Remark 3.2 (*Simple suspended particles*)
We assume that the suspended particles are simple, i.e., they are either rigid, viscous, or gaseous. They are monodispersed (of the same size) and at low concentration. Attempts will be made to consider polydispersivity and high concentrations, whenever possible (of course, with additional assumptions to be mentioned appropriately).

3.2 How Small Is Small?

We first consider a particle of size a, moving with velocity U in a Newtonian viscous liquid of density ρ_s, viscosity η_s. Typical sizes of small physical particles are illustrated in Fig. 3.5. If the Reynolds number (for a portray of Reynolds, see Fig. 2.5), based on the particle size and its velocity, defined by

$$Re = \frac{\rho U a}{\eta_s}, \tag{3.1}$$

is small, then we have a Stokes flow (Batchelor [16], Happel and Brenner [14], Kim and Karrila [15]), whose governing equations at the microscale are

$$\nabla \cdot \mathbf{u} = 0, \quad -\nabla P + \eta_s \nabla^2 \mathbf{u} = 0, \tag{3.2}$$

where $\mathbf{u}$ is the fluid velocity and P is the pressure. These Stokes equations are linear and instantaneous in the driving forces and/or driving boundaries, and that have major

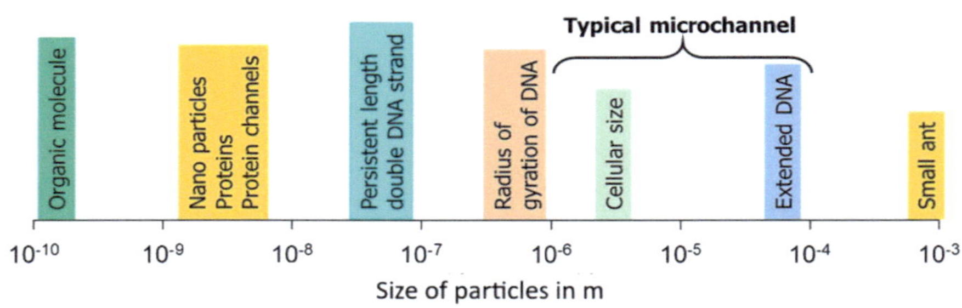

Fig. 3.5 Typical sizes of small physical particles—how small a particle is to be considered small?

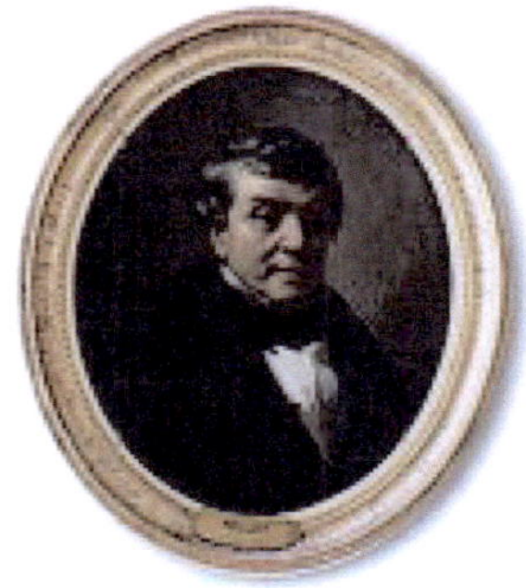

Fig. 3.6 Jean Claude Eugène Péclet (1793–1857) was a French physicist. The Péclet number was named after him. (Public domain painting of unknown author, source: Ecole Centrale de Paris)

important implications on the behavior of the suspension. These will be discussed in a later chapter, §5. Note that although Re in the microscale is small, the Reynolds number at the macroscale (based on L) can be large, as

$$Re_{\text{macro}} = \frac{L}{a} Re_{\text{micro}}. \tag{3.3}$$

In addition, if a suspended particle is small enough, it will experience tiny impulses imparted by collisions with solvent molecules that will lead to its *diffusion*, that is, it will experience *Brownian forces*. This particle is called a *Brownian particle*.

Remark 3.3 (*Diffusion*)
Diffusion is a net motion of particles due to their random motion (Brownian forces).

The parameter that determines whether diffusion effects, or Brownian forces, are significant and must be included in the equation of motion for the particles is the Péclet number (Fig. 3.6), Pe,

$$Pe = \frac{\eta_s U a^2}{kT}, \tag{3.4}$$

where a typical shear rate in the system is $\dot{\gamma} = U/a$, and kT is the Boltzmann temperature. In a large Pe flow, convection will dominate, diffusion effects, or Brownian forces, need not be considered, and conversely. For instances, a particle of the size of an ant in water at 300°K, moving at a speed of one body length per second will have $Re = 0.1$ and $Pe = 2 \times 10^9$: Stokes equation without Brownian forces will be a good model for this. However, the same flow for a 10 μm particle will have $Re = 10^{-5}$ and $Pe = 2 \times 10^3$; Stokes flow remains a good model for its motion; diffusion effects/Brownian forces may be considered, depending on the problem. For a micro-sized particle, Stokes flow is an excellent model ($Re = 10^{-7}$), but diffusion/Brownian forces must also be considered ($Pe = 2$).

3.3 Langevin Equation

3.3.1 Brownian Force

In formulating all the relevant principles governing the motion of a Langevin system, we consider a generic system of *Brownian particles*. These Brownian particles experience tiny impulses, represented by a non-differentiable force, called *complementary force* by Langevin [7],[1] now known as Brownian force, denoted by $\mathbf{F}^{(b)}(t)$. Langevin considered the motion of a Brownian particle in its Newton's second law of motion under a viscous force and the Brownian force, the latter was treated as a "normal" force. The Newtonian equation of motion for the particle under $\mathbf{F}^{(b)}$, is now known as the *Langevin equation* for the particle.[2] In his words, his treatment of a Brownian particle is "infinitely more simpler" than Einstein.

It was known to Langevin that the Brownian force has zero mean and is stationary and isotropic in its statistics, that is, its statistics are independent of its origin, its mean autocorrelation between two time instants of time goes to zero as the time lapse between the two time instants becomes large. We model this behavior mathematically by writing

$$\left\langle \mathbf{F}^{(b)}(t) \right\rangle = 0, \tag{3.5}$$

$$\left\langle \mathbf{F}^{(b)}\left(t'\right)\mathbf{F}^{(b)}\left(t''\right) \right\rangle = 2\delta\left(t' - t''\right)\mathbf{f}, \tag{3.6}$$

where $\delta(s)$ is the Dirac delta function, and $< \cdot >$ denotes the *ensemble average*, or simply the *average*, of the quantity $(\cdot)$. Some useful information on ensemble average and Dirac delta function, and its derivative, can be found in the remarks below.

Remark 3.4 (*Ensemble average*)
If $\mathbf{Q}(\mathbf{X})$ is a quantity depending on a stochastic process $\mathbf{X}(t)$, then the average of $\mathbf{Q}$ given by (time dependence on t is suppressed for brevity here)

$$\langle \mathbf{Q} \rangle = \int_{\Omega} \mathbf{Q}(\mathbf{X})\phi(\mathbf{X})d\mathbf{X}, \tag{3.7}$$

where $\phi(\mathbf{X})$ is the probability density function, or simply the probability distribution of $\mathbf{X} \in \Omega$, Ω is the space of all possible values for $\mathbf{X}$, $d\mathbf{X}$ is the (volume) differential element, such that $\phi(\mathbf{X})d\mathbf{X}$ is the probability of where $\phi(\mathbf{X})$ is the probability density function, or simply the probability distribution of $\mathbf{X}$, and $d\mathbf{X}$ is the (volume) differ-

[1] A translation of Langevin's original paper from French to English can be found in Lemons and Gythiel [17].

[2] Langevin's insight into the modeling of Brownian force heralds in new branches of mathematics and physics (stochastic process and differential equation, Wiener/Ornstein–Uhlenbeck process, Markov process, mathematical white noise, to name a few).

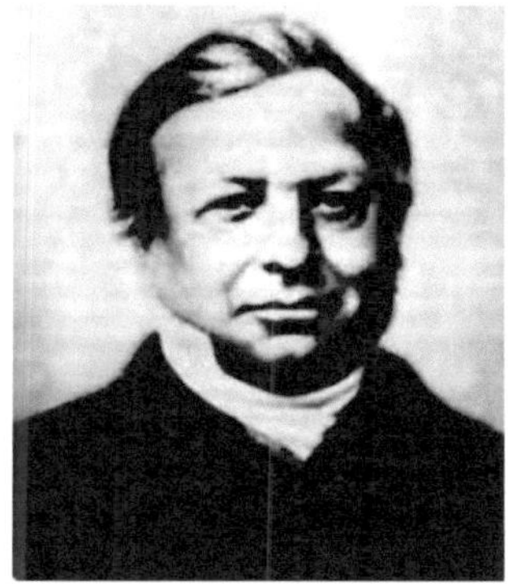

Fig. 3.7 Joseph Liouville (1809–1882) was a French mathematician. His main contributions include Liouville numbers, Sturm–Liouville method of solving differential equations, Liouville theorem Eq. (3.9) in Hamiltonian mechanics. (Public domain photograph by unknown author)

ential element, such that $\phi(\mathbf{X})d\mathbf{X}$ is the probability of $\mathbf{X}$ taking on a value within the differential volume $d\mathbf{X}$.

Remark 3.5 For our purposes, a stochastic process is a family of random variables $X(t)$ indexed by time t, with $X(t)$ the observed value for the random variable X at time t. The totality of $\{X(t), \ t \in \mathbb{R}\}$ is said to be a random function or a stochastic process.

Remark 3.6 (*Conservation of probability: Liouville equation*)
The probability density distribution must satisfy the normalization condition (all the probability must sum up to 1)

$$\int_{\Omega} \phi(\mathbf{X}, t)\, d\mathbf{X} = 1, \tag{3.8}$$

an application of the Reynolds theorem to this yields

$$\frac{\partial \phi}{\partial t} + \frac{\partial}{\partial \mathbf{X}} \cdot \left(\dot{\mathbf{X}}\phi\right) = 0, \tag{3.9}$$

where $\dot{\mathbf{X}}$ is the formal velocity of the process $\mathbf{X}$. Equation (3.9) is a statement of conservation of probability, and usually known as *Liouville equation,* named after the French mathematician Joseph Liouville (1809–1882). A portray of Liouville can be found in Fig. 3.7.

Remark 3.7 (*Dirac delta function*)
The *Dirac delta function* is the first *generalized function* $\delta(x)$ introduced by Dirac, his portray is found in Fig. 3.8. This generalized function satisfies

$$\int_{-\infty}^{\infty} \delta(x)G(x)dx = G(0), \tag{3.10}$$

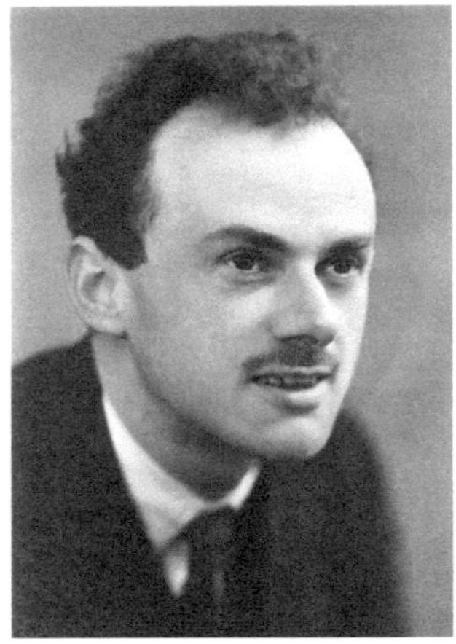

Fig. 3.8 Paul Adrien Maurice Dirac (1902–1984) was a English mathematician and theoretical physicist. He is truly a giant in Physics besides Einstein. He is considered as the Father of quantum mechanics. He was awarded the 1933 Nobel Prize together with Erwin Schrödinger. The Dirac delta function was named after him. (Public domain photograph by Nobel Foundation (1933))

for any continuous function $G(x)$. See Lighthill [18] for a good exposition on generalized functions. The limits $\pm\infty$ on the integral (also below in Eq. (3.11)) may be replaced with a finite interval covering point $x = 0$.

Remark 3.8 (*Derivative of the Dirac delta function*)
Using integration by parts, the *derivative of the Dirac delta function*, itself is a generalized function, $\delta'(x)$, can be thus defined by

$$\int_{-\infty}^{\infty} \delta'(x)G(x)dx = -G'(0), \tag{3.11}$$

for any continuous and differentiable function $G(x)$.

Returning to the statistics of the Brownian forces, Eqs. (3.5–3.6), it is clear that $2\mathbf{f}$ is the *strength* of the Brownian force; it is defined by

$$2\mathbf{f} = \int_{-\infty}^{\infty} \left\langle \mathbf{F}^{(b)}(t+s)\,\mathbf{F}^{(b)}(t) \right\rangle ds. \tag{3.12}$$

Again, the limits $\pm\infty$ can be replaced by a finite interval covering point $s = 0$.

3.3.2 A Generic Langevin System

A system of Brownian particles is a collection of a (small) number of Brownian particles, connected together by their interactions or by their constraints, some examples are shown in Fig. 3.9: a rigid-rod dumbbell consisting of two Brownian particles freely to move, but maintain a constant distance between them, or a system of Brownian particles connected by elastic springs between two adjacent particles.

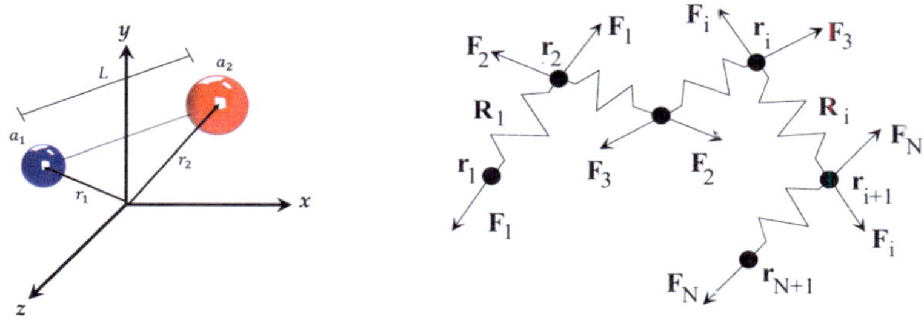

(a) A rigid-rod dumbbell

(b) A polymer chain

Fig. 3.9 Some examples of Langevin systems

A Brownian particle located at $\mathbf{x}_i$ in the system moves according to its Newton's second law of motion under a retarding viscous force (which is $-6\pi\eta_s a(\dot{\mathbf{x}}_i - \mathbf{u})$, for a sphere of radius a moving with velocity $\dot{\mathbf{x}}_i$ relative to the fluid velocity $\mathbf{u}$, in a viscous fluid of viscosity η_s), a restoring force from the neighboring particles $\mathbf{x}_j$ in the system (of the form $K_{ij}(\mathbf{x}_j - \mathbf{x}_i)$), and a Brownian force $\mathbf{F}_i^{(b)}$.

The canonical form for the equations of motion for this Langevin system is therefore

$$\underbrace{m\ddot{\mathbf{x}}}_{\text{ma}} = \underbrace{-\,\boldsymbol{\zeta}\dot{\mathbf{x}}}_{\text{viscous}} \underbrace{-\,\mathbf{K}\mathbf{x}}_{\text{restoring}} \underbrace{+\,\mathbf{F}^{(b)}(t)}_{\text{Brownian}}, \tag{3.13}$$

where the terms labeled "ma" is the mass × acceleration in Newton's second law, "viscous" represents the viscous resistance forces in a viscous fluid, "restoring" represents the restoring forces from the neighboring particles due to their constraints, and "Brownian" represents the Brownian forces on the system. Here $\{\mathbf{x}, \dot{\mathbf{x}}\}$ is the *state-space vector*, the collection of the positions and velocities of the particles of the system, such that $\mathbf{m}\dot{\mathbf{x}}$ is its momentum, $\frac{1}{2}\mathbf{m} : \dot{\mathbf{x}}\dot{\mathbf{x}}$ is its kinetic energy, $\mathbf{m}$ is its inertia tensor, $\boldsymbol{\zeta}$ is the viscous frictional tensor, $\mathbf{K}$ represents the stiffness tensor due to the constraints between the particles, and $\mathbf{F}^{(b)}(t)$ is a vector of all the Brownian forces of the statistics indicated by (3.5–3.6). $\mathbf{m}$, $\boldsymbol{\zeta}$ and $\mathbf{K}$ may be dependent on $\mathbf{x}$, but in almost all cases they are constant. There is no loss of generality in assuming that both $\mathbf{m}$ and $\boldsymbol{\zeta}$ are symmetric and invertible. We must also supply initial conditions to Eq. (3.13), and, without loss of generality, we can assume that the system starts with zero initial conditions for both $\mathbf{x}$ and $\dot{\mathbf{x}}$.

There are three time scales in the Langevin system (3.13):

1. τ_r: the relaxation time scale of the system; it is the longest time scale. This time scale is of $O\left(\left|\boldsymbol{\zeta}\mathbf{K}^{-1}\right|\right)$ and is of order seconds for a typical aqueous polymer solution;
2. τ_i: the inertial relaxation time scale of the system, it is much shorter than the relaxation time scale. This time scale is of the order $\left(\left|\mathbf{m}\boldsymbol{\zeta}^{-1}\right|\right)$. If a is the size of a particle, then $\mathbf{m}$ scales as a^3 (density × volume), while $\boldsymbol{\zeta}$ (Stokes friction

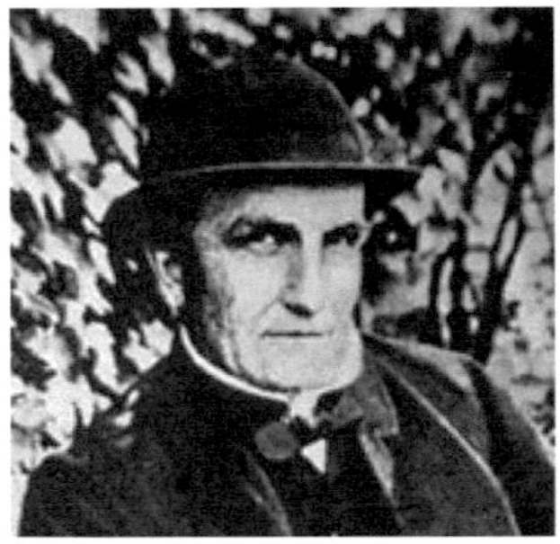

Fig. 3.10 John James Waterston (1811–1883) was a Scottish physicist. His main contributions were in the kinetic theory of gases, but we should remember him for his Equipartition of Energy Principle paper, submitted for publication in 1845, but only posthumously re-published by Lord Rayleigh in full in 1892. (Public domain photograph from Curious Edinburgh.)

factor) scales as a. Depending on how a is estimated, this time scale may be of $O(10^{-2} - 10^{-4})$s;

3. τ_c: the fluctuation/correlation time scale of the Brownian force—this is the shortest time scale, and is of the same order as the relaxation time scale of a solvent molecule; for water it is $O(10^{-13})$s.

Depending on the time scale of interest, the Langevin system Eq. (3.13) may be further simplified. We return to this later.

Remark 3.9 (*Equipartition of Energy Principle*)
For a particle at equilibrium in a fluid of temperature T, the *Equipartition of Energy Principle* states that its mean kinetic energy is $\frac{1}{2}kT$, where k is the Boltzmann constant,

$$\lim_{t\to\infty} \langle \dot{\mathbf{x}}(t)\, \dot{\mathbf{x}}(t)\rangle = kT\mathbf{m}^{-1}. \tag{3.14}$$

This is because of the velocity of the particle is Maxwellian distributed [19]. The limit of infinity means $t \gg \tau_c$.

The Equipartition of Energy Principle was original proposed by Waterston [20] (Fig. 3.10) in a manuscript submitted to the Royal Society in 1845 but was rejected. He then published a version of this principle in *British Association Reports* in 1851, and so established a priority date over Maxwell, who discussed this principle in a meeting of the British Association in 1859 [21], and Boltzmann [22]. The lost manuscript submitted to the Royal Society was discovered by Lord Rayleigh (who was then the Secretary of the Society), and was re-published in full in 1893. The morale of this story, paraphrased in the words of Lord Rayleigh is that, if you are "a young author who believes himself capable of great things", then you "would usually do well to secure favorable recognition of the scientific world by work whose scope is limited, and whose value is easily judged, before embarking upon higher flights!"

3.3.3 Fluctuation–Dissipation Theorem

Now, returning to our Eq. (3.13), and it is sufficient for our purpose to consider only events on the inertial time scale τ_i. Then, $\mathbf{m}(\mathbf{x})$ and $\boldsymbol{\zeta}(\mathbf{x})$ can be replaced by their local values, regarded as constant. Furthermore, the state vector can be re-defined to eliminate $\mathbf{Kx}$ so that our Langevin equation (3.13) becomes a linear equation in the velocity,

$$\ddot{\mathbf{x}} + \mathbf{m}^{-1}\boldsymbol{\zeta}\dot{\mathbf{x}} = \mathbf{m}^{-1}\mathbf{F}^{(b)}(t), \tag{3.15}$$

subjected to the initial rest state $\dot{\mathbf{x}}(0) = \mathbf{0} = \mathbf{x}(0)$.

Remark 3.10 (*Fundamental Matrix*)

1. For every pair of commutative second-order tensors $\mathbf{A}$ and $\mathbf{B}$, $\mathbf{AB} = \mathbf{BA}$, we have

$$e^{\mathbf{A}}e^{\mathbf{B}} = e^{\mathbf{A}+\mathbf{B}}. \tag{3.16}$$

   The proof relies on the series representation of an exponential function.
2. Consequently, since $\mathbf{A}$ clearly commutes with itself,

$$e^{\mathbf{A}}e^{-\mathbf{A}} = \mathbf{I}, \tag{3.17}$$

3. If $\mathbf{A}$ is a constant,

$$\frac{d}{dt}e^{\mathbf{A}} = \mathbf{A}e^{t\mathbf{A}} = e^{t\mathbf{A}}\mathbf{A}. \tag{3.18}$$

4. Consequently

$$\frac{d}{dt}\left(e^{\mathbf{A}t}\mathbf{v}\right) = e^{\mathbf{A}t}\left(\dot{\mathbf{v}} + \mathbf{A}\mathbf{v}\right). \tag{3.19}$$

   The tensor (matrix) $e^{t\mathbf{A}}$ is sometimes known as the *fundamental matrix* of the equation $\dot{\mathbf{x}} + \mathbf{Ax} = 0$.

Identify $\mathbf{A} = \mathbf{m}^{-1}\boldsymbol{\zeta}$ and $\mathbf{v} = \dot{\mathbf{x}}$ in Eq. (3.19), one finds, using Eq. (3.19),

$$\frac{d}{dt}\left(e^{\mathbf{A}t}\dot{\mathbf{x}}\right) = e^{\mathbf{m}^{-1}\boldsymbol{\zeta}t}\mathbf{m}^{-1}\mathbf{F}^{(b)}(t) \tag{3.20}$$

leading to the formal solution to Eq. (3.15),

$$\dot{\mathbf{x}}(t) = \int_0^t \exp\left\{\mathbf{m}^{-1}\boldsymbol{\zeta}\left(t'-t\right)\right\}\mathbf{m}^{-1}\mathbf{F}^{(b)}\left(t'\right)dt'. \tag{3.21}$$

This is only a formal solution, because the Brownian force is not a well-behaved function, and we are not expect to use this to generate the velocity; however, we can use it to generate the expectation for the kinetic energy, and this will be done next. Now since

$$\langle \dot{\mathbf{x}}(t)\,\dot{\mathbf{x}}(t)\rangle == \int_0^t \int_0^t \exp\left\{\mathbf{m}^{-1}\boldsymbol{\zeta}\left(t'-t\right)\right\}\mathbf{m}^{-1}\left\langle \mathbf{F}^{(b)}\left(t'\right)\mathbf{F}^{(b)}\left(t''\right)\right\rangle \cdot \mathbf{m}^{-1}\exp\left\{\boldsymbol{\zeta}\mathbf{m}^{-1}\left(t''-t\right)\right\}dt'dt'', \tag{3.22}$$

The strength of the Brownian force can be used in (3.22), and the delta function can be integrated out to yield

$$\langle \dot{\mathbf{x}}(t)\dot{\mathbf{x}}(t)\rangle = 2\int_0^t \exp\left\{\mathbf{m}^{-1}\boldsymbol{\zeta}\left(t'-t\right)\right\}\mathbf{m}^{-1}\mathbf{f}\mathbf{m}^{-1}\exp\left\{\boldsymbol{\zeta}\mathbf{m}^{-1}\left(t'-t\right)\right\}dt'. \tag{3.23}$$

We then integrate the integral on the right of (3.23) by parts, $\int u'v = [uv] - \int uv'$, with u' identified with $\exp\left(\mathbf{m}^{-1}\boldsymbol{\zeta}\left(t'-t\right)\right)$, $u = \boldsymbol{\zeta}^{-1}\mathbf{m}\exp\left(\mathbf{m}^{-1}\boldsymbol{\zeta}\left(t'-t\right)\right)$, and v with $\exp\left(\boldsymbol{\zeta}\mathbf{m}^{-1}\left(t'-t\right)\right)$, leading to v' as $\boldsymbol{\zeta}\mathbf{m}^{-1}\exp\left(\boldsymbol{\zeta}\mathbf{m}^{-1}\left(t'-t\right)\right)$. We then have, for this integral,

$$\begin{aligned}\langle \dot{\mathbf{x}}(t)\dot{\mathbf{x}}(t)\rangle &= 2\boldsymbol{\zeta}^{-1}\mathbf{m}\exp\left\{\mathbf{m}^{-1}\boldsymbol{\zeta}\left(t'-t\right)\right\}\mathbf{m}^{-1}\mathbf{f}\mathbf{m}^{-1}\exp\left\{\boldsymbol{\zeta}\mathbf{m}^{-1}\left(t'-t\right)\right\}\Big|_0^t \\ &\quad - 2\int_0^t \boldsymbol{\zeta}^{-1}\mathbf{m}e^{\mathbf{m}^{-1}\boldsymbol{\zeta}(t'-t)}\mathbf{m}^{-1}\mathbf{f}\mathbf{m}^{-1}\mathbf{m}\boldsymbol{\zeta}^{-1}e^{\boldsymbol{\zeta}\mathbf{m}^{-1}(t'-t)}dt'.\end{aligned} \tag{3.24}$$

The form of the integral on the right of (3.24) is recognized to be in the same form as $\langle \dot{\mathbf{x}}(t)\dot{\mathbf{x}}(t)\rangle$ in Eq. (3.22), and upon evaluation of the first term on the right of (3.24), we obtain

$$\langle \dot{\mathbf{x}}(t)\dot{\mathbf{x}}(t)\rangle = 2\boldsymbol{\zeta}^{-1}\mathbf{f}\mathbf{m}^{-1} - \boldsymbol{\zeta}^{-1}\mathbf{m}\,\langle \dot{\mathbf{x}}(t)\dot{\mathbf{x}}(t)\rangle\,\boldsymbol{\zeta}\mathbf{m}^{-1}. \tag{3.25}$$

Finally from the principle of equipartition of energy (3.14) (3.25) yields the *Fluctuation–Dissipation Theorem*,

$$\mathbf{f} = kT\boldsymbol{\zeta}. \tag{3.26}$$

In another words, the strength of the Brownian forces cannot be arbitrarily assigned independently; it is inherited from the mobility of the Brownian system, and any dependence on the configuration of $\mathbf{f}$ must also come from that of $\boldsymbol{\zeta}$. Note that the fluctuation–dissipation theorem (3.26) holds at finite mass; all that is needed is that we focus on the inertial time scale τ_i and that $\tau_i \gg \tau_c$.

There are many other types of fluctuation–dissipation theorems, in resistance and electrical noise, in light absorption and thermal radiation; there is even a version of this in quantum mechanics. The general proof of the theorem was given in Callen and Welton [23].

Remark 3.11 (*A Summary*) Very often we are interested in the limit of $\mathbf{m} = 0$, and reinstate the restoring forces, the system Langevin equations are summarized as follows

$$\dot{\mathbf{x}} + \zeta^{-1}\mathbf{K}\mathbf{x} = \zeta^{-1}\mathbf{F}^{(b)}(t), \tag{3.27}$$

$$\left\langle \mathbf{F}^{(b)} \right\rangle = 0, \ \left\langle \mathbf{F}^{(b)}(t+s)\,\mathbf{F}^{(b)}(t) \right\rangle = 2kT\zeta\delta(s), \tag{3.28}$$

where the Fluctuation–Dissipation theorem has been used in the statistics of the Brownian forces. This is the default form of our Langevin equation for the rest of this Lecture Note.

3.3.4 Average Quantities

In most cases, we do not need the full statistics of the Langevin state variables, only their mean quantities. These can be easily found using their Langevin equations (3.27–3.28). For example, the two quantities of interest are the *drift velocity*, $v_k = \langle \Delta x_k/\Delta t \rangle$, and the *diffusivity (tensor)*,[3] $D_{mn} = \langle \Delta x_m \Delta x_n/(2\Delta t) \rangle$. In these definitions, the limit $\Delta t \to \infty$ is implied.

Drift Velocity

For the drift velocity and by taking the differential of the Langevin equation (3.27),

$$\zeta_{ij}\Delta x_j + K_{ij}x_j\Delta t = \int_0^{\Delta t} F_i^{(b)}(t)dt. \tag{3.29}$$

Note that we *do not* differentiate $F_i^{(b)}(t)$, since this function is not differentiable everywhere; rather its integral over Δt is taken, since its integral is well-defined.[4] From (3.29), we find that the drift velocity is given by, noting that Brownian statistics (3.28),

$$v_i = \left\langle \frac{\Delta x_i}{\Delta t} \right\rangle = -\zeta_{ij}^{-1} K_{jk} x_k. \tag{3.30}$$

---

[3] The reason for the naming will be soon obvious.

[4] This is the most useful "trick" in Langevin analysis.

Diffusivity Tensor

Next, also from (3.29),

$$\begin{aligned}\zeta_{ij}\Delta x_j \Delta x_l \zeta_{kl} &= \left(-K_{ij}x_j\Delta t + \int_0^{\Delta t} F_i^{(b)}(t)\,dt\right)\left(-K_{kl}x_l\Delta t + \int_0^{\Delta t} F_k^{(b)}(t)\,dt\right) \\ &= \text{terms of } O\left(\Delta t^2\right) + \text{terms linear in } \mathbf{F}(b) \\ &+ \int_0^{\Delta t} dt' \int_0^{\Delta t} F_i^{(b)}(t')F_k^{(b)}(t'')dt''. \end{aligned} \tag{3.31}$$

Now, noting the statistics of the Brownian forces (3.28),

$$\begin{aligned}\int_0^{\Delta t} dt' \int_0^{\Delta t} \left\langle F_i^{(b)}(t')F_k^{(b)}(t'')\right\rangle dt'' &= 2f_{ik}\int_0^{\Delta t} dt' \int_0^{\Delta t} \delta\left(t''-t'\right)dt'' \\ &= 2f_{ik}\Delta t. \end{aligned} \tag{3.32}$$

With the result (3.32), Eq. (3.31) can now be averaged, neglecting $O\left(\Delta t^2\right)$, and noting that terms linear in $\mathbf{F}(b)$ do not contribute to this average,

$$\zeta_{ij}\left\langle \Delta x_j \Delta x_l\right\rangle \zeta_{kl} = 2f_{ik}\Delta t. \tag{3.33}$$

With the fluctuation–dissipation theorem (3.26), we finally arrive at the diffusivity tensor,

$$\mathbf{D} = \frac{\Delta\mathbf{x}\Delta\mathbf{x}}{2\Delta t} = \boldsymbol{\zeta}^{-1}\mathbf{f}\boldsymbol{\zeta}^{-1} = kT\boldsymbol{\zeta}^{-1}. \tag{3.34}$$

There are other definitions of diffusivity tensor. One is

$$\mathbf{D} = \lim_{t\to\infty}\frac{1}{2}\frac{d}{dt}\left\langle \mathbf{x}(t)\,\mathbf{x}(t)\right\rangle, \tag{3.35}$$

and the other,

$$\mathbf{D} = \lim_{t\to\infty}\frac{1}{2}\int_0^t \left\langle \dot{\mathbf{x}}(t)\,\dot{\mathbf{x}}(t-\tau) + \dot{\mathbf{x}}(t-\tau)\,\dot{\mathbf{x}}(t)\right\rangle d\tau. \tag{3.36}$$

In these definitions, $t \to \infty$ means $t \gg \tau_c$.

3.3.5 *Fokker–Plack/Kolmogorov/Smoluchowski Diffusion Equation*

The Langevin system is a stochastic process, which is considered solved only when the probability density distribution is specified. This diffusion equation is associated

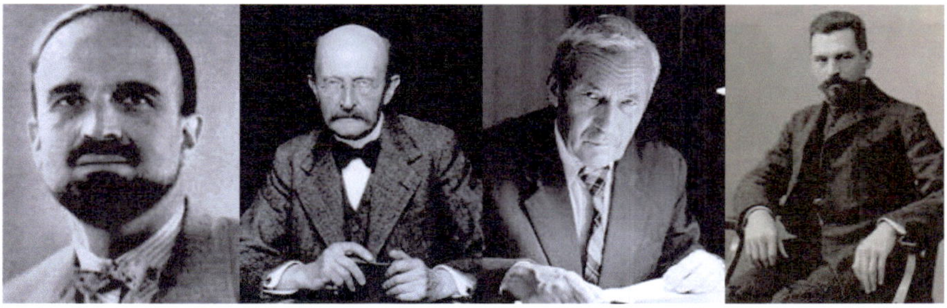

Fig. 3.11 From left to right: Adriaan Daniël Fokker (1887–1972), a Dutch physicist, with contributions in statistical mechanics and relativity. He was the inventor of the *Fokker* organ, named after him, which he designed and built (Photograph provided in Snelders [24]); Max Karl Ernst Ludwig Planck (1858–1947), a German physicist, known for the Planck constant and for the originator of quantum theory, for which he was awarded the 1918 Nobel Prize in Physics (Public domain photograph by Hugo Erfurth (1874–1948)); Andrey Nikolaevich Kolmogorov (1903–1987), a Soviet mathematician, with contributions in many areas of mathematics and physics, including turbulence (Photograph provided in Manokhin [25]); and Marian Smoluchowski (1872–1917), a Polish physicist, with major contributions in stochastic processes (Public domain photograph, Nowości Illustrowane)

with various names, Fokker [26], Planck [27], Kolmogorov [28], von Smoluchowski [29], see Fig. 3.11 for brief histories of the scientists concerned. Chandrasekhar [30] provided an excellent overview of stochastic problems. Fokker–Planck equation is usually associated with the complete Langevin system, with inertia tensor included, and Smoluchowski is associated with the system where the mass tensor is put to zero. In the Fokker-Planck case, the probability density distribution $\phi(\mathbf{x}, \dot{\mathbf{x}})$ is in the *phase space* $\{\mathbf{x}, \dot{\mathbf{x}}\}$, and in the Smoluchowski case, in the *configuration space* $\{\mathbf{x}\}$, $\phi(\mathbf{x})$.

The development considered here is for the case of $\mathbf{m} = 0$, for pedagogical purposes, and the diffusion equation in configuration space is strictly speaking the Smoluchowski equation.

Although we often are interested in mean quantities, we show in this section how to derive the diffusion equation from Langevin equation. Steps in deriving the Fokker–Planck equation in phase space $\{\mathbf{x}, \dot{\mathbf{x}}\}$ are outlined in Problems (3.3–3.4).

We start with the Langevin equation (3.27), then a differential in the state vector is given by

$$\Delta\mathbf{x} = \mathbf{x}(t + \Delta t) - \mathbf{x}(t) = -\boldsymbol{\zeta}^{-1}\mathbf{K}\mathbf{x}\Delta t + \int^{\Delta t} \zeta^{-1}\mathbf{F}^{(b)}(t)\, dt \tag{3.37}$$

where $\int^{\Delta t}$ is a short-hand notation for $\int_t^{\Delta t}$. Note that the integral on the right of (3.37) is $O\left(\sqrt{\Delta t}\right)$. Now, for any function $G(\mathbf{x})$ of the state variable $\mathbf{x}$,

$$\Delta G = \frac{\partial G}{\partial t}\Delta t = G(\mathbf{x} + \Delta\mathbf{x}) - G(\mathbf{x}) = \Delta\mathbf{x}.\frac{\partial G}{\partial \mathbf{x}} + \frac{1}{2}\Delta\mathbf{x}\Delta\mathbf{x} : \frac{\partial^2 G}{\partial\mathbf{x}\partial\mathbf{x}} + \ldots \tag{3.38}$$

Next, identify $\Delta\mathbf{x}$ with the right side of (3.37), we have

$$\begin{aligned}\Delta G &= \left(-\zeta^{-1}\mathbf{Kx}\Delta t + \zeta^{-1}\int^{\Delta t}\mathbf{F}^{(b)}(t)dt\right).\frac{\partial G}{\partial \mathbf{x}}\\ &+ \frac{1}{2}\zeta^{-1}\left(-\mathbf{Kx}\Delta t + \int^{\Delta t}\mathbf{F}^{(b)}(t)dt\right)\zeta^{-1}\left(\mathbf{Kx}\Delta t + \int^{\Delta t}\mathbf{F}^{(b)}(t)dt\right) : \frac{\partial^2 G}{\partial\mathbf{x}\partial\mathbf{x}} + \ldots\\ &= \text{terms linear in } \mathbf{F}^{(b)}(t) - \zeta^{-1}\mathbf{Kx}\Delta t.\frac{\partial G}{\partial \mathbf{x}}\\ &+ \frac{1}{2}\zeta^{-1}\int^{\Delta t}dt'\int^{\Delta t}dt''\mathbf{F}^{(b)}(t')\mathbf{F}^{(b)}(t'')\,\zeta^{-1} : \frac{\partial^2 G}{\partial\mathbf{x}\partial\mathbf{x}} + \ldots\end{aligned} \tag{3.39}$$

The double integral on the right of (3.39) can be evaluated with the help of the statistics of the Brownian forces (3.28),

$$\frac{1}{2}\boldsymbol{\zeta}^{-1}\int^{\Delta t}dt'\int^{\Delta t}dt''\left\langle\mathbf{F}^{(b)}(t')\mathbf{F}^{(b)}(t'')\right\rangle\boldsymbol{\zeta}^{-1} = kT\zeta^{-1}\Delta t. \tag{3.40}$$

As a function of time t, $\Delta G = \Delta t\partial G/\partial t$ to $O(\Delta t)$. Using this in the average of (3.39) together with result (3.40) yields

$$\left\langle\frac{\partial G(\mathbf{x})}{\partial t}\right\rangle = \left\langle-\boldsymbol{\zeta}^{-1}\mathbf{Kx}.\frac{\partial G}{\partial\mathbf{x}} + kT\boldsymbol{\zeta}^{-1} : \frac{\partial G}{\partial\mathbf{x}\partial\mathbf{x}}\right\rangle. \tag{3.41}$$

Now, if $\phi(\mathbf{x}, t)$ the probability density distribution of the process, then

$$\begin{aligned}\langle G\rangle &= \int G\phi(\mathbf{x}, t)\\ \left\langle\frac{\partial G(\mathbf{x})}{\partial t}\right\rangle &= \frac{\partial}{\partial t}\int G(\mathbf{x})\,\phi d\mathbf{x}d\mathbf{x}\\ \left\langle-\zeta^{-1}\mathbf{Kx}.\frac{\partial G}{\partial\mathbf{x}} + kT\zeta^{-1} : \frac{\partial^2 G}{\partial\mathbf{x}\partial\mathbf{x}}\right\rangle &= \int\left(-\zeta^{-1}\mathbf{Kx}.\frac{\partial G}{\partial\mathbf{x}} + kT\zeta^{-1} : \frac{\partial^2 G}{\partial\mathbf{x}\partial\mathbf{x}}\right)\phi d\mathbf{x}.\end{aligned} \tag{3.42}$$

These results (3.41–3.42) hold for any function $G(\mathbf{x}, t)$—in particular, for $G(\mathbf{x}, t) = \delta(\mathbf{x} - \mathbf{X})$, for any particular state variable $\mathbf{X}$, and noting that, from the properties of Dirac delta function (3.10–3.11), we have

$$\begin{aligned}\int\delta(\mathbf{x} - \mathbf{X})\,\phi(\mathbf{x})\,d\mathbf{x} &= \phi(\mathbf{X}),\\ \int\frac{\partial}{\partial\mathbf{x}}(\delta(\mathbf{x} - \mathbf{X}))\,\phi(\mathbf{x})\,d\mathbf{x} &= -\frac{\partial}{\partial\mathbf{X}}\phi(\mathbf{X}),\end{aligned}$$

$$\left\langle -\zeta^{-1}\mathbf{Kx}.\frac{\partial G}{\partial \mathbf{x}}\right\rangle = \int \left(-\zeta^{-1}\mathbf{Kx}.\frac{\partial}{\partial \mathbf{x}}\delta\left(\mathbf{x}-\mathbf{X}\right)\right)\phi(\mathbf{x})d\mathbf{x}$$
$$= \frac{\partial}{\partial \mathbf{X}}.\left(\zeta^{-1}\mathbf{KX}\phi\left(\mathbf{X},t\right)\right),$$

$$\left\langle kT\zeta^{-1}:\frac{\partial^2 G}{\partial \mathbf{x}\partial \mathbf{x}}\right\rangle = \int \left(kT\zeta^{-1}:\frac{\partial^2}{\partial \mathbf{x}\partial \mathbf{x}}\delta\left(\mathbf{x}-\mathbf{X}\right)\right)\phi\left(\mathbf{x}\right)d\mathbf{x}$$
$$= \frac{\partial}{\partial \mathbf{X}}.\left(kT\zeta^{-1}.\frac{\partial}{\partial \mathbf{X}}\phi\left(\mathbf{X}\right)\right).$$

These results can be used in (3.41–3.42) to finally arrive at the Fokker–Planck Kolmogorov Smoluchowski, or simply diffusion equation in configuration space (changing the state variable to $\mathbf{x}$),

$$\frac{\partial}{\partial t}\phi\left(\mathbf{x},t\right) = \frac{\partial}{\partial \mathbf{x}}.\left(kT\boldsymbol{\zeta}^{-1}\frac{\partial}{\partial \mathbf{x}}\phi\left(\mathbf{x},t\right) + \boldsymbol{\zeta}^{-1}\mathbf{Kx}\phi\left(\mathbf{x},t\right)\right). \tag{3.43}$$

Remark 3.12 (*Diffusion Equation*) From our definitions of drift velocity (3.30) and diffusivity (3.34), the diffusion equation in configuration space can be written in an equivalent form:

$$\frac{\partial \phi}{\partial t} = \lim_{\Delta t \to 0}\frac{\partial}{\partial \mathbf{x}}\cdot\left[\frac{\langle \Delta\mathbf{x}\Delta\mathbf{x}\rangle}{2\Delta t}\cdot\frac{\partial \phi}{\partial \mathbf{x}} - \frac{\langle \Delta\mathbf{x}\rangle}{\Delta t}\phi\right]. \tag{3.44}$$

This justifies our definitions in Sect. 3.3.4; see also Chandrasekhar [30].

3.3.6 Smoothed-Out Brownian Force

The conservation of probability demands that the probability density distribution satisfy the Liouville equation (3.9). Compared to the diffusion equation (3.43), one finds that the equivalent velocity of this Liouville system must be

$$\dot{\mathbf{x}} = -\zeta^{-1}\cdot\mathbf{Kx} - kT\boldsymbol{\zeta}^{-1}\cdot\frac{\partial \ln \phi}{\partial \mathbf{x}}, \tag{3.45}$$

in order to satisfied the Liouville equation identically. That is,

$$\boldsymbol{\zeta}\dot{\mathbf{x}} + \mathbf{Kx} = -kT\frac{\partial \ln \phi}{\partial \mathbf{x}}, \tag{3.46}$$

which expresses the balance between viscous force, restoring force, and a *smoothed-out* Brownian force, or *time smoothed-out* Brownian force [31], defined by

$$\mathbf{F}^{(b)}(t) = -kT\frac{\partial \ln \phi}{\partial \mathbf{x}}. \tag{3.47}$$

There is a voluminous amount of literature using this smoothed-out Brownian force—it certainly affords a quick and convenient way to incorporate the Brownian force into the modeling of complex liquids, and it is a familiar tool in Chemical Engineering.

Problems

Problem 3.1 The first part of this problem can be used to find path lines in a constant velocity gradient field; the second part is used in finding the formal solution to the velocity of a massless Langevin particle.

1. Consider a steady velocity field given by ($\mathbf{L}$ is a constant velocity gradient),

$$\dot{\mathbf{x}} = \mathbf{L}\mathbf{x}, \ \ \mathbf{x}(t=0) = \mathbf{x}_0. \tag{3.48}$$

Show that the solution to this is

$$\mathbf{x}(t) = \boldsymbol{\Phi}(t)\mathbf{x}_0, \tag{3.49}$$

where $\boldsymbol{\Phi}$ is called the *fundamental matrix* of the system. Further show that the fundamental matrix is in fact the deformation gradient, and it is given by

$$\boldsymbol{\Phi}(t) = e^{t\mathbf{L}}. \tag{3.50}$$

Depending on the form of $\mathbf{L}$, this may, or may not be actually exponential in time.

2. Investigate the solution to

$$\dot{\mathbf{x}} + \mathbf{A}\mathbf{x} = \mathbf{F}, \ \ \mathbf{x}(t=0) = \mathbf{x}_0. \tag{3.51}$$

Problem 3.2 Show that the diffusivity definitions (3.35) and (3.36) all lead to the result (3.34).

Problem 3.3 Consider the Langevin equation (3.13). Define $\mathbf{u} = \dot{\mathbf{x}}$, and re-write this in the incremental form, where $\tau_c \ll \Delta t \ll \tau_i$,

$$\Delta\mathbf{u} = -(\boldsymbol{\beta}\mathbf{u} + \mathbf{H})\Delta t + \mathbf{B}(\Delta t), \tag{3.52}$$

where $\boldsymbol{\beta} = \mathbf{m}^{-1}\boldsymbol{\zeta}$, $\mathbf{H} = \mathbf{m}^{-1}\mathbf{K}\mathbf{x}$ and

$$\mathbf{B}(\Delta t) = \mathbf{m}^{-1} \int_t^{t+\Delta t} \mathbf{F}^{(b)}(t). \tag{3.53}$$

Show that, with the help of statistics (3.28),

$$\langle \mathbf{B}(\Delta t) \rangle = 0, \tag{3.54}$$

$$\langle \mathbf{B}(\Delta t)\mathbf{B}(\Delta t) \rangle = 2kT\mathbf{m}^{-1}\boldsymbol{\zeta}\mathbf{m}^{-1}\Delta t. \tag{3.55}$$

Further, show that

$$\langle \Delta\mathbf{u} \rangle = -(\boldsymbol{\beta}\mathbf{u} + \mathbf{H})\Delta t, \tag{3.56}$$

$$\langle \Delta\mathbf{u}\Delta\mathbf{u} \rangle = 2kT\mathbf{m}^{-1}\boldsymbol{\zeta}\mathbf{m}^{-1}\Delta t + O\left(\Delta t^2\right). \tag{3.57}$$

Problem 3.4 First, we provide a short discussion on *Markov process*.[5] The central idea behind this process is that what happens at any instant of time depends on the current instantaneous state of the system, but not on its previous history—and this is indeed the property of a Langevin (Brownian) process. We can write, with the state of the process at time t is $\{\mathbf{u}, \mathbf{x}\}$, where $\mathbf{u} = \dot{\mathbf{x}}$ is the velocity of the system,

$$\phi(\mathbf{u}, \mathbf{x}, t + \Delta t) = \int \phi(\mathbf{u} - \Delta\mathbf{u}, \mathbf{x} - \Delta\mathbf{x}, t)\psi(\mathbf{u} - \Delta\mathbf{u}, \mathbf{x} - \Delta\mathbf{x}; \Delta\mathbf{u}, \Delta\mathbf{x})d(\Delta\mathbf{u})d(\Delta\mathbf{x}), \tag{3.58}$$

where $\psi(\mathbf{u}, \mathbf{x}; \Delta\mathbf{u}, \Delta\mathbf{x})$ is the *transition probability* that $\{\mathbf{u}, \mathbf{x}\}$ will have a an increment $\{\Delta\mathbf{u}, \Delta\mathbf{x}\}$ in the next duration Δt time interval. The fact that $\mathbf{u}$ is the velocity demands that

$$\psi(\mathbf{u}, \mathbf{x}; \Delta\mathbf{u}, \Delta\mathbf{x}) = \Psi(\mathbf{u}, \mathbf{x}; \Delta\mathbf{u})\delta(\Delta\mathbf{x} - \mathbf{u}\Delta t). \tag{3.59}$$

1. Show that the integral in (3.58) in $d(\Delta\mathbf{x})$ can be performed to yield

$$\phi(\mathbf{u}, \mathbf{x}, t + \Delta t) = \int \phi(\mathbf{u} - \Delta\mathbf{u}, \mathbf{x} - \mathbf{u}\Delta t, t)\Psi(\mathbf{u} - \Delta\mathbf{u}, \mathbf{x} - \mathbf{u}\Delta t; \Delta\mathbf{u})d(\Delta\mathbf{u}). \tag{3.60}$$

2. Then show that

$$\phi(\mathbf{u}, \mathbf{x} + \mathbf{u}\Delta t, t + \Delta t) = \int \phi(\mathbf{u} - \Delta\mathbf{u}, \mathbf{x}, t)\Psi(\mathbf{u} - \Delta\mathbf{u}, \mathbf{x}; \Delta\mathbf{u})d(\Delta\mathbf{u}). \tag{3.61}$$

3. Show that the left side of (3.61), LHS, can be expanded in a Taylor's series as, up to $O\left(\Delta t, \Delta\mathbf{u}^2\right)$,

$$LHS = \phi(\mathbf{u}, \mathbf{x}, t) + \Delta t\frac{\partial}{\partial t}\phi(\mathbf{u}, \mathbf{x}, t) + \mathbf{u}\Delta t.\frac{\partial}{\partial \mathbf{x}}\phi(\mathbf{u}, \mathbf{x}, t). \tag{3.62}$$

[5] A portray of Andrey Andreyevich Markov (1856–1922) can be found in Fig. 4.3.

4. Show that the right side of (3.61), RHS, can be expanded in a Taylor's series as, up to $O\left(\Delta t, \Delta\mathbf{u}^2\right)$,

$$RHS = \int d(\Delta\mathbf{u}) \left[\phi(\mathbf{u},\mathbf{x},t) - \Delta\mathbf{u}\frac{\partial}{\partial\mathbf{u}}\phi(\mathbf{u},\mathbf{x},t) + \frac{1}{2}\Delta\mathbf{u}\Delta\mathbf{u} : \frac{\partial^2}{\partial\mathbf{u}\partial\mathbf{u}}\phi(\mathbf{u},\mathbf{x},t)\right]$$
$$\times \left[\Psi(\mathbf{u},\mathbf{x};\Delta\mathbf{u}) - \Delta\mathbf{u}\frac{\partial}{\partial\mathbf{u}}\Psi(\mathbf{u},\mathbf{x};\Delta\mathbf{u}) + \frac{1}{2}\Delta\mathbf{u}\Delta\mathbf{u} : \frac{\partial^2}{\partial\mathbf{u}\partial\mathbf{u}}\Psi(\mathbf{u},\mathbf{x};\Delta\mathbf{u})\right]. \quad (3.63)$$

5. Expanding (3.63), noting that

$$\int \Psi(\mathbf{u},\mathbf{x};\Delta\mathbf{u}) d(\Delta\mathbf{u}) = 1,$$
$$\int \Delta\mathbf{u}\Psi(\mathbf{u},\mathbf{x};\Delta\mathbf{u}) d(\Delta\mathbf{u}) = \langle\Delta\mathbf{u}\rangle,$$
$$\int \Delta\mathbf{u}\Delta\mathbf{u}\Psi(\mathbf{u},\mathbf{x};\Delta\mathbf{u}) d(\Delta\mathbf{u}) = \langle\Delta\mathbf{u}\Delta\mathbf{u}\rangle,$$
$$\int \Delta\mathbf{u}\frac{\partial}{\partial\mathbf{u}}.\Psi(\mathbf{u},\mathbf{x};\Delta\mathbf{u}) d(\Delta\mathbf{u}) = \frac{\partial}{\partial\mathbf{u}}.\langle\Delta\mathbf{u}\rangle,$$
$$\int \Delta\mathbf{u}\Delta\mathbf{u} : \frac{\partial^2}{\partial\mathbf{u}\partial\mathbf{u}}\Psi(\mathbf{u},\mathbf{x};\Delta\mathbf{u}) d(\Delta\mathbf{u}) = \frac{\partial^2}{\partial\mathbf{u}\partial\mathbf{u}} : \langle\Delta\mathbf{u}\Delta\mathbf{u}\rangle,$$

and then equating $LHS = RHS$, to find the following diffusion equation in phase space, or the Fokker–Planck equation,

$$\frac{\partial\phi}{\partial t} + \mathbf{u}.\frac{\partial\phi}{\partial\mathbf{x}} = \frac{\partial}{\partial\mathbf{u}}.\left\{\frac{\langle\Delta\mathbf{u}\Delta\mathbf{u}\rangle}{2\Delta t}.\frac{\partial\phi}{\partial\mathbf{u}} - \left[\frac{\langle\Delta\mathbf{u}\rangle}{\Delta t} - \frac{\partial}{\partial\mathbf{u}}.\frac{\langle\Delta\mathbf{u}\Delta\mathbf{u}\rangle}{2\Delta t}\right]\phi\right\}. \quad (3.64)$$

Allowing $\Delta t \to 0$, and using the results obtained in Problem (3.3) to finally arrive at the Fokker–Planck equation in phase space:

$$\frac{\partial\phi}{\partial t} + \mathbf{u}.\frac{\partial\phi}{\partial\mathbf{x}} = \frac{\partial}{\partial\mathbf{u}}.\left\{kT\mathbf{m}^{-1}\boldsymbol{\zeta}\mathbf{m}^{-1}.\frac{\partial\phi}{\partial\mathbf{u}} + \mathbf{m}^{-1}\left(\boldsymbol{\zeta}\mathbf{u} + \mathbf{K}\mathbf{x}\right)\phi\right\}. \quad (3.65)$$

References

1. R. Brown, A brief account of microscopical observations made in the months of June, July and August 1827, on the particles contained in the pollen of plants; and on the general existence of active molecules in organic and inorganic bodies. Philos. Mag. **4**, 161–173 (1828)
2. R. Brown, Additional remarks on active molecules. Philos. Mag. **6**, 161–166 (1829)
3. L. Cohen, The history of noise. IEEE Signal Process. Mag. **22**, 20–45 (2005)
4. L. Cohen, What did Brown do? Phys. Fluids **37**, 037154 (2025)

5. A Einstein, *Investigations on the Theory of the Brownian Movement*, ed. by R. Fürth, Trans. A.D. Cowper (Dover, New York, 1988)
6. J. Perrin, Mouvement brownien et r alit mol culaire. Annales de Chimie et de Physique 8th series **18**, 1–114 (1909)
7. P. Langevin, Sur la théorie du mouvement brownien. C R Acad Sci (Paris) **146**, 530–533 (1908)
8. M.D. Graham, *Microhydrodynamics, Brownian Motion, and Complex Fluids* (Cambridge University Press, Cambridge, 2018)
9. R.I. Tanner, K. Walters, *Rheology: An Historical Perspective* (Elsevier Science B.V., Amtersdam, 1998)
10. E. Upton, Marie curie once had two duels fought over her after an affair with a married man. https://www.todayifoundout.com/index.php/2013/09/marie-curie-once-had-two-duels-fought-over-her-after-an-affair-with-a-married-man/ (2013)
11. R. Huilgol, N. Phan-Thien, *Fluid Mechanics of Viscoelasticity: General Principles, Constitutive Modelling, Analytical and Numerical Techniques* (Elsevier, Amsterdam, 1997)
12. R.B. Bird, R.C. Armstrong, O. Hassager, *Dynamics of Polymeric Liquids. Vol. 1: Fluid Mechanics*, 2nd edn. (Wiley, New York, 1987)
13. R.I. Tanner, *Engineering Rheology*, revised edition edn. (Oxford University Press, Oxford, 1992)
14. J. Happel, H. Brenner, *Low Reynolds Number Hydrodynamics* (Noordhoff International Publishing, Leyden, 1973)
15. S. Kim, S.J. Karrila, *Microhydrodynamics: Principles and Selected Applications* (Dover, Unabridged Edition, New York, 2005)
16. G.K. Batchelor, *An Introduction to Fluid Dynamics* (Cambridge University Press, Cambridge, 1967)
17. D.S. Lemons, A. Gythiel, Paul Langevin's 1908 paper on the theory of brownian motion [sur la théorie du mouvement brownien, c. r. acad. sci. (paris) 146, 530–533 (1908)]. Am. J. Phys. **65**, 1179–1181 (1997)
18. M.J. Lighthill, *An Introduction to Fourier Analysis and Generalised Functions* (Cambridge University Press, Cambridge, 1958)
19. D.A. McQuarrie, *Statistical Mechanics*, 2nd edn. (University Science Books, New York, 2000)
20. J.J. Waterston, On the physics of media that are composed of free and elastic molecules in a state of motion. This paper was submitted to the Royal Society in 1846, but rejected and lost. It was recovered by Lord Rayleigh and published in full posthumously. Philos. Trans. **A183**, 1–79 (1893)
21. J.C. Maxwell, Paper read by prof. Maxwell at a meeting of the British Association at Aberdeen on 21 september 1859. The Scientific Papers of James Clerk Maxwell New York: Dover, ed W D Niven **1**, 377–409 (2003)
22. L. Boltzmann, Einige allgemeine sätze über wärmegleichgewicht. Wiener Berichte **63**, 679–711 (1871)
23. H.B. Callen, T.A. Welton, Irreversibility and generalized noise. Phys. Rev. **83**(1), 34–40 83:34–40 (1951)
24. H. Snelders, Fokker, adriaan dani l (1887-1972). https://resources.huygens.knaw.nl/bwn1880-2000/lemmata/bwn3/fokkerad (2013)
25. V. Manokhin, Andrey kolmogorov: Master of uncertainty and order. https://valeman.medium.com/andrey-kolmogorov-master-of-uncertainty-and-order-1080618e1afe (2025)
26. A.D. Fokker, Die mittlere energie rotierender elektrischer dipole im strahlungsfeld. Ann Physik **384**, 810–820 (1914)
27. M. Planck, Über einen satz der statistischen dynamik und seine erweiterung in der quantentheorie. Sitzungsberichte der Preussischen Akademie der Wissenschaften zu Berlin **24**, 324–341 (1917)
28. A. Kolmogorov, Über die analytischen methoden in der wahrscheinlichkeitstheorie [on analytical methods in the theory of probability]. Math. Ann. **104**, 415–458 (1931)
29. M. von Smoluchowski, Über brownsche molekularbewegung unter einwirkung usserer kr fte und deren zusammenhang mit der verallgemeinerten diffusionsgleichung. Ann Physik **104**, 1103–1112 (1915)

30. S. Chandrasekhar, Stochatics problems in physics and astronomy. Rev. Mod. Phys. **15**, 1–89 (1943)
31. R.B. Bird, C.F. Curtiss, R.C. Armstrong, O. Hassager, *Dynamics of Polymeric Liquids. Vol. 2: Kinetic Theory*, 2nd edn. (Wiley, New York, 1991)

Chapter 4
Polymer Chains and Lopsided Dumbbells

Mainly About Dumbbells

The analysis proceeds in three main steps, realizing that there are two widely separated length scales in the problem, a macrolength scale L representative of the size of the apparatus, and a microlength scale a representative of the size of a microstructure feature, $a \ll L$,

1. Step 1. Identify the most relevant features of the microstructure fluid in question, and come up with an idealized micromechanic model. This may often be a suspension of particles, droplets or bubbles, or an entangled network of strands, for instance. Develop the Langevin equations for the simplified model;
2. Step 2. Connect the macro-observable stress tensor contributed by the microstructure (this is our "particle-contributed" stress) to the average quantities derived from the Langevin equations;
3. Step 3. Look for a close-form constitutive equation if possible. In many cases closure may not be possible, then look for closure approximations from the quality of fitting to the experimental results in the step below;
4. Step 4. Fit the model's predictions in some simple flows, and often a lack of fits may be traced to some missing physics in the modeling process. Here *AI* may be a good avenue for the modeling loop, see, for example, Lennon et al. [1].

Plenty of reading materials for this section exist, for example, Bird et al. [2], Graham [3], Huilgol and Phan-Thien [4], Larson [5], Lodge [6], Morrison [7], Phan-Thien and Mai-Duy [8], Tanner [9], Tanner and Walters [10], to name a few.

© The Author(s), under exclusive license to Springer Nature Singapore Pte Ltd. 2026

D. Pan et al., *Langevin Analysis of Microstructured Fluids*,
SpringerBriefs in Applied Sciences and Technology,
https://doi.org/10.1007/978-981-95-2318-4_4

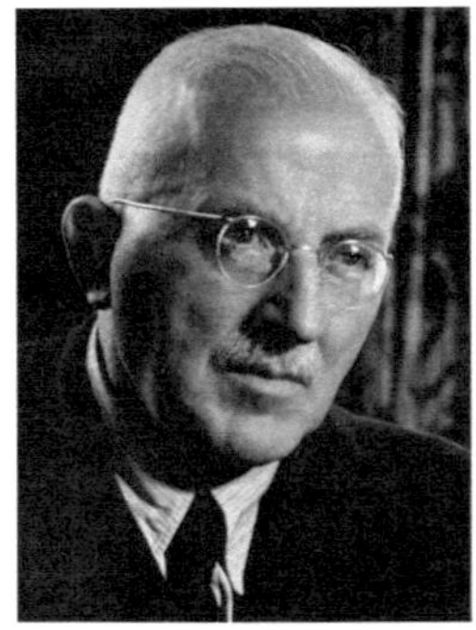

Fig. 4.1 Hermann Staudinger (1881–1965) was a German organic chemist. He demonstrated the existence of long-chain, not an aggregate of smaller-sized, molecules. The word *makromolekül* was due to him. He was awarded the 1953 Nobel Prize in Chemistry. (Public domain photograph, Nobel Foundation (1953))

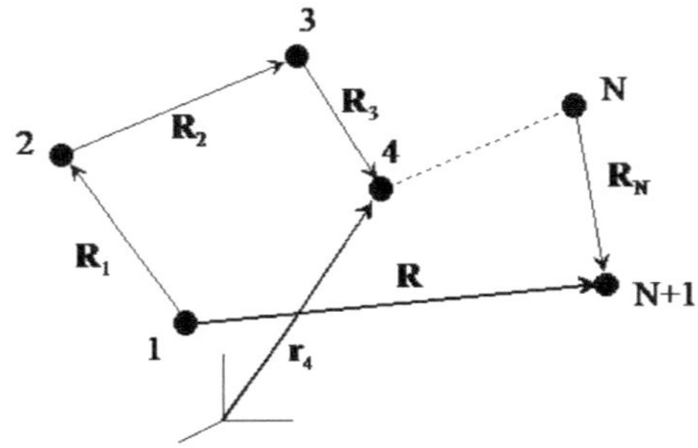

Fig. 4.2 A cartoon drawing of a freely-rotating ideal chain for a polymer chain

4.1 Polymer Chain

The idea of long-chain molecules, not just aggregates of smaller-sized molecules, took a long time for scientific acceptance: Staudinger (1881–1965) was the first who demonstrated this (Fig. 4.1); for this important discovery, he was awarded the 1953 Nobel Prize in Chemistry, for his "discoveries in the field of macromolecular chemistry", when the opposition had faded away. Now, we routinely speak of a *polymer* macromolecular molecule, which makes up of many repeating *monomer* units, typically of 10^5 or more units. It is this extraordinary long chain structure, its flexibility, its many possible configurations that endowed the polymers their unique properties. See Tanner and Walters [10] for a fascinating history of macromolecular concepts.

4.1.1 Freely-Rotating Ideal Chain in Random Walk

Here, our main aim is to model a dilute polymeric solution by *freely-rotating ideal chains* in a viscous fluid (Fig. 4.2).

Remark 4.1 The *freely-rotating* chain is perhaps the simplest model of a polymer chain. It consists of a number of fixed-length *phantom* links (of no physical dimension), or *bond vector* $\mathbf{R}_i$, all of the same *bond length* b, connected end-to-end in a linear fashion, freely-rotating at their ends.

Each bond vector,[1] $\mathbf{R}_i$, $i = 1, \ldots, N$ (there are N of them) can take all allowable configuration with uniform probability. A bond vector i is also uncorrelated with another bond vector j, $i \neq j$. Thus

$$\langle \mathbf{R}_i \rangle = 0, \quad \langle \mathbf{R}_i \mathbf{R}_j \rangle = b^2 \delta_{ij}. \tag{4.1}$$

Now the end-to-end vector of the chain is

$$\mathbf{R} = \sum_{j=1}^{N} \mathbf{R}_j. \tag{4.2}$$

Thus the chain has zero end-to-end vector in the mean:

$$\langle \mathbf{R} \rangle = \sum_{j=1}^{N} \langle \mathbf{R}_j \rangle = \mathbf{0}. \tag{4.3}$$

This is not a useful result and is expected, since all the bond vectors are phantom, isotropic and possess all available configuration in space with uniform probability. For the mean square end-to-end,

$$\langle \mathbf{R} \cdot \mathbf{R} \rangle = \left\langle R^2 \right\rangle = \sum_{j=1}^{N} \sum_{k=1}^{N} \left\langle \mathbf{R}_j \cdot \mathbf{R}_k \right\rangle = \sum_{j=1}^{N} \left\langle \mathbf{R}_j \cdot \mathbf{R}_j \right\rangle + \sum_{j=1}^{N} \sum_{k \neq j}^{N} \left\langle \mathbf{R}_j \cdot \mathbf{R}_k \right\rangle. \tag{4.4}$$

The last double summation on the right of (4.4) is nil, in view of (4.1). Thus

$$\left\langle R^2 \right\rangle = N b^2. \tag{4.5}$$

Remark 4.2 A measure of the curled-up size of a chain is expected to scale with $\sqrt{N} b$. Various non-freely-rotating chains (of fixed angle constraint between neighboring bond vectors) have been considered [11], with the result

$$\left\langle R^2 \right\rangle = K N b^2, \tag{4.6}$$

where K is a constant depending on the geometry constraint. Since N is large, the fully stretched length of a chain $Nb \gg \sqrt{KN} b$: it is difficult to stretch a polymer

---

[1] Sometimes known as a Kuhn segment [11].

chain to its full length. Flows that can do this are called *strong*; otherwise they are called *weak* [9].

4.1.2 Diffusion Equation

The end-to-end vector for a chain, Eq. (4.2), is a stochastic process, with $\phi(\mathbf{R}, N)$ represents the probability density distribution function for a chain of N bond vectors, with end-to-end vector $\mathbf{R}$.

Now, let's consider a chain of N segments, with an end-to-end vector of $\mathbf{R} - \mathbf{b}$. The probability of $N + 1$ segments having an end-to-end vector $\mathbf{R}$ is precisely the probability of the last segment ($N + 1$) having a bond vector $\mathbf{b}$, conditional on the first N segments having an end-to-end vector of $\mathbf{R} - \mathbf{b}$:

$$\phi\left(\mathbf{R}; N+1\right) = \int \phi\left(\mathbf{R} - \mathbf{b}; N\right) \psi_b\left(\mathbf{b}\right) d\mathbf{b}, \tag{4.7}$$

where $\psi_b(\mathbf{b})$ is the probability, or the transition probability, of having a bond vector $\mathbf{b}$. This is precisely the property of Markov processes (Fig. 4.3), see our short discussion in Problem 3.4 and also Lin [12] for a good discussion on Markov processes. Note that $\mathbf{b}$ is completely independent of the current state, and what happens at any given instant depends only on the instantaneous state of the system, not on its previous history.

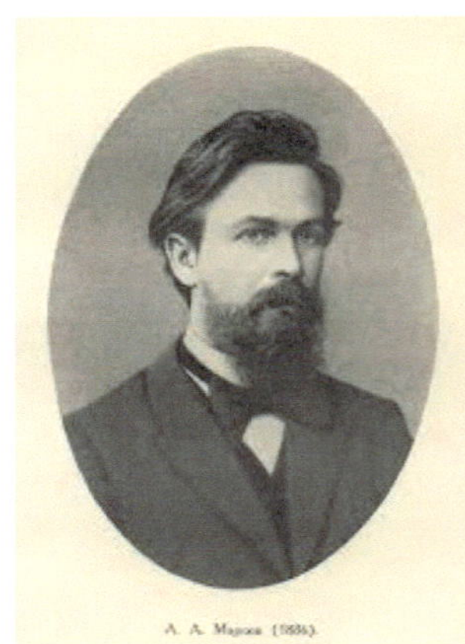

Fig. 4.3 Andrey Andreyevich Markov (1856–1922) was a Russian mathematician, best known for his contributions in stochastic process. *Markov process, Markov chain* were named after him. He believed in chances, not in God, and he had requested his own excommunication, after Leo Tolstoy's excommunication from the Russian Orthodox Church—the Church complied. (Public domain photograph by unknown author)

Now, Eq. (4.7) can be expanded in a Taylor's series for $|\mathbf{b}| \ll |\mathbf{R}|$,

$$\phi(\mathbf{R};\mathbf{N}) + \frac{\partial}{\partial \mathbf{N}}\phi(\mathbf{R};\mathbf{N}) + \ldots = \int d\mathbf{b}\psi_b(\mathbf{b}) \times \left[\phi(\mathbf{R};\mathbf{N}) - \mathbf{b}\cdot\nabla\phi(\mathbf{R};\mathbf{N}) + \frac{\mathbf{1}}{\mathbf{2!}}\mathbf{bb}:\nabla\nabla\phi(\mathbf{R};\mathbf{N}) + \cdots\right]. \tag{4.8}$$

Note that $\psi_b(\mathbf{b})$ is the probability density distribution for the bond vector; furthermore is an isotropic vector (having no preferred direction in space), thus

$$\int \psi_b(\mathbf{b})\,d\mathbf{b} = 1, \quad \int \mathbf{b}\psi_b(\mathbf{b})\,d\mathbf{b} = \mathbf{0}, \quad \int \mathbf{bb}\psi_b(\mathbf{b})\,d\mathbf{b} = \frac{b^2}{3}\mathbf{I}. \text{ (why?)}$$

These yield the following diffusion equation for the chain,

$$\frac{\partial}{\partial N}\phi(\mathbf{R};N) = \frac{b^2}{6}\nabla^2\phi(\mathbf{R};N). \tag{4.9}$$

Note that the steps in the derivation leading to Eq. (4.9) are very similar to those of Problem (3.4). Prescribing an initial condition for the chain $\mathbf{R}$ is equivalent to assigning a delta function to the probability:

$$\lim_{N\to 0}\phi(\mathbf{R};N) = \delta(\mathbf{R}). \tag{4.10}$$

The solution to (4.9) subjected to this initial condition is called the *Gaussian distribution*, named after Gauss (for a portray, see Fig. 1.4),

$$\phi(\mathbf{R};N) = \left(\frac{3}{2\pi N b^2}\right)^{3/2}\exp\left(-\frac{3R^2}{2Nb^2}\right). \tag{4.11}$$

This solution returns a finite probability at large bond length (larger than the fully stretched length Nb) and thus is not physical. A better treatment yields the *Langevin probability distribution*, which vanishes for $R \geq Nb$ as required by the physics [11].

4.1.3 Rouse Model for Polymer Chain

In the Rouse model proposed by Rouse [13], a polymer chain in a viscous solvent is modeled by $(N+1)$ viscous points of resistance (called *beads*,[2] located at

[2] The beads have negligible mass—more correctly, the inertial time formed by the viscous drag and the mass is small compared to the relaxation time of its Langevin system, see the discussion in Sect. 3.3.2.

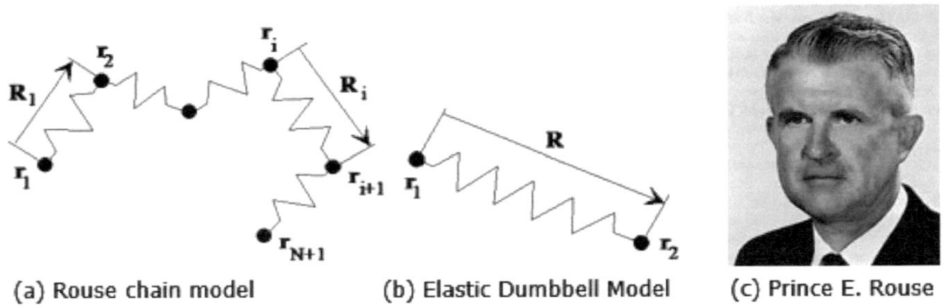

Fig. 4.4 **a** *Rouse model* for a polymer chain consists of N points with Stokes resistance, connected to neighboring beads by linear springs; **b** The simplest version of Rouse model is the *dumbbell model*, with two beads connected by a linear spring; **c** Princ E. Rouse (1917–2003) was an American physicist, his description of the now-known as "Rouse dynamics" has earned him the Bingham Medal in 1966. (Public domain photograph, source: Los Alamos National Laboratory)

$\mathbf{r}_i, i = 1, \ldots, N + 1$, connected by N linear springs (Fig. 4.4a). Since the springs are phantom having no physical dimension, there is no hydrodynamic interaction among the beads, nor chain self entanglement (hydrodynamic interactions and entanglements between different chains are not considered because of the dilute assumption). This model has now been invariably the starting discussion point in polymer texts. Reducing the number of segments to just one, one has the ubiquitous pedagogic *dummbell model* (Fig. 4.4b), consisting of two beads connected by a linear spring; its discussion is found in almost all Rheology textbooks, e.g., [2]. We shall return to the dumbbell model later.

The forces acting on the chain include

1. *Hydrodynamic forces*: as the Reynolds number based on the size of the bead or the segment is negligibly small, Stokes resistances localized at the beads can be used to model this. Thus the hydrodynamic interactions can be represented by Stokes drag/damping forces at the beads:

$$\mathbf{F}_i^{(d)} = \zeta\left(\mathbf{u}_i - \dot{\mathbf{r}}_i,\right), \tag{4.12}$$

where $\dot{\mathbf{r}}_i - \mathbf{u}_i$ is the relative velocity of the bead to the fluid velocity $\mathbf{u}_i$ at the bead, and ζ is the Stokes resistance factor; it is $6\pi\eta_s a$ for a solvent viscosity of η_s, and for a spherical bead of radius a. This hydrodynamic interaction model (4.12) is referred to as *free-draining assumption*, it neglects hydrodynamics interactions among the beads, and any directional preference of the segment; we shall not discuss these here, but refer to Bird et al. [2], Huilgol and Phan-Thien [4] for more comprehensive treatments.

2. *Tension in the chain segment*: a chain segment is composed of several monomer units, having a large number of configurations. At rest it tends to adopt a coiled-up configuration; a force is required to pullthe segment apart due to fewer configu-

rations available (i.e., lower entropy). This force is related to the *free energy* of the segment, $\Phi_r\left(\mathbf{r}_j\right)$, given by Flory [11]

$$\Phi_r\left(\mathbf{r}_j\right) = A\left(T\right) - kT \ln \phi\left(\mathbf{r}_j\right) \tag{4.13}$$

where $A(T)$ is a function of the temperature, and $\phi\left(\mathbf{r}_j\right)$ is the probability distribution for the segment. The entropic force on the segment is

$$\mathbf{F}_i^{(s)} = -\frac{\partial \Phi_r}{\partial \mathbf{r}_i} = kT\frac{\partial \ln \phi}{\partial \mathbf{r}_i}. \tag{4.14}$$

For a Gaussian chain of N segments, bond length b, where the distribution is Gaussian (4.11), the entropic force to maintain a end-to-end separation vector $\mathbf{R}$ is

$$\mathbf{F} = \frac{3kT}{Nb^2}\mathbf{R}. \tag{4.15}$$

Applied to the individual segment of the Rouse model, containing n sub-units, each of bond length b, then the force on bead i is

$$\mathbf{F}_i^{(s)} = \frac{3kT}{nb^2}\left(\mathbf{r}_{i+1} - \mathbf{r}_i + \mathbf{r}_{i-1} - \mathbf{r}_i\right) = \frac{3kT}{nb^2}\left(\mathbf{R}_i - \mathbf{R}_{i-1}\right). \tag{4.16}$$

This implies that the adjacent beads are connected by linear springs of stiffness

$$H = \frac{3kT}{nb^2}. \tag{4.17}$$

A better distribution taking into account of the finite segment length leads to the *inverse Langevin spring law*, Bird et al. [2].

3. *Brownian forces*: finally, the beads are subjected to numerous tiny impulses from the solvent molecules. These impulses are modeled by Brownian forces $\mathbf{F}_i^{(b)}(t)$, with statistics (3.28).

We leave the development of a Langevin system for a chain for the next sections—it will be more useful pedagogically to accomplish this for the more simpler dumbbell models.

4.1.4 Stress Contributed by Polymer Chains

Continuing with our modeling effort, in Step 2 we wish to relate the macro-observable stress tensor to the mean quantities derived from the micromechanics.

There are different ways to accomplish this. In the probabilistic approach, the probability of a polymer chain straddling a surface contributing to the traction on the surface (and thus the contributed stress) can be calculated leading to an expression

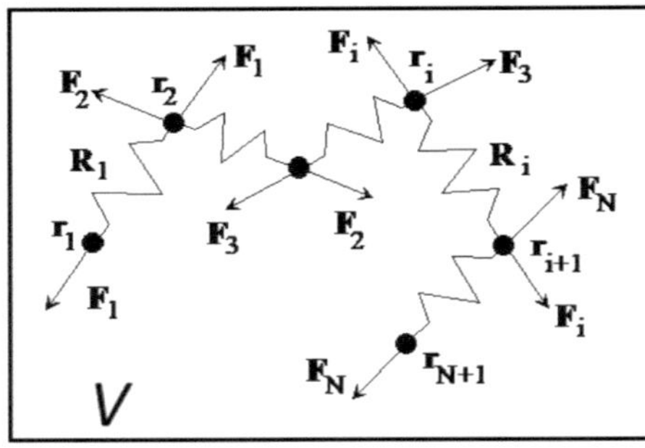

Fig. 4.5 A representative volume V containing one polymer chain, $V = V_s \cup \sum_p V_p$, where V_s is the volume occupied by the solvent, and $\sum_p V_p$ is the total volume occupied by the polymer chain, with V_p the volume of a bead

for the contributed stress [2, 9]. In another approach, the free energy of the chain can be calculated, together with the work done in relation to the dissipation from which the polymer-contributed stress can be derived, Larson [5]. In this Lecture, we present a mechanic approach based on volume average due to Landau and Lifshitz [14] and Batchelor [15].

Let V be a *representative volume*, a volume containing enough particles/polymer chains to make it statistically significant. $V = V_s \cup \sum_p V_p$ consists of the solvent volume V_s and the polymer volume $\cup \sum_p V_p$. Since we only deal with dilute systems here, V can be chosen to contain exactly one polymer chain, see Fig. 4.5, there is no nearby chain; however, we still use the sum $\sum_p$ over the chains p for a slightly more general result. V_p can be regarded as the total volume of beads on chain p, at this level of approximation. The volume concentration of the polymer is

$$\varphi = \frac{1}{V} \sum_p V_p. \tag{4.18}$$

On the length scale of the apparatus, one sees a *homogenized medium*, where the effective stress is the *volume average stress* $\langle \mathbf{T} \rangle$ over this representative volume,

$$\langle \mathbf{T} \rangle = \frac{1}{V} \int_V \mathbf{T} dV = \underbrace{\frac{1}{V} \int_{V_s} \mathbf{T} dV}_{\text{solvent}} + \underbrace{\frac{1}{V} \sum_p \int_{V_p} \mathbf{T} dV}_{\text{polymer}}. \tag{4.19}$$

Here, $\mathbf{T}^{(s)}$ and $\mathbf{T}^{(p)}$ are the stresses in the solvent and the polymer, respectively. This consists of a *solvent contribution* (the term labeled "solvent"), a *polymer contribution* (the term labeled "polymer").

The solvent contribution can be written as

$$\frac{1}{V} \int_{V_s} \mathbf{T}^{(s)} dV = \frac{1}{V} \int_V \mathbf{T}^{(s)} dV - \frac{1}{V} \sum_p \int_{V_p} \mathbf{T}^{(s)} dV. \tag{4.20}$$

The first term on the right of (4.20) is the solvent average stress[3]:

$$\frac{1}{V}\int_V \mathbf{T}^{(s)} dV = -p_1\mathbf{I} + 2\eta_s\mathbf{D}, \tag{4.21}$$

where p_1 is a hydrodynamic pressure, η_s is the solvent viscosity, and $\mathbf{D} = \frac{1}{2}\left(\mathbf{L} + \mathbf{L}^T\right)$ is the strain rate tensor, $\mathbf{L} = (\nabla\mathbf{u})^T$ the velocity gradient tensor,[4] and $\mathbf{u}$ the fluid velocity.

The Newtonian assumption can be used in the second term on the right of (4.21) and divergence theorem can be applied to yield

$$\begin{aligned}\frac{1}{V}\sum_p \int_{V_p} \mathbf{T}^{(s)} dV &= \frac{1}{V}\sum_p \int_{V_p} \left[-p\mathbf{I} + \eta_s\left(\nabla\mathbf{u} + \nabla\mathbf{u}^T\right)\right] dV \\ &= -p_2\mathbf{I} + \frac{\eta_s}{V}\sum_p \int_{S_p} (\mathbf{un} + \mathbf{nu})\, dS. \end{aligned} \tag{4.22}$$

At this level of approximation, the beads are regarded as rigid particles, the fluid velocity is uniform on a particle surface and divergence theorem can be applied again:

$$\int_{S_p} \mathbf{un} dS = \mathbf{u}\int_{S_p} \mathbf{n} dS = \mathbf{0}.$$

Thus, the solvent contribution is simply the Newtonian expression (4.21), with a different hydrodynamic pressure.

Returning to the polymer contribution to the effective stress (term labeled "polymer" in Eq. (4.19)), we note that, no matter what the polymer material, the force balance condition $\partial T_{ij}/\partial x_j = 0$ holds in the beads, where T_{ij} is the stress tensor in the polymer volume V_p; from this condition $T_{ik} = \partial\left(T_{ij}x_k\right)/\partial x_j$. Thus the polymer-contributed stress is, after an application of the divergence theorem,

$$\frac{1}{V}\sum_p \int_{V_p} \mathbf{T} dV = \frac{1}{V}\sum_p \int_{S_p} \mathbf{xT}\cdot\mathbf{n} dS = \nu \int_{S_p} \mathbf{xT}\cdot\mathbf{n} dS. \tag{4.23}$$

where ν is the *number density* of the polymer chains (chains per unit volume), S_p is the surface of a generic chain V_p, with $\mathbf{n}$ its normal outward unit vector. Now the integral over the generic chain can be replaced by a sum of integrals over the beads:

$$\int_{S_p} \mathbf{xT}\cdot\mathbf{n} dS = \sum_i \int_{\text{bead } i} \mathbf{xT}\cdot\mathbf{n} dS. \tag{4.24}$$

---

[3] The solvent is always assumed Newtonian.

[4] Note the transpose operation in the definition; in Cartesian tensor, $L_{ij} = \nabla_j u_i = (\nabla\mathbf{u})^T_{ij}$.

On bead i, the position vector can be approximated as the position of bead i, $\mathbf{r}_i$, and can be taken outside the integral; the remaining integral, $\int_{S_p} \mathbf{T} \cdot \mathbf{n} dS$ returns the drag force on the bead, $\mathbf{F}_i^{(d)} = -\zeta\,(\mathbf{P}_i - \mathbf{u}_i)$. This drag force is balanced by the sum of the *connector forces* $\mathbf{F}_{i,i-1} + \mathbf{F}_{i,i+1}$, and the Brownian force $\mathbf{F}_i^{(b)}$. Here $\mathbf{F}_{i,j}$ is the connector force on i by the neighboring node j, $j = i \pm 1, 1 \geq j \geq N+1$, and $\mathbf{F}_{i,j} = -\mathbf{F}_{j,i}$ (special consideration is required for beads $i = 1, N+1$). The connector forces arise from the constraints between the neighboring beads. Thus

$$\begin{aligned}
\sum_i \mathbf{x}_i \int_{\text{bead } i} \mathbf{T}\mathbf{n} dS &= \sum_i \mathbf{r}_i \left(-\mathbf{F}_{i,i-1} - \mathbf{F}_{i,i+1} - \mathbf{F}_i^{(b)}\right) \\
&= \mathbf{r}_1 \mathbf{F}_{1,2} + \mathbf{r}_2 \left(\mathbf{F}_{1,2} - \mathbf{F}_{2,3}\right) + \ldots + \mathbf{r}_{N=1} \mathbf{F}_{N+1} - \sum_{i+1}^{N+1} \mathbf{r}_i \mathbf{F}_i^{(b)} \\
&= \sum_{i=1}^{N} \mathbf{R}_i \mathbf{F}_i^{(c)} - \sum_{i=1}^{N+1} \mathbf{r}_i \mathbf{F}_i^{(b)},
\end{aligned} \tag{4.25}$$

where we have re-labeled $\mathbf{F}_i^{(c)} = \mathbf{F}_{i,i+1}$, $i = 1, \ldots, N$, the connector force on bead i be bead $i+1$, and define the i segment by

$$\mathbf{R}_i = \mathbf{r}_{i+1} - \mathbf{r}_i, \; i = 1, \ldots, N. \tag{4.26}$$

From Problem (4.2) we learn that the Brownian contributed stress is simply a hydrostatic stress, which can be lumped into the hydrostatic pressure. Thus the polymer-contributed stress is

$$\mathbf{S}^{(p)} = \nu \sum_{i=1}^{N} \left\langle \mathbf{R}_i \mathbf{F}_i^{(c)} \right\rangle = \nu \sum_{i=1}^{N} \langle H_i \mathbf{R}_i \mathbf{R}_i \rangle. \tag{4.27}$$

Here, the neighboring beads are connected by a spring of stiffness H. This special form for the polymer-contributed stress, Eq. (4.27), is named after Kramers [16], Bird et al. [2], see Fig. 4.6. Thus, the observable effective stress can be related to microstructure as

$$\langle \mathbf{T} \rangle = -p\mathbf{I} + \mathbf{S}^{(s)} + \mathbf{S}^{(p)} = -p\mathbf{I} + 2\eta_s \mathbf{D} + \nu \sum_{i=1}^{N} \langle H_i \mathbf{R}_i \mathbf{R}_i \rangle. \tag{4.28}$$

We have accomplished our goal in Step 2, relating the macro-observable stress to the microstructure mean quantities. It is possible to derive the constitutive equation for the Kramers expression (4.27) in Step 3, but we shall not pause to do that; rather we will concentrate on even a further simplification of the polymer chain to dumbbells.

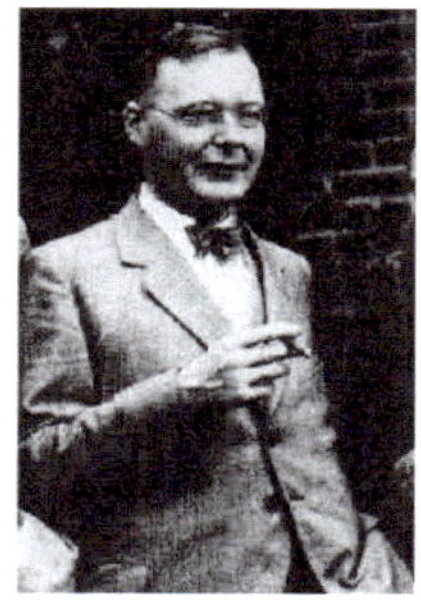

Fig. 4.6 Hendrik Anthony (Hans) Kramers (1894–1952) was a Dutch physicist, with major contributions in quantum mechanics. He is well-remembered in Rheology for the Kramers expression for the stress. (Public domain photograph)

4.2 Lopsided Dumbbell

For pedagogical purposes, we now focus on a simpler representation of a polymer chain, the *dumbbell model*. Figure 4.7 is a sketch of a lopsided rigid dumbbell, consisting of two unequal-sized bead located at $\mathbf{r}_1$ radius a_1, and $\mathbf{r}_2$ radius a_2, respectively; they are connected by a rigid phantom rod. If the rigid rod is replaced by an elastic spring, then an elastic dumbbell results—the elastic dumbbell model for a polymer chain was first proposed by Kuhn [18], and is a ubiquitous model discussed in all texts in polymer rheology, Bird et al. [2], Tanner [9]. This section is patterned after Phan-Thien et al. [17, 19].

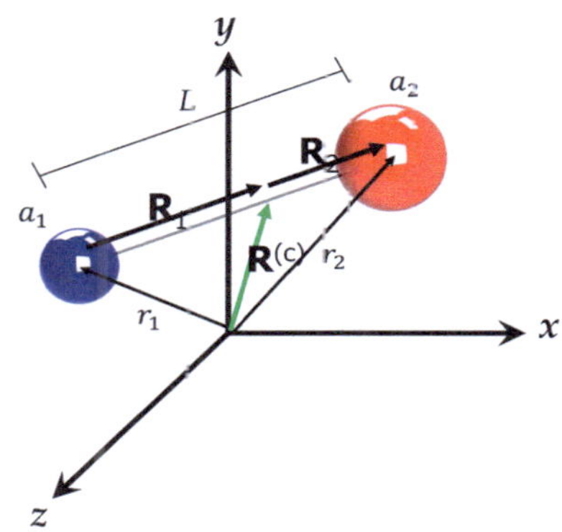

Fig. 4.7 A rigid dumbbell model consists of two-unequal-sized spheres connected by a rigid phantom rod. For an elastic lopsided dumbbell, replace the rigid connector rod by an elastic spring, [17]

4.2.1 Geometric Consideration

As the dumbbell's beads move in a viscous fluid of viscosity η_s in a zero Reynolds number flow, they feel a viscous Stokes frictional factor of $\zeta_i = 6\pi\eta_s a_i$; we may regard the ratio of the radii, or

$$\alpha \equiv \frac{\zeta_2}{\zeta_1} = \frac{6\pi\eta_s a_2}{6\pi\eta_s a_1} = \frac{a_2}{a_1} \tag{4.29}$$

as a definition of *lopsidedness*. It is not important which bead is the larger, and we may as well assume that bead 2 is larger than bead 1, as illustrated in Fig. 4.7.

We define the *center of resistance* $\mathbf{R}^{(c)}$ as

$$\mathbf{R}^{(c)} = \frac{\zeta_1}{\zeta_1+\zeta_2}\mathbf{r}_1 + \frac{\zeta_2}{\zeta_1+\zeta_2}\mathbf{r}_2. \tag{4.30}$$

The center of resistance divides the end-to-end vector $\mathbf{R} = \mathbf{r}_2 - \mathbf{r}_1$ in the ratio of $\zeta_1 : \zeta_2$. Indeed, define $bf R_i$ by

$$\mathbf{r}_1 = \mathbf{R}^{(c)} - \mathbf{R}_1,\ \mathbf{r}_2 = \mathbf{R}^{(c)} + \mathbf{R}_2,\ \mathbf{R} = \mathbf{R}_1 + \mathbf{R}_2, \tag{4.31}$$

then $\mathbf{R}_i$ is parallel to $\mathbf{R}$, and

$$\begin{aligned}
\mathbf{R}_1 &= -\mathbf{r}_1 + \mathbf{R}^{(c)} = -\mathbf{r}_1 + \frac{\zeta_1}{\zeta_1+\zeta_2}\mathbf{r}_1 + \frac{\zeta_2}{\zeta_1+\zeta_2}\mathbf{r}_2\\
&= -\frac{\zeta_2}{\zeta_1+\zeta_2}\mathbf{r}_1 + \frac{\zeta_2}{\zeta_1+\zeta_2}\mathbf{r}_2\\
&= \frac{\zeta_2}{\zeta_1+\zeta_2}\mathbf{R}
\end{aligned} \tag{4.32}$$

$$\begin{aligned}
\mathbf{R}_2 &= \mathbf{r}_2 - \mathbf{R}^{(c)} = \mathbf{r}_2 - \frac{\zeta_1}{\zeta_1+\zeta_2}\mathbf{r}_1 - \frac{\zeta_2}{\zeta_1+\zeta_2}\mathbf{r}_2\\
&= -\frac{\zeta_1}{\zeta_1+\zeta_2}\mathbf{r}_1 + \frac{\zeta_1}{\zeta_1+\zeta_2}\mathbf{r}_2\\
&= \frac{\zeta_1}{\zeta_1+\zeta_2}\mathbf{R}.
\end{aligned} \tag{4.33}$$

Thus

$$\zeta_1\mathbf{R}_1 = \zeta_2\mathbf{R}_2. \tag{4.34}$$

To make progress, we shall assume either an elastic or a rigid connector; there are some common elements between the two cases, but repeating information between the two cases may be good pedagogically.

4.2.2 Elastic Dumbbell

4.2.2.1 Langevin Equations

First, we assume an elastic connector, with spring stiffness $H = 3kT/(nb^2)$ (*cf.* (4.17)), and with the Langevin equations,

$$\begin{aligned} m_1\ddot{\mathbf{r}}_1 &= \zeta_1(\mathbf{u}_1 - \dot{\mathbf{r}}_1) + H(\mathbf{r}_2 - \mathbf{r}_1) + \mathbf{F}_1^{(b)}(t), \\ m_2\ddot{\mathbf{r}}_2 &= \zeta_2(\mathbf{u}_2 - \dot{\mathbf{r}}_2) + H(\mathbf{r}_1 - \mathbf{r}_2) + \mathbf{F}_2^{(b)}(t). \end{aligned} \tag{4.35}$$

Here, the Brownian forces $\mathbf{F}_i^{(b)}(t)$ have the following statistics, *cf.* (3.28),

$$\begin{aligned} \langle \mathbf{F}_j^{(b)}(t)\rangle &= 0, \\ \langle \mathbf{F}_1^{(b)}(t+s)\,\mathbf{F}_2^{(b)}(t)\rangle &= 0, \\ \langle \mathbf{F}_1^{(b)}(t+s)\,\mathbf{F}_1^{(b)}(t)\rangle &= 2kT\zeta_1\delta(s)\,\mathbf{I}, \\ \langle \mathbf{F}_2^{(b)}(t+s)\,\mathbf{F}_2^{(b)}(t)\rangle &= 2kT\zeta_2\delta(s)\,\mathbf{I}. \end{aligned} \tag{4.36}$$

Once again, there are three time scales in the system (4.35), the relaxation time scale $\tau_r = O\left(\zeta_i H^{-1}\right)$, the inertial time scale $\tau_i = O\left(m\zeta_i^{-1}\right)$, and the fluctuation time scale τ_c of the Brownian forces. Note that, as $m_i \approx \frac{4}{3}\pi\rho_b a_i^3$, and $\zeta_i = 6\pi\eta_s a_i$, $\tau_i = O(\rho_b a_i^2/\eta_s)$, where ρ_b is the density of the bead's material, and $\tau_r = 2\pi\eta_s a_i nb^2/(kT)$. Thus, as $\tau_i/\tau_r \to 0$, the beads' inertia in Eq. (4.35) can be neglected; these equations can be combined to yield the equations of motion for the center of resistance and for the end-to-end vector

$$(\zeta_1 + \zeta_2)\,\dot{\mathbf{R}}^{(c)} = \zeta_1\mathbf{u}_1 + \zeta_2\mathbf{u}_2 + \mathbf{F}^{(b,c)}(t), \tag{4.37}$$

$$\zeta_2\dot{\mathbf{R}} = \zeta_2(\mathbf{u}_2 - \mathbf{u}_1) - H(1+\alpha)\,\mathbf{R} + \mathbf{F}^{(b,R)}(t), \tag{4.38}$$

where $\mathbf{F}^{(b,c)}(t)$, $\mathbf{F}^{(b,R)}(t)$ are the Brownian forces acting on the center of resistance and the end-to-end vector:

$$\mathbf{F}^{(b,c)}(t) = \mathbf{F}_1^{(b)}(t) + \mathbf{F}_2^{(b)}(t), \tag{4.39}$$

$$\mathbf{F}^{(b,R)}(t) = \mathbf{F}_2^{(b)}(t) - \alpha\mathbf{F}_1^{(b)}(t). \tag{4.40}$$

Their statistics can be found from (4.36):

$$\begin{aligned} \langle \mathbf{F}^{(b,c)}(t)\rangle &= 0 \\ \langle \mathbf{F}^{(b,c)}(t+s)\,\mathbf{F}^{(b,c)}(t)\rangle &= 2kT(\zeta_1+\zeta_2)\,\delta(s)\,\mathbf{I}, \end{aligned} \tag{4.41}$$

$$\begin{aligned} \langle \mathbf{F}^{(b,R)}(t)\rangle &= 0 \\ \langle \mathbf{F}^{(b,R)}(t+s)\,\mathbf{F}^{(b,R)}(t)\rangle &= 2kT\zeta_2(1+\alpha)\,\delta(s)\,\mathbf{I}. \end{aligned} \tag{4.42}$$

4.2.2.2 Velocity Expansion About $\mathbf{R}^{(c)}$

Next, the velocities that appear in (4.37)–(4.38) need to be evaluated. A Taylor's series expansion of the fluid velocity about the center of resistance yields

$$\mathbf{u}_1 = \mathbf{u}^{(c)} - \mathbf{R}^{(1)} \cdot \nabla \mathbf{u}^{(c)} + \frac{1}{2}\mathbf{R}^{(1)}\mathbf{R}^{(1)} : \nabla\nabla\mathbf{u}^{(c)} + HOT,$$
$$\mathbf{u}_2 = \mathbf{u}^{(c)} + \mathbf{R}^{(2)} \cdot \nabla \mathbf{u}^{(c)} + \frac{1}{2}\mathbf{R}^{(2)}\mathbf{R}^{(2)} : \nabla\nabla\mathbf{u}^{(c)} + HOT, \tag{4.43}$$

where HOT are terms of higher orders, and the superscript (c) refers to an evaluation at the center of resistance. The velocities appearing in (4.37)–4.38) can be evaluated, neglecting HOT,

$$\zeta_1\mathbf{u}_1 + \zeta_2\mathbf{u}_2 = (\zeta_1 + \zeta_2)\,\mathbf{u}^{(c)} + \frac{1}{2}\left[\zeta_1\mathbf{R}^{(1)}\mathbf{R}^{(1)} + \zeta_2\mathbf{R}^{(2)}\mathbf{R}^{(2)}\right] : \nabla\nabla\mathbf{u}^{(c)} \tag{4.44}$$

and

$$\mathbf{u}_2 - \mathbf{u}_1 = \mathbf{LR} + \frac{1}{2}\left[\mathbf{R}^{(2)}\mathbf{R}^{(2)} - \mathbf{R}^{(1)}\mathbf{R}^{(1)}\right] : \nabla\nabla\mathbf{u}^{(c)}, \tag{4.45}$$

where $\mathbf{L} = \nabla\mathbf{u}^{(c)T}$ is the velocity gradient evaluated at the center of resistance. Neglecting quadratic and higher-order terms, we have the Langevin equations for the center of resistance and the end-to-end vector:

$$\dot{\mathbf{R}}^{(c)} = \mathbf{u}^{(c)} + (\zeta_1 + \zeta_2)^{-1}\,\mathbf{F}^{(b,c)}(t), \tag{4.46}$$
$$\dot{\mathbf{R}} = \mathbf{LR} - (1+\alpha)\,\zeta_2^{-1}H\mathbf{R} + \zeta_2^{-1}\mathbf{F}^{(b,R)}(t), \tag{4.47}$$

where the statistics of the random forces are given in Eqs. (4.41–4.42).

4.2.2.3 Average Motions

Now, from (4.46), we learn that the dumbbell center of resistance moves just like a fluid particle:

$$\langle\dot{\mathbf{R}}^{(c)}\rangle = \mathbf{u}^{(c)}. \tag{4.48}$$

Remark 4.3 The dumbbell center of resistance departs from a fluid particle moving on a streamline in a non-homogeneous flow,[5] and is given by (*cf.*, see Problem (4.126)),

$$\langle\dot{\mathbf{R}}^{(c)}\rangle - \mathbf{u}^{(c)} = \frac{\zeta_1\zeta_2}{2\,(\zeta_1 + \zeta_2)^2}\langle\mathbf{RR}\rangle : \nabla\nabla\mathbf{u}^{(c)}. \tag{4.49}$$

---

[5] Homogeneous flows have constant velocity gradient.

From (4.47), the average motion of the end-to-end vector is

$$\langle\dot{\mathbf{R}}\rangle = \underbrace{\mathbf{L}\langle\mathbf{R}\rangle}_{\text{stretching}} - \underbrace{\left(\zeta_1^{-1} + \zeta_2^{-1}\right) H \langle\mathbf{R}\rangle}_{\text{restoring}}, \tag{4.50}$$

subject to an initial condition

$$\mathbf{R}(0) = \mathbf{R}_0. \tag{4.51}$$

Whether $\mathbf{R}(t)$ increases unboundedly in time depends on the two competing terms on the right side of (4.50), a flow-induced stretching term (labeled "stretching"), and a restoring term due to the spring forces (labeled "restoring").

We now define a time parameter, called the *relaxation time*, by

$$\lambda = \frac{\zeta_1\zeta_2}{2\left(\zeta_1 + \zeta_2\right) H}, \tag{4.52}$$

then (4.50) can be written as

$$\langle\dot{\mathbf{R}}\rangle = \mathbf{L}\langle\mathbf{R}\rangle - (2\lambda)^{-1}\langle\mathbf{R}\rangle. \tag{4.53}$$

The solution to this, subject to initial condition (4.51) has been explored in Problem 4.4,

$$\langle\mathbf{R}\rangle = e^{-t/2\lambda} e^{\mathbf{L}t}\mathbf{R}_0. \tag{4.54}$$

Remark 4.4 A flow is strong and effective in stretching the dumbbell, if one of the eigenvalues of $\mathbf{L}$ satisfies

$$\text{eigen}\,(\mathbf{L}) > \frac{1}{2\lambda}. \tag{4.55}$$

4.2.2.4 Smoluchowski Diffusion Equation

Since the motion in $\mathbf{R}^{(c)}$, it is not much of interest and ma be integrated out of the probability distribution; it is of more interest in the $\mathbf{R}$ motion, Eq. (4.47), and we now proceed to derive the Smoluchowski diffusion equation for $\mathbf{R}$, refer to Sect. 3.3.5, Remark 3.12. The steps involve calculating the drift velocity and the diffusivity. This is done by working with the differential version of (4.47),

$$\Delta\mathbf{R} = \left(\mathbf{L}\mathbf{R} - (1+\alpha)\,\zeta_2^{-1} H\mathbf{R}\right)\Delta t + \zeta_2^{-1}\int^{\Delta t} dt\,\mathbf{F}^{(b,R)}(t)\,, \tag{4.56}$$

where $\int^{\Delta t}$ is a short-hand notation for $\int_t^{t+\Delta t}$. From this, we find the drift velocity is given by

$$\lim_{\Delta t \to 0} \frac{\langle \Delta \mathbf{R} \rangle}{\Delta t} = \mathbf{LR} - \frac{1}{2\lambda}\mathbf{R}, \tag{4.57}$$

where the relaxation time λ is as given in (4.52).

Now the product $\Delta\mathbf{R}\Delta\mathbf{R}$ involves terms linear in $\int^{\Delta t} dt \mathbf{F}^{(b,R)}(t)$ (which do not contribute to its average), terms of $O(\Delta t)^2$ (to be neglected); thus to $O(\Delta t)$,

$$\begin{aligned}\langle \Delta\mathbf{R}\Delta\mathbf{R} \rangle &= \zeta_2^{-2} \int^{\Delta t} \int^{\Delta t} \left\langle \mathbf{F}^{(b,R)}(t)\, \mathbf{F}^{(b,R)}(t') \right\rangle dt dt' \\ &= 2kT(1+\alpha)\zeta_2^{-1} \int^{\Delta t} \int^{\Delta t} \delta(t-t')\, dt dt' \mathbf{I} \\ &= 2kT\left(\zeta_2^{-1} + \zeta_1^{-1}\right) \Delta t \mathbf{I}.\end{aligned} \tag{4.58}$$

Thus, the Smoluchowski diffusion equation for the process $\mathbf{R}$ is

$$\begin{aligned}\frac{\partial \phi}{\partial t} &= \lim_{\Delta t \to 0} \frac{\partial}{\partial \mathbf{R}} \cdot \left[\frac{\langle \Delta\mathbf{R}\Delta\mathbf{R}\rangle}{2\Delta t} \frac{\partial \phi}{\partial \mathbf{R}} - \frac{\langle \Delta \mathbf{R} \rangle}{\Delta t} \phi \right] \\ &= \frac{\partial}{\partial \mathbf{R}} \cdot \left[kT\left(\zeta_1^{-1} + \zeta_2^{-2}\right) \frac{\partial \phi}{\partial \mathbf{R}} - \left(\mathbf{L}\langle\mathbf{R}\rangle - (2\lambda)^{-1}\langle \mathbf{R}\rangle\right)\phi \right].\end{aligned} \tag{4.59}$$

If we now define the *effective* friction factor ζ by

$$\zeta = \frac{2\zeta_1\zeta_2}{\zeta_1 + \zeta_2} \iff \frac{2}{\zeta} = \frac{1}{\zeta_1} + \frac{1}{\zeta_2}, \tag{4.60}$$

the *i.e., harmonic mean* of the two friction factors, then

$$\frac{\partial \phi}{\partial t} = \frac{\partial}{\partial \mathbf{R}} \cdot \left[\frac{2kT}{\zeta} \frac{\partial \phi}{\partial \mathbf{R}} - \left(\mathbf{L}\langle \mathbf{R} \rangle - \frac{2H}{\zeta} \langle \mathbf{R} \rangle \right) \phi \right], \tag{4.61}$$

which is identical to the diffusion equation for a *symmetric dumbbell* with a friction factor ζ.

Remark 4.5 The Langevin equation is considered solved when the probability density distribution function is specified. This implies that all the results derived for a symmetric elastic dumbbell can be taken over for a lopsided dumbbell, simply with the replacement of the friction factor for the symmetric dumbbell by the harmonic mean of the friction factors on the lopsided dumbbell. Since the friction factor is proportional to the radius, one can also simply replace the lopsided dumbbell with an equivalent symmetric dumbbell with beads' radius of

$$a = \frac{2a_1 a_2}{a_1 + a_2} \iff \frac{2}{a} = \frac{1}{a_1} + \frac{1}{a_2}. \tag{4.62}$$

Abdel-Khalik and Bird [20] arrived at this conclusion for a lopsided rigid dumbbell.

4.2.2.5 Stress and Configuration Tensors

For a dumbbell, the average stress is simply, from (4.27–4.28),

$$\mathbf{T} = -p\mathbf{I} + \mathbf{S}^{(s)} + \mathbf{S}^{(p)} = -p\mathbf{I} + 2\eta_s \mathbf{D} + \nu H \langle \mathbf{RR} \rangle, \tag{4.63}$$

where p is the hydrodynamics pressure, $\mathbf{S}^{(s)} = 2\eta_s \mathbf{D}$ is the viscous solvent stress, $\mathbf{D} = \frac{1}{2}\left(\nabla \mathbf{u}^T + \nabla \mathbf{u}\right)$ is the strain rate tensor, $\mathbf{S}^{(p)} = \nu H \langle \mathbf{RR} \rangle$ is the polymer-contributed stress, and ν is the number density of dumbbells.

$\langle \mathbf{RR} \rangle$ is called the *configuration tensor*; for an elastic dumbbell suspension, it is simply proportional to the polymer-contributed stress. The evolution equation for $\langle \mathbf{RR} \rangle$ is also the evolution equation for the polymer-contributed stress, or the *constitutive equation*. To develop this evolution equation we can either use the Smoluchowski diffusion equation (4.61) and then form the relevant averages, or use the Langevin equation (4.47) directly—our choice here is the latter. From the Langevin equation (4.47),

$$\begin{aligned} \frac{d}{dt}(\mathbf{RR}) &= \mathbf{R}\dot{\mathbf{R}} + \dot{\mathbf{R}}\mathbf{R} \\ &= \mathbf{L}.\mathbf{RR} + \mathbf{RR}.\mathbf{L}^T \\ &- 2(1+\alpha)\zeta_2^{-1} H \mathbf{RR} + \zeta_2^{-1}\left(\mathbf{R}\mathbf{F}^{(b,R)}(t) + \mathbf{F}^{(b,R)}(t)\mathbf{R}\right). \end{aligned} \tag{4.64}$$

Oldroyd (see Fig. 4.8) [21] introduced the *upper convected derivative*

$$\frac{\delta}{\delta t}(\cdot) = \frac{d}{dt}(\cdot) - \mathbf{L}(\cdot) - (\cdot)\mathbf{L}^T. \tag{4.65}$$

With this definition, the evolution of the conformation tensor is

$$\frac{\delta}{\delta t}\langle \mathbf{RR} \rangle + 2(1+\alpha)\frac{H}{\zeta_2}\langle \mathbf{RR} \rangle = \frac{1}{\zeta_2}\left\langle \mathbf{R}\mathbf{F}^{(b,R)} + \mathbf{F}^{(b,R)}\mathbf{R}\right\rangle. \tag{4.66}$$

The terms on the right side of (4.66) can be evaluated by using the widely different time scale between a kinematic quantity $Q(\mathbf{R}, t)$ and the fluctuating time scale of the Brownian forces to equate the average at time t to that of time Δt, where Δt

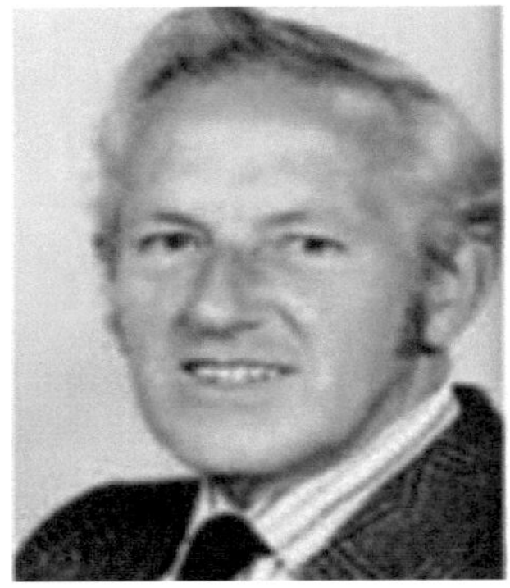

Fig. 4.8 James Gardner Oldroyd (1921–1982) was a British mathematician and well-known rheologist. His seminal paper [21] laid down the general principles in formulating constitutive relations. A fascinating account was given in [10], Sect. 4.2.

is small in the relaxation time scale τ_r, but large compared to the fluctuating time scale τ_c:

$$\left\langle Q(\mathbf{R},t)\mathbf{F}^{(b,R)}(t)\right\rangle = \left\langle Q(\mathbf{R},\Delta t)\mathbf{F}^{(b,R)}(\Delta t)\right\rangle. \tag{4.67}$$

Thus

$$\begin{aligned}\left\langle \mathbf{R}\mathbf{F}^{(b,R)}\right\rangle &= \left\langle \mathbf{R}\,(\Delta t)\,\mathbf{F}^{(b,R)}\,(\Delta t)\right\rangle \\ &= \zeta_2^{-1}\int_0^{\Delta t} dt \left\langle \mathbf{F}^{(b,R)}\,(t)\,\mathbf{F}^{(b,R)}\,(\Delta t)\right\rangle \\ &= kT\,(1+\alpha)\,\mathbf{I}.\end{aligned} \tag{4.68}$$

Here, terms linear in $\mathbf{F}^{(b,R)}$ do not contribute to the average and therefore not included here. Terms $O(\Delta t^2)$ are also neglected, and the statistics (4.42) have been used, where the $\int_0^{\Delta t}$ on the symmetric Dirac delta function returns a value of $1/2$. Then

$$\frac{\delta}{\delta t}\langle \mathbf{RR}\rangle + 2\frac{\zeta_1+\zeta_2}{\zeta_2\zeta_1}H\,\langle \mathbf{RR}\rangle = 2kT\frac{(\zeta_1+\zeta_2)}{\zeta_1\zeta_2}\mathbf{I}. \tag{4.69}$$

Using the equivalent friction factor (4.60), and the relaxation time (4.52), one finally ends up with

$$\lambda\frac{\delta}{\delta t}\langle \mathbf{RR}\rangle + \langle \mathbf{RR}\rangle = \frac{1}{3}R_e^2\mathbf{I}, \tag{4.70}$$

where

$$R_e^2 = \frac{kT}{H} = nb^2 \tag{4.71}$$

is the equilibrium mean square of the dumbbell, *cf.* (4.17). Since the polymer stress is proportional to $\langle \mathbf{RR}\rangle$, Eq. (4.63), one immediately finds the constitutive equation for the polymer stress:

$$\lambda \left(\frac{d}{dt}\mathbf{S}^{(p)} - \mathbf{L}\mathbf{S}^{(p)} - \mathbf{S}^{(p)}\mathbf{L}^T \right) + \mathbf{S}^{(p)} = G\mathbf{I}, \tag{4.72}$$

where

$$G = \frac{1}{3}\nu n b^2 H = \nu kT. \tag{4.73}$$

Equation (4.72) is one of a few rare cases where an exact closed-form constitutive equation can be derived. It is named *Upper Convected Maxwell* (UCM) model by Oldroyd [21], after Maxwell linear viscoelastic relation derived by Maxwell for the dynamical theory of gases [22].

Remark 4.6 Problem (4.5) shows that an equivalent form to the UCM model is

$$\tau^{(p)} + \lambda \frac{\delta}{\delta t}\tau^{(p)} = 2\eta_p \mathbf{D}, \tag{4.74}$$

where

$$\eta_p = G\lambda = \frac{\nu\zeta n b^2}{12} = \frac{1}{2}\pi \nu a n b^2 \eta_s \tag{4.75}$$

is the polymer-contributed viscosity, a is the equivalent size of the beads, and

$$\mathbf{S}^{(p)} = G\mathbf{I} + \tau^{(p)}. \tag{4.76}$$

Note that $\mathbf{S}^{(p)}$ is proportional to $\langle \mathbf{RR} \rangle$, thus it is positive definite, and $\boldsymbol{\tau}^{(p)}$ may not. $\mathbf{S}^{(p)}$ may be preferred in numerical implementation; the lack of positive definiteness may be taken as an impending numerical instability.

Remark 4.7 By combining the solvent stress $\mathbf{S}^{(s)}$ and $\boldsymbol{\tau}^{(p)}$ into

$$\mathbf{S} = \mathbf{S}^{(s)} + \tau^{(p)} = 2\eta_s \mathbf{D} + \tau^{(p)}, \tag{4.77}$$

results in the *Oldroyd-B* model

$$\mathbf{S} + \lambda_1 \frac{\delta \mathbf{S}}{\delta t} = 2\eta \left(\mathbf{D} + \lambda_2 \frac{\delta \mathbf{D}}{\delta t} \right) \tag{4.78}$$

where $\lambda_1 = \lambda$ is the *relaxation time*, $\eta = \eta_s + \eta_p$ is the total viscosity, $\lambda_2 = \lambda\eta_s/\eta$ is the *retardation time*. Oldroyd [21] called this *fluid B*.

Remark 4.8 The integral equivalent to the UCM model (4.72) can be shown to be

$$\mathbf{S}^{(p)}(t) = \frac{G}{\lambda}\int_{-\infty}^{t} e^{(s-t)/\lambda}\mathbf{C}_t(s)^{-1}\, ds = G\mathbf{I} + \tau^{(p)}. \tag{4.79}$$

This is done by taking its time derivative and using the result in Problem (4.7). This integral constitutive relation is a typical example of fading memory: recent past deformation has more say than distant past (due to the negative exponential kernel in the integral). It is called the Lodge rubber-like liquid model [6], derived for a network of polymer strands, a model meant for concentrated polymer solutions and melts. It is remarkable that two models for two distinct microstructures, a dilute suspension of dumbbells and a concentrated network of polymer strands, share a common constitutive framework.

4.2.2.6 Simple Flows

Here, we summarize the predictions of a dilute suspension of elastic dumbbells in some simple flows.

Simple shear flows are a class of flows called *viscometric flows* [23]; they form the basis for measuring *viscometric functions* for the fluids: viscosity (shear stress/shear rate, $S_{12}/\dot{\gamma}$, first normal stress difference ($N_1 = S_{11} - S_{22}$) and second normal stress difference ($N_2 = S_{22} - S_{33}$). From Problem (4.8), we find that the Oldroyd-B model predicts a constant viscosity

$$\eta = \eta_s + \eta_p, \tag{4.80}$$

a first normal stress difference

$$N_1 = 2\eta_p \lambda \dot{\gamma}^2 \tag{4.81}$$

quadratic in the shear rate, and a zero second normal stress difference

$$N_2 = S_{22} - S_{33} = 0. \tag{4.82}$$

The viscosity in almost all polymer solutions decreases with shear rate, and thus the Oldroyd-B model is not good quantitatively; however, it provides a good qualitative trend, and for certain polymer liquids, known as *Boger fluids,* the model actually provided good predictions [24].

In a **small amplitude oscillatory shear** (SAOS) flow, where the shear strain is

$$\gamma = \gamma_0 \sin(\omega t), \quad \gamma_0 \ll 1, \tag{4.83}$$

the shear rate is

$$\dot{\gamma} = \dot{\gamma}_0 \cos(\omega t), \quad \dot{\gamma}_0 = \omega \gamma_0. \tag{4.84}$$

In this small strain, the flow is in the linear viscoelastic regime, and the shear stress is also sinusoidal, but neither in phase with the strain nor with the strain rate,

$$S_{12} = S' \sin \omega t + S'' \cos \omega t. \tag{4.85}$$

The part that is in phase with the strain (S') is used to define the storage modulus (G'), or the storage viscosity (η'') (this is the "elastic" part in "viscoelastic"),

$$G' = \frac{S'}{\gamma_0}, \quad \eta'' = \frac{S'}{\dot{\gamma}_0}, \quad G' = \omega\eta'', \tag{4.86}$$

and the part that is in phase with the strain rate is used to define the loss modulus (G''), or the dynamic viscosity (η') (this is the "viscous" part in "viscoelastic"),

$$G'' = \frac{S''}{\gamma_0}, \quad \eta' = \frac{S''}{\dot{\gamma}_0}, \quad G'' = \omega\eta'. \tag{4.87}$$

Remark 4.9 Working with complex number, the *complex viscosity*, η^*, defined as

$$\eta^* = \eta' - i\eta''. \tag{4.88}$$

The complex viscosity is a response of the shear stress to a complex shear rate, see Problem 4.9.

Flow along the centerline of a stretching filament can be approximated by **elongational flow**, where the velocity gradient is $[\mathbf{L}] = \text{diag}\left(\dot{\varepsilon}, -\dot{\varepsilon}/2, -dot\varepsilon/2\right),$. In this flow, the *elongational viscosity* is defined as

$$\eta_E = \frac{S_{11} - S_{22}}{\dot{\varepsilon}} = 3\eta_s + \frac{3\eta_p}{(1 - 2\lambda\dot{\varepsilon})(1 + \lambda\dot{\varepsilon})}. \tag{4.89}$$

Remark 4.10 The Oldroyd-B model predicts a finite elongational viscosity only when the elongational rate satisfies $-1 < \lambda\dot{\varepsilon} < 1/2$, see Problem 4.10.

The Trouton ratio, defined as η_E/η, increases from the Newtonian value of 3, when $\dot{\varepsilon} = 0$ and becomes unbounded when $\lambda\dot{\varepsilon}$ approaches either -1 of $1/2$.

4.2.2.7 Variants of Elastic Dumbbell Model

Various modifications of the standard elastic dumbbell model have been made. The obvious shortcoming of the dumbbell model is the linear spring that allows the dumbbell to be stretched indefinitely in a strong elongational flow, leading to a run-away stress. The simple fix is to turn the spring into a non-linear spring, with a finite extensibility, and there are several models for this.

Inverse Langevin spring force Here the connector force between the beads is, instead of the linear force law (4.17), Flory [11],

$$\mathbf{F} = \frac{kT}{b}\mathbf{p}\mathcal{L}^{-1}\left(\frac{R}{nb}\right), \quad \mathbf{p} = \frac{\mathbf{R}}{R},$$

where the *inverse Langevin* function is defined as $\mathcal{L}^{-1}(x) = \coth x - 1/x$.

Warner spring force: The inverse Langevin spring force may be inconvenient, its approximation, the *Warner spring force*, may be simpler to implement, Bird et al. [2]

$$\mathbf{F} = \frac{3kT}{nb^2}\mathbf{R}\left(1 - \frac{R^2}{nb^2}\right)^{-1}.$$

Finite extensible nonlinear elastic (FENE): Another modification of the Warner spring may be easier to implement numerically, the FENE model (and its invariants), Bird et al. [2], Tanner [9],

$$\mathbf{F} = K\mathbf{R}\left(1 - \left\langle\frac{R^2}{L^2}\right\rangle\right)^{-1}.$$

These nonlinear springs induce shear thinning in the viscosity and normal stress differences, and allow for a finite elongation viscosity at high elongational rate, Bird et al. [2], Tanner [9].

Rouse model: In this model (Fig. 4.4), N linear elastic dumbbells are connected end-to-end providing a better description for a polymer chain. The end result is a spectrum of UCM model, allowing flexibility of fitting SAOS data.

4.2.3 Rigid-Rod Dumbbell

Rigid dumbbell model is well-studied, as a starting point in kinetic macromolecular theory, for example, Bird et al. [2]. It could be a simple model for a rigid rod, where the interactions with the solvent take place at the two ends ("beads") of the rod. Examples of real systems with rod-like microstructures may include tobacco mosaic virus [2], lipid encapsulation of mRNA into vaccin [25] (a transmission electron microscope image is given in Fig. 4.9); other physical examples were cited in Phan-Thien et al. [17]; this section is patterned after this.

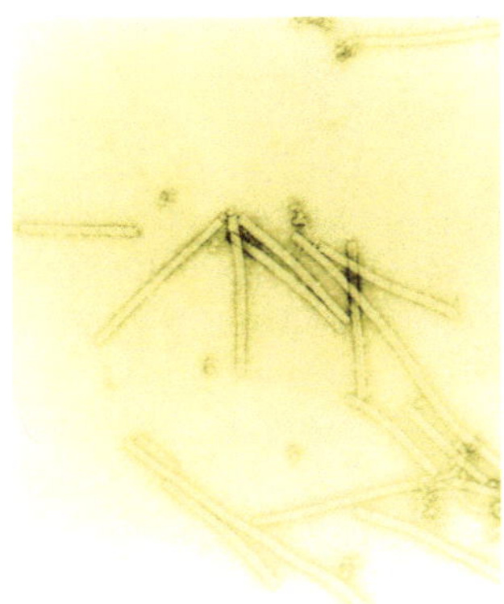

Fig. 4.9 Tobacco mosaic virus made visible in a transmission electron microscope, X 160,000. Its diameter is $\approx$ 20nm, and length $\approx$ 300nm, aspect ratio 15, source: Tobacco Mosiac Virus—Simple English Wikipedia, the free encyclopedia, https://sl.bing.net/bDS0yq4Xlym

We consider a dilute suspension of lopsided rigid dumbbells in a Newtonian fluid, a sketch of the problem is given in Fig. 4.7. All the definitions of beads' position, center of resistance, end-to-end vector, Stokes friction factors, and all the geometric results from the previous section, Sect. 4.2.1, are carried to this section. The only difference to the elastic dumbbell is that the connector between the two beads is a phantom rigid rod. We will repeat some of the equations in Sect. 4.2.2 for pedagogical purposes.

4.2.3.1 Langevin Equations

The equations of motion for the two beads are

$$\begin{aligned} m_1\ddot{\mathbf{r}}_1 &= \zeta_1\left(\mathbf{u}_1-\dot{\mathbf{r}}_1\right)+\mathbf{F}^{(c)}+\mathbf{F}_1^{(b)}(t), \\ m_2\ddot{\mathbf{r}}_2 &= \zeta_2\left(\mathbf{u}_2-\dot{\mathbf{r}}_2\right)-\mathbf{F}^{(c)}+\mathbf{F}_2^{(b)}(t). \end{aligned} \tag{4.90}$$

where $\mathbf{F}^{(c)}$ is the connector force that arises from the inextensibility of the connector rod. Other terms in the Langevin equation (4.90) have the same meaning as before. The Brownian forces $\mathbf{F}_i^{(b)}(t)$ have the same statistics as stated in Eq. (4.36). We furthermore define the unit vector along $\mathbf{R}$ as

$$\mathbf{R}=L\mathbf{p}. \tag{4.91}$$

Note that $\mathbf{R}\cdot\mathbf{R}=L^2$, and $\mathbf{p}\cdot\mathbf{p}=1$; this fact will be used to provide the constraint force $\mathbf{F}^{(c)}$ in Eq. (4.90).

Next, neglecting inertia, the Langevin equations in terms of the center of resistance and the end-to-end vector become

$$\begin{aligned} \left(\zeta_1+\zeta_2\right)\dot{\mathbf{R}}^{(c)} &= \zeta_1\mathbf{u}_1+\zeta_2\mathbf{u}_2+\mathbf{F}^{(b\ c)}(t), \\ \zeta_2\dot{\mathbf{R}} = \zeta_2\left(\mathbf{u}_2-\mathbf{u}_1\right) &- \frac{\zeta_1+\zeta_2}{\zeta_1}\mathbf{F}^{(c)}+\mathbf{F}^{(b,\mathbf{R})}(t), \end{aligned} \tag{4.92}$$

where the Brownian forces on $\mathbf{R}^{(c)}$ and $\mathbf{R}$ are given by (4.39–4.40), with the statistics determined by (4.41–4.42)

4.2.3.2 Constraint Connector Force

The rigidity of the rod demands that

$$\mathbf{R}\cdot\dot{\mathbf{R}}=0=\mathbf{p}\cdot\dot{\mathbf{R}}=\mathbf{p}\cdot\dot{\mathbf{p}}, \tag{4.93}$$

thus,

$$\mathbf{L}:\mathbf{Rp}-\frac{\zeta_1+\zeta_2}{\zeta_1\zeta_2}\mathbf{p}\cdot\mathbf{F}^{(c)}+\zeta_2^{-1}\mathbf{p}\cdot\mathbf{F}^{(b,\mathbf{R})}(t)=0. \tag{4.94}$$

Because $\mathbf{F}^{(c)}$ is parallel to $\mathbf{p}$, it can be expressed as

$$\mathbf{F}^{(c)}=\frac{\zeta_1\zeta_2}{\zeta_1+\zeta_2}\mathbf{L}:\mathbf{Rpp}+\frac{\zeta_1}{\zeta_1+\zeta_2}\mathbf{pp}\cdot\mathbf{F}^{(b,\mathbf{R})}(t). \tag{4.95}$$

It is noted that replacing the two friction factors ζ_1 and ζ_2 by their harmonic mean $\zeta=2\zeta_1\zeta_2/(\zeta_1+\zeta_2)$, Eq. (4.60), or equivalently, replacing the two radii a_i with their harmonic mean $a=2a_1a_2/(a_1+a_2)$ (see Remark 4.5), the connector force, and hence the Langevin equations, take the same form as a symmetric dumbbell [2].

Remark 4.11 In other words, the results for a symmetric dumbbell with equivalent harmonic mean friction factor can be carried over to the lopsided dumbbell. This was noted by Abdel-Khalik and Bird [20]; it was also valid for lopsided elastic dumbbell, Sect. 4.2.2 [19].

Using the result (4.95) in the $\mathbf{R}$-mode Langevin to obtain

$$\dot{\mathbf{R}}=\mathbf{L}\cdot\mathbf{R}-\mathbf{L}:\mathbf{ppR}+\zeta_2^{-1}(\mathbf{I}-\mathbf{pp})\,\mathbf{F}^{(b,\mathbf{R})}(t). \tag{4.96}$$

The filter $(\mathbf{I}-\mathbf{pp})$ on the Brownian force $\mathbf{F}^{(b,\mathbf{R})}(t)$ effectively allows only its components normal to $\mathbf{p}$ participate in the motion, as demanded by the rigidity of the rod (it can only affect rotational motion of the rod). $(\mathbf{I}-\mathbf{pp})\,\mathbf{F}^{(b,\mathbf{R})}(t)$ is justifiably called the rotational Brownian force.

4.2.3.3 Smoluchowski Diffusion Equation

Apart from calculating the mean motion and the migration of dumbbells in a flow, the $\mathbf{R}^{(c)}$-motion is not much of interest to us; hence it is discarded for now, and we concentrate on deriving the Smoluchowski diffusion equation for the $\mathbf{R}$-process. First we write down the differential form of (4.96),[6]

$$\Delta\mathbf{R}=(\mathbf{L}\cdot\mathbf{R}-\mathbf{L}:\mathbf{ppR})\,\Delta t+\zeta_2^{-1}\int_t^{t+\Delta t}dt\,(\mathbf{I}-\mathbf{pp})\,\mathbf{F}^{(b,\mathbf{R})}(t). \tag{4.97}$$

Thus, the drift velocity of the process is

$$\frac{\langle\Delta\mathbf{R}\rangle}{\Delta t}=\mathbf{L}\cdot\mathbf{R}-\mathbf{L}:\mathbf{ppR}. \tag{4.98}$$

[6] The reason for choosing to work with the integral, rather than the differential, of the Brownian motion should be now obvious to you.

The product $\Delta\mathbf{R}\Delta\mathbf{R}$ contains terms of $O(\Delta t^2)$, which can be neglected, terms linear in $\mathbf{F}^{(b,\mathbf{R})}(t)$, which have zero means and do not contribute to the diffusivity; finally, we obtain

$$\begin{aligned}\frac{\langle \Delta R_i \Delta R_j \rangle}{2\Delta t} &= \frac{\zeta_2^{-2}}{2\Delta t}\int_t^{t+\Delta t}\int_t^{t+\Delta t} dt d\tau \left(\delta_{ik} - p_i p_k\right)\left(\delta_{jm} - p_j p_m\right) \\ &\qquad \cdot \left\langle F_k^{(b,\mathbf{R})}(t)\, F_m^{(b,\mathbf{R})}(\tau)\right\rangle \\ &= kT\frac{\zeta_1+\zeta_2}{\zeta_1\zeta_2}\left(\delta_{ij} - p_i p_j\right). \end{aligned} \tag{4.99}$$

Thus the Smoluchowski diffusion for the process $\mathbf{R}$ is

$$\frac{\partial\phi}{\partial t} = \frac{\partial}{\partial\mathbf{R}}\cdot\left[kT\frac{\zeta_1+\zeta_2}{\zeta_1\zeta_2}\left(\mathbf{I}-\mathbf{pp}\right)\frac{\partial\phi}{\partial\mathbf{R}} - \left(\mathbf{LR} - \mathbf{L}:\mathbf{ppR}\right)\phi\right], \tag{4.100}$$

where $\phi(\mathbf{R}, t)$ is the probability distribution function for the process $\mathbf{R}$. In terms of the equivalent harmonic-mean friction factor ζ, and for the process $\mathbf{p} = \mathbf{R}/L$,

$$\frac{\partial\phi}{\partial t} = \frac{\partial}{\partial\mathbf{p}}\cdot\left[\frac{2kT}{\zeta L^2}\left(\mathbf{I}-\mathbf{pp}\right)\frac{\partial\phi}{\partial\mathbf{p}} - \left(\mathbf{Lp} - \mathbf{L}:\mathbf{ppp}\right)\phi\right], \tag{4.101}$$

which is precisely the diffusion equation for a symmetric rigid dumbbell of friction factor ζ [2]. Of course, the result (4.100) can be obtained directly from the symmetric dumbbell diffusion using the equivalent friction factor, Remark 4.11.

4.2.3.4 Average Motion and Configuration Tensor

If the flow is homogeneous, i.e., $\mathbf{L}$ is constant, $\nabla\nabla\mathbf{u}^{(r)}$ and HOT are identically zero, the dumbbell's center of resistance drifts just like a particle of fluid,

$$\langle \dot{\mathbf{R}}^{(c)} \rangle = \langle \mathbf{u}^{(c)} \rangle = \mathbf{L}\langle \mathbf{R}^{(c)} \rangle = \mathbf{u}\left(\langle \mathbf{R}^{(c)} \rangle\right). \tag{4.102}$$

A migration from the streamline of the center of resistance is therefore induced by a non-homogeneous flow field (or by external forces on the beads). Problem 4.3 has considered this for an elastic dumbbell—it is the same for a rigid-rod dumbbell.

Next, for the average orientation vector,

$$\langle \dot{\mathbf{p}} \rangle = \mathbf{L}\cdot\langle \mathbf{p} \rangle - \mathbf{L}:\langle \mathbf{ppp} \rangle. \tag{4.103}$$

Note that this does not involve a material time constant, unlike in the elastic dumbbell case—the only time constant comes from the shear rate ($\mathbf{L}$). To solve for the average orientation, third- and higher-order statistics in $\mathbf{p}$ are required, a classical closure problem.

For the configuration tensor $\langle \mathbf{RR} \rangle$, we first note

$$\frac{d}{dt}\langle \mathbf{RR} \rangle = \left\langle \mathbf{R}\dot{\mathbf{R}} + \dot{\mathbf{R}}\mathbf{R} \right\rangle = \mathbf{L} \cdot \langle \mathbf{RR} \rangle + \langle \mathbf{RR} \rangle \cdot \mathbf{L}^T - 2\mathbf{L} : \langle \mathbf{ppRR} \rangle$$
$$+ \zeta_2^{-1} \left\langle \mathbf{R}\left(\mathbf{I} - \mathbf{pp}\right) \mathbf{F}^{(b,\mathbf{R})}(t) + \left(\mathbf{I} - \mathbf{pp}\right) \mathbf{F}^{(b,\mathbf{R})}(t)\, \mathbf{R} \right\rangle. \quad (4.104)$$

Because of the widely different time scales between any kinematic entity $Q(t)$ the Brownian force,

$$\left\langle \mathbf{Q}(t)\mathbf{F}^{(b,\mathbf{R})}(t) \right\rangle = \left\langle \mathbf{Q}(\Delta t)\mathbf{F}^{(b,\mathbf{R})}(\Delta t) \right\rangle, \quad (4.105)$$

where Δt is very large compared to the fluctuating time scale, but very small compared to the time scale of interest. For instance, in the term $\left\langle R_i(t)\, F_j^{(b,\mathbf{R})}(t) \right\rangle = \left\langle R_i(\Delta t)\, F_j^{(b,\mathbf{R})}(\Delta t) \right\rangle$, the differential form (4.97) can be used for $R_i(\Delta t)$, and the product involves neglected terms $O(\Delta t^2)$, and terms linear in the Brownian forces, which do not contribute to the average, and we find

$$\left\langle R_i(\Delta t)\, F_j^{(b,\mathbf{R})}(\Delta t) \right\rangle = \zeta_2^{-1} \left\langle (\delta_{ik} - p_i p_k) \int_0^{\Delta t} F_k^{(b,\mathbf{R})}(t)\, F_j^{(b,\mathbf{R})}(\Delta t)\, dt \right\rangle$$
$$= kT\,(1+\alpha) \left\langle \delta_{ij} - p_i p_j \right\rangle. \quad (4.106)$$

Similarly,

$$\left\langle \left[R_i p_j p_k F_k^{(b,\mathbf{R})} \right]_{\Delta t} \right\rangle = \zeta_2^{-1} \left\langle p_i p_j\,(\delta_{km} - p_k p_m) \int_0^{\Delta t} F_k^{(b,\mathbf{R})}(t)\, F_m^{(b,\mathbf{R})}(\Delta t)\, dt \right\rangle$$
$$= 2kT\,(1+\alpha) \left\langle p_i p_j \right\rangle. \quad (4.107)$$

The results (4.106–4.107) can be used in Eq. (4.104) to yield

$$\frac{d}{dt}\langle \mathbf{RR} \rangle - \mathbf{L} \cdot \langle \mathbf{RR} \rangle - \langle \mathbf{RR} \rangle \cdot \mathbf{L}^T + 2\mathbf{L} : \langle \mathbf{ppRR} \rangle$$
$$+ \frac{6kT\,(1+\alpha)}{\zeta_2 L^2} \langle \mathbf{RR} \rangle = \frac{2kT\,(1+\alpha)}{\zeta_2} \mathbf{I}. \quad (4.108)$$

Now, define the time constant

$$\lambda = \frac{\zeta_2 L^2}{6kT\,(1+\alpha)} = \frac{\zeta_1 \zeta_2 L^2}{6kT\,(\zeta_1 + \zeta_2)} = \frac{\zeta L^2}{12kT}, \quad (4.109)$$

where ζ is the equivalent harmonic-mean friction factor from Eq. (4.60), we finally arrive at the constitutive equation for the configuration tensor,

$$\lambda \left\{ \frac{d}{dt}\langle \mathbf{pp}\rangle - \mathbf{L}\cdot\langle \mathbf{pp}\rangle - \langle \mathbf{pp}\rangle\cdot\mathbf{L}^T + 2\mathbf{L} : \langle \mathbf{pppp}\rangle \right\} + \langle \mathbf{pp}\rangle = \frac{1}{3}\mathbf{I}, \tag{4.110}$$

or equivalently,

$$\lambda \frac{\delta}{\delta t}\langle \mathbf{pp}\rangle + 2\lambda\mathbf{L} : \langle \mathbf{pppp}\rangle + \langle \mathbf{pp}\rangle = \frac{1}{3}\mathbf{I}. \tag{4.111}$$

At equilibrium, $\langle \mathbf{pp}\rangle = \mathbf{I}/3$, an isotropic tensor as it should be.

Remark 4.12 The solution to $\langle \mathbf{pp}\rangle$ requires the solution of $\langle \mathbf{pppp}\rangle$, and so on. To close this infinite system, at some stage, a closure approximation is made, expressing the current moment by a combination of previous moments. This is the classical closure problem in many branches of science.

4.2.3.5 Stress Tensor

To find the polymer-contributed stress tensor, we return to (4.25) and specialize it to a dumbbell case with $N = 2$:

$$\begin{aligned} \mathbf{S}^{(p)} &= \nu\left\langle \mathbf{r}_1\left(-\mathbf{F}^{(c)} - \mathbf{F}_1^{(b)}\right) + \mathbf{r}_2\left(\mathbf{F}^{(c)} - \mathbf{F}_2^{(b)}\right)\right\rangle \\ &= \nu\left\langle \mathbf{RF}^{(c)} - \mathbf{r}_1\mathbf{F}_1^{(b)} - \mathbf{r}_2\mathbf{F}_2^{(b)}\right\rangle. \end{aligned} \tag{4.112}$$

Here we could directly find the contributions from the Brownian forces to the polymer-contributed stress, using their statistics and the beads' Langevin equations. However, in this form the Brownian forces play the role of external forces, and therefore it may be of interest to simplify (4.112) further.

Now, using the results from our geometric consideration in (4.112), (4.31–4.33),

$$\begin{aligned} \mathbf{S}^{(p)} &= \nu\left\langle \mathbf{RF}^{(c)}\right\rangle - \nu\left\langle \mathbf{R}^{(c)}\left(\mathbf{F}_1^{(b)} + \mathbf{F}_2^{(b)}\right)\right\rangle - \nu\left\langle \mathbf{R}_2\mathbf{F}_2^{(b)} - \mathbf{R}_1\mathbf{F}_1^{(b)}\right\rangle \\ &= \nu\left\langle \mathbf{RF}^{(c)}\right\rangle - \nu\left\langle \mathbf{R}^{(c)}\left(\mathbf{F}_1^{(b)} + \mathbf{F}_2^{(b)}\right)\right\rangle - \nu\left\langle \frac{\zeta_1}{\zeta_1+\zeta_2}\mathbf{RF}_2^{(b)} - \frac{\zeta_2}{\zeta_1+\zeta_2}\mathbf{RF}_1^{(b)}\right\rangle. \end{aligned} \tag{4.113}$$

In (4.113b), the first on the right is the contribution from the dumbbell (called "contribution from intramolecular forces"), the second from the motion of the center of resistance due to the Brownian forces, and the third, "contributions from external forces". These expressions are given in Bird et al. [2] for the symmetric dumbbell case where $\zeta_1 = \zeta_2$.

Now, using or "trick" (4.105), and from the Langevin equation for the center of resistance (4.92a), and keeping only non-trivial terms in the average,[7]

---

[7] Note that the integral $\int_0^{\Delta t}$ of the symmetric delta Dirac function returns a value of 1/2 only.

$$
\begin{aligned}
\left\langle \mathbf{R}^{(c)}\mathbf{F}_2^{(b)} \right\rangle &= \left\langle (\zeta_1 + \zeta_2)^{-1} \int_0^{\Delta t} \mathbf{F}^{(b,c)}(t)\, \mathbf{F}_2^{(b)}(\Delta t)\, dt \right\rangle \\
&= \left\langle (\zeta_1 + \zeta_2)^{-1} \int_0^{\Delta t} \left(\mathbf{F}_1^{(b)}(t) + \mathbf{F}_2^{(b)}(t) \right) \mathbf{F}_2^{(b)}(\Delta t)\, dt \right\rangle \\
&= kT\, (\zeta_1 + \zeta_2)^{-1}\, \zeta_2 \mathbf{I}. \qquad (4.114)
\end{aligned}
$$

Similarly,

$$
\left\langle \mathbf{R}^{(c)}\mathbf{F}_1^{(b)} \right\rangle = kT\, (\zeta_1 + \zeta_2)^{-1}\, \zeta_1 \mathbf{I}. \qquad (4.115)
$$

Thus, the contributions from the Brownian forces via the motion of the center of resistance is

$$
\left\langle \mathbf{R}^{(c)} \left(\mathbf{F}_1^{(b)} + \mathbf{F}_2^{(b)} \right) \right\rangle = kT\mathbf{I}. \qquad (4.116)
$$

This term seems absent from Bird et al.'s treatment [2] in that a no-drift assumption was made.

Next, from the **R**-Langevin equation (4.96),

$$
\begin{aligned}
\left\langle \mathbf{R}\mathbf{F}_2^{(b)} \right\rangle &= \left\langle \zeta_2^{-1} (\mathbf{I} - \mathbf{pp}) \int_0^{\Delta t} \mathbf{F}^{(b,\mathbf{R})}(t)\, \mathbf{F}_2^{(b)}(\Delta t)\, dt \right\rangle \\
&= \left\langle \zeta_2^{-1} (\mathbf{I} - \mathbf{pp}) \int_0^{\Delta t} \left(\mathbf{F}_2^{(b)}(t) - \alpha \mathbf{F}_1^{(b)} \right) \mathbf{F}_2^{(b)}(\Delta t)\, dt \right\rangle \\
&= kT\, (\mathbf{I} - \mathbf{pp}), \qquad (4.117)
\end{aligned}
$$

and

$$
\begin{aligned}
\left\langle \mathbf{R}\mathbf{F}_1^{(b)} \right\rangle &= \left\langle \zeta_2^{-1} (\mathbf{I} - \mathbf{pp}) \int_0^{\Delta t} \mathbf{F}^{(b,\mathbf{R})}(t)\, \mathbf{F}_1^{(b)}(\Delta t)\, dt \right\rangle \\
&= \left\langle \zeta_2^{-1} (\mathbf{I} - \mathbf{pp}) \int_0^{\Delta t} \left(\mathbf{F}_2^{(b)}(t) - \alpha \mathbf{F}_1^{(b)} \right) \mathbf{F}_1^{(b)}(\Delta t)\, dt \right\rangle \\
&= -kT\, (\mathbf{I} - \mathbf{pp}). \qquad (4.118)
\end{aligned}
$$

Thus, the contribution from the external Brownian forces is

$$
\begin{aligned}
\frac{\zeta_1}{\zeta_1 + \zeta_2} \left\langle \mathbf{R}\mathbf{F}_2^{(b)} - \alpha \mathbf{R}\mathbf{F}_1^{(b)} \right\rangle &= \frac{\zeta_1}{\zeta_1 + \zeta_2} kT\, (\mathbf{I} - \mathbf{pp}) \left(1 + \frac{\zeta_2}{\zeta_1} \right) \\
&= kT\, (\mathbf{I} - \mathbf{pp}). \qquad (4.119)
\end{aligned}
$$

Finally, the intramolecular contribution:

$$\left\langle \mathbf{RF}^{(c)} \right\rangle = \frac{\zeta L^2}{2} \langle \mathbf{L} : \mathbf{pppp} \rangle + \frac{\zeta_1}{\zeta_1 + \zeta_2} \left\langle \mathbf{Rpp}.\mathbf{F}^{(b,\mathbf{R})} \right\rangle . \tag{4.120}$$

To find the contribution from the last term on the right of (4.120), we note

$$\begin{aligned} \frac{d}{dt} \left(R_i p_k p_l \right) = A_{ikl} &+ \zeta_2^{-1} \left(\delta_{im} - p_i p_m \right) p_k p_l F_m^{(b,\mathbf{R})} (t) \\ &+ \zeta_2^{-1} p_i p_l \left(\delta_{km} - p_k p_m \right) F_m^{(b,\mathbf{R})} (t) \\ &+ \zeta_2^{-1} p_i p_k \left(\delta_{lm} - p_l p_m \right) F_m^{(b,\mathbf{R})} (t) . \end{aligned}$$

Thus

$$\begin{aligned} \left\langle R_i p_j p_k F_k^{(b,\mathbf{R})} \right\rangle = &\left\langle \zeta_2^{-1} \left(\delta_{im} - p_i p_m \right) p_j p_k \int_0^{\Delta t} F_m^{(b,\mathbf{R})} (t) \, F_k^{(b,\mathbf{R})} (\Delta t) \, dt \right\rangle \\ &+ \left\langle \zeta_2^{-1} p_i p_k \left(\delta_{jm} - p_j p_m \right) \int_0^{\Delta t} F_m^{(b,\mathbf{R})} (t) \, F_k^{(b,\mathbf{R})} (\Delta t) \, dt \right\rangle \\ &+ \left\langle \zeta_2^{-1} p_i p_j \left(\delta_{km} - p_k p_m \right) \int_0^{\Delta t} F_m^{(b,\mathbf{R})} (t) \, F_k^{(b,\mathbf{R})} (\Delta t) \, dt \right\rangle , \end{aligned}$$

$$\begin{aligned} \left\langle R_i p_j p_k F_k^{(b,\mathbf{R})} \right\rangle = &\, kT \frac{\zeta_1 + \zeta_2}{\zeta_1} \delta_{km} \left(\delta_{im} - p_i p_m \right) p_j p_k \\ &+ kT \frac{\zeta_1 + \zeta_2}{\zeta_1} \delta_{km} p_i p_k \left(\delta_{jm} - p_j p_m \right) \\ &+ kT \frac{\zeta_1 + \zeta_2}{\zeta_1} \delta_{km} p_i p_j \left(\delta_{km} - p_k p_m \right) \end{aligned}$$

Simplifying,

$$\left\langle R_i p_j p_k F_k^{(b,\mathbf{R})} (\Delta t) \right\rangle = 2kT \frac{\zeta_1 + \zeta_2}{\zeta_1} p_i p_j . \tag{4.121}$$

Putting all the results together,

$$\begin{aligned} \mathbf{S}^{(p)} &= \frac{\nu \zeta L^2}{2} \langle \mathbf{L} : \mathbf{pppp} \rangle + 2\nu kT \langle \mathbf{pp} \rangle - \nu kT \mathbf{I} - \nu kT \left(\mathbf{I} - \langle \mathbf{pp} \rangle \right) \\ &= \frac{\nu \zeta L^2}{2} \langle \mathbf{L} : \mathbf{pppp} \rangle + 3\nu kT \langle \mathbf{pp} \rangle - 2\nu kT \mathbf{I} . \end{aligned} \tag{4.122}$$

In addition, we note that from (4.111),

$$-\frac{\nu\zeta}{4}\frac{\delta}{\delta t}\langle\mathbf{pp}\rangle = \frac{\nu\zeta}{4\lambda}\left(2\lambda\mathbf{L}:\langle\mathbf{pppp}\rangle + \langle\mathbf{pp}\rangle - \frac{1}{3}\mathbf{I}\right),$$
$$= \frac{\nu\zeta}{2}\mathbf{L}:\langle\mathbf{pppp}\rangle + \frac{3\nu kT}{L^2}\left(\langle\mathbf{pp}\rangle - \frac{1}{3}\mathbf{I}\right). \tag{4.123}$$

Remark 4.13 The expression (4.122) is referred to as the Kramers expression for the stress. From (4.123), and to within an unimportant isotropic stress,

$$\mathbf{S}^{(p)} = -\frac{\nu\zeta}{4}\frac{\delta}{\delta t}\langle\mathbf{RR}\rangle. \tag{4.124}$$

This is called the Giesekus expression for the stress, Bird et al. [2].

In summary, the constitutive relation for the polymer-contributed stress consists of (4.111) and (4.122), or (4.124). Note that our stress results, Eq. (4.122), differs from the expression given by Bird et al. [2] by an unimportant isotropic stress—it was given as $\nu kT\mathbf{I}$ instead of $2\nu kT\mathbf{I}$ here; the unimportant difference is due to the Brownian contribution through the motion of the center of resistance, Eq. (4.116). Abdel-Khalik and Bird [20] also noticed this unimportant difference due to a no-drift assumption was made. Clearly, we are plagued with the closure problem for even a dilute suspension of rigid dumbbells. Despite this, there have been a large number of solved problems for the rigid dumbbell suspension, a good collection of these can be found in Bird et al. [2].

Problems

Problem 4.1 Show that the solution to the diffusion equation (4.9) subjected to the initial condition (4.10) is indeed the Gaussian distribution (4.11).

Problem 4.2 Show that the contributed stress from the Brownian forces in Eq. (4.25) results in a hydrostatic stress:

$$-\sum_{i=1}^{N+1}\mathbf{r}_i\mathbf{F}_i^{(b)} = -kT(N+1)\mathbf{I}. \tag{4.125}$$

Problem 4.3 Show that the migration of the center of resistance of an elastic dumbbell from the streamline is given by

$$\langle\dot{\mathbf{R}}^{(c)}\rangle = \mathbf{u}^{(c)} + \frac{\zeta_1\zeta_2}{2\left(\zeta_1+\zeta_2\right)^2}\langle\mathbf{RR}\rangle : \nabla\nabla\mathbf{u}^{(c)}, \tag{4.126}$$

which reduces to the symmetric dumbbell expression

$$\langle \dot{\mathbf{R}}^{(c)} \rangle = \mathbf{u}^{(c)} + \frac{1}{8} \langle \mathbf{RR} \rangle : \nabla\nabla \mathbf{u}^{(c)}, \tag{4.127}$$

when $\zeta_1 = \zeta_2$.

Problem 4.4 Show that the solution to (4.53) subject to the initial condition (4.51) is

$$\langle \mathbf{R} \rangle = e^{-t/2\lambda} e^{\mathbf{L}t} \mathbf{R}_0. \tag{4.128}$$

Thus, deduce that $\langle \mathbf{R} \rangle$ decays or grows unboundedly, depends on the eigenvalues of $\mathbf{L} - \mathbf{I}/2\lambda$. Show that, if one of the eigenvalue

$$\text{eigen}\,(\mathbf{L}) > \frac{1}{2\lambda}, \tag{4.129}$$

then $\langle \mathbf{R} \rangle$ is a run-away process exponentially in time.

Problem 4.5 Show that the UCM form (4.74) is equivalent to (4.72).

Problem 4.6 Show that, when combining $\mathbf{S}^{(s)}$ and $\boldsymbol{\tau}^{(p)}$ into $\mathbf{S}$ as indicated in Eq. (4.77), the Oldroyd-B constitutive equation (4.78) results.

Problem 4.7 Recall the right relative Cauchy–Green tensor, $\mathbf{C}_t\,(t - s) = \mathbf{F}_t\,(s)^T\,\mathbf{F}_t\,(s)$, where $\mathbf{F}_t\,(s)$ is the relative deformation gradient, see Sect. 2.2.3 Find the inverse of $\mathbf{C}_t\,(t - s)$ and show that

$$\dot{\mathbf{C}}_t\,(s)^{-1} = \mathbf{L}\,(t)\,\mathbf{C}_t\,(s)^{-1} + \mathbf{C}_t\,(s)^{-1}\,\mathbf{L}\,(t)^T. \tag{4.130}$$

Problem 4.8 In a simple shear flow with velocity $\mathbf{u} = (\dot{\gamma} y, 0, 0)$ and constant shear rate $\dot{\gamma}$, and assuming zero initial conditions for the polymer stresses, write down all the Oldroyd-B stress components, show that the non-trivial stresses, subject to zero initial conditions, are

$$\tau_{12}^{(p)} = \eta_p \dot{\gamma} \left(1 - e^{-t/\lambda}\right) \tag{4.131}$$

$$\tau_{11}^{(p)} = 2\eta_p \lambda \dot{\gamma}^2 \left(1 - e^{-t/\lambda}\right) - 2\eta_p t \dot{\gamma}^2 e^{-t/\lambda}. \tag{4.132}$$

Thus at steady state, the model predicts a constant viscosity, a quadratic first normal stress difference in $\dot{\gamma}$, and zero second normal stress difference:

$$\begin{aligned} S_{12} &= S_{12}^{(s)} + \tau_{12}^{(p)} = \left(\eta_s + \eta_p\right) \dot{\gamma} \\ N_1 &= S_{11} - S_{22}, \quad N_2 = S_{22} - S_{33} \\ \eta &= \eta_s + \eta_p, \quad N_1 = 2\eta_p \lambda \dot{\gamma}^2, \quad N_2 = 0. \end{aligned} \tag{4.133}$$

Problem 4.9 Consider a shear flow with the shear rate $\dot{\gamma} = \dot{\gamma}_0 \Re\left(e^{i\omega t}\right)$, where $\Re$ denotes the real part, write down the stress component equations from Eq. (4.77), look for the steady solution

$$\tau_{12}^{(p)} = \Re\left(S_0 e^{i\omega t}\right), \quad \tau_{11}^{(p)} = \Re\left(N_0 e^{2i\omega t}\right). \tag{4.134}$$

Find the expressions for S_0 and N_0, and show that

$$\eta^* = \eta_s + \frac{\eta_p}{1 + i\lambda\omega}, \tag{4.135}$$

$$\eta' = \eta_s + \frac{\eta_p}{1 + \lambda^2\omega^2}, \quad \eta'' = \frac{\eta_p \lambda\omega}{1 + \lambda^2\omega^2}, \tag{4.136}$$

$$G' = \frac{G\lambda^2\omega^2}{1 + \lambda^2\omega^2}, \quad G'' = \eta_s\omega + \frac{G\lambda\omega}{1 + \lambda^2\omega^2}. \tag{4.137}$$

Problem 4.10 In an uniaxial elongational flow where the velocity gradient is

$$[\mathbf{L}] = \operatorname{diag}\left(\dot{\varepsilon}, -\dot{\varepsilon}/2, -\dot{\varepsilon}/2\right), \tag{4.138}$$

where $\dot{\varepsilon}$ is the elongational rate, show that the stresses for the Oldroyd-B fluid, subject to zero initial conditions, are

$$\tau_{11}^{(p)} = \frac{2\eta_p\dot{\varepsilon}}{1 - 2\lambda\dot{\varepsilon}}\left(1 - e^{-(1-2\lambda\dot{\varepsilon})t/\lambda}\right), \tag{4.139}$$

$$\tau_{22}^{(p)} = \tau_{33}^{(p)} = -\frac{\eta_p\dot{\varepsilon}}{1 + \lambda\dot{\varepsilon}}\left(1 - e^{-(1+\lambda\dot{\varepsilon})t/\lambda}\right). \tag{4.140}$$

Deduce that, if either $\lambda\dot{\varepsilon} \geq 1/2$ or $\lambda\dot{\varepsilon} \leq -1$, then at least one component of the stress grows unboundedly. Show that, $-1 < \lambda\dot{\varepsilon} < 1/2$, the steady state elongational viscosity of the Oldroyd-B model is

$$\eta_E = \frac{S_{11} - S_{22}}{\dot{\varepsilon}} = 3\eta_s + \frac{3\eta_p}{(1 - 2\lambda\dot{\varepsilon})(1 + \lambda\dot{\varepsilon})}. \tag{4.141}$$

Problem 4.11 1. Show detailed work leading to result (4.99).
2. Show detailed working leading to results (4.106–4.107). Thus show that (4.108) follows from (4.104).

Problem 4.12 Show the detailed work leading to (4.123–4.124).

Problem 4.13 Rouse chain made up of $N + 1$ beads connected by N linear elastic spring. Find the constitutive equation for a dilute suspension of Rouse chains.

References

1. K.R. Lennon, G.H. McKinley, J.W. Swan, Scientific machine learning for modeling and simulating complex fluids. PNAS **120**, e2304669120 (2023)
2. R.B. Bird, C.F. Curtiss, R.C. Armstrong, O. Hassager, Dynamics of Polymeric Liquids. Vol. 2: Kinetic Theory, 2nd edn. (Wiley, New York, 1991)
3. M.D. Graham, *Microhydrodynamics, Brownian Motion, and Complex Fluids* (Cambridge University Press, Cambridge, 2018)
4. R. Huilgol, N. Phan-Thien, *Fluid Mechanics of Viscoelasticity: General Principles, Constitutive Modelling, Analytical and Numerical Techniques* (Elsevier, Amsterdam, 1997)
5. R.G. Larson, *Constitutive Equations for Polymer Melts and Solutions* (Butterworth Publishers, Boston, 1988)
6. A.S. Lodge, *Elastic Liquids* (Academic Press, New York, 1964)
7. F.A. Morrison, *Understanding Rheology: Topic in Chemical Engineering* (Oxford Oxford University Press, Oxford, 2001)
8. N. Phan-Thien, N. Mai-Duy, *Understanding Viscoelasticity: An Introduction to Rheology*, 3rd edn. (Springer International Publishing AG, Berlin, 2017)
9. R.I. Tanner, *Engineering Rheology*, revised edition edn. (Oxford University Press, Oxford, 1992)
10. R.I. Tanner, K. Walters, *Rheology: An Historical Perspective* (Elsevier Science B.V, Amtersdam, 1998)
11. P.J. Flory, *Statistical Mechanics of Chain Molecules* (Wiley Interscience, New York, 1969)
12. Y.K. Lin, *Probabilistic Theory of Structural Dynamics* (McGraw-Hill, New York, 1967)
13. P.E. Rouse, A theory of the linear viscoelastic properties of dilute solutions of coiling polymers. J. Chem. Phys. **21**, 1272–1280 (1953)
14. L.D. Landau, E.M. Lifshitz, *Fluid Mechanics*, revised edition edn. (Pergamon Press, New York, 1959)
15. G.K. Batchelor, The stress system in a suspension of force-free particles. J. Fluid Mech. **41**, 545–570 (1970)
16. H.A. Kramers, Het gedrag van macromoleculen in een stroomende vloeistof. Physica **11**, 1–19 (1945)
17. N. Phan-Thien, D. Pan, M.A. Kanso, A.J. Giacomin, Lopsided rigid dumbbell rheology from Langevin equation: a graduate tutorial. Phys. Fluids **36**, 091801 (2024)
18. W. Kuhn, Über die gestalt fadenförmiger moleküle in lösungen. Kolloid Z. **68**, 2–15 (1934)
19. N. Phan-Thien, M.A. Kanso, A.J. Giacomin, Lopsided elastic dumbbell suspension. Phys. Fluids **35**, 071707 (2024)
20. S.I. Abdel-Khalik, R.B. Bird, Letter to the Editor: Rheology of lopsided-dumbbell suspensions. Appl. Sci. Res. 268–270 (1975)
21. J.G. Oldroyd, On the formulation of rheological equations of state. Proc. Roy. Soc. Lond. A **200**, 523–541 (1950)
22. J.C. Maxwell, Paper read by prof. Maxwell at a meeting of the British Association at Aberdeen on 21 September 1859. The Scientific Papers of James Clerk Maxwell New York: Dover, ed. by W.D. Niven, vol. 1, pp. 377–409 (2003)
23. A.C. Pipkin, *Lectures on Viscoelasticity Theory*, 2nd edn. (Springer, Berlin, 1986)
24. D.V. Boger, A highly elastic constant-viscosity fluid. J. Non-Newton. Fluid Mech. **3**, 87–91 (1977)
25. M.L. Brader, S.J. Williams, J.M. Banks, H. Wong, H. Zhou, L. Jin, Encapsulation state of messenger rna inside lipid nanoparticles. Biophys. J. **120**(14), 2756–2770 (2021)

Chapter 5
Dilute Suspensions

About Dilute Particle Suspensions

A suspension is a *composite* fluid composed of a solvent in which there are many suspended particles—again, there are widely separated length scales in the fluid, the particle length scale a, and the apparatus length scale L, $a \ll L$. When the solvent is Newtonian, we speak of *Newtonian* or *viscous suspension*, and when it is viscoelastic, *viscoelastic suspension*. The particles can either be rigid, *particle suspension*, fluid droplets, *droplet suspension*, or gaseous bubbles *bubble suspension*.

Suspensions abound in nature and man-made materials, all have distinctive microstructure.

An example of man-made suspensions is bread dough, made by mixing wheat flour in water (together with some leavening agent and salt), Fig. 5.1. Its microstructure consists of crossed-linked network of glutens (chain-like structure), starch granules $\sim 14\,\mu\text{m}$ lentil shape (A-type) plus $\sim 4\,\mu\text{m}$ spherical shape (B-type). Due to the viscoelastic nature of the glutens network, bread dough is a viscoelastic suspension. In fact, it is more solid-like, or rubberlike in its response. In a relevant constitutive equation for this, stresses should be expected to correlate with the strain, not strain rate; in addition, yield stress may be expected.

Most biological fluids are suspensions; an example is human blood, Fig. 5.2. It is a suspension of highly deformable red blood cells (mainly), biconcave in shape $\sim 8\,\mu\text{m}$, of $\sim 45\%$ in volume concentration; the rest of suspended particles are white blood cells (ruffed spheres) and platelets (oblate spheroids), of $\sim 0.3\%$, in a solvent called plasma, itself a mildly viscoelastic fluid.

From these few examples, and many more that we can see around, it is apparent that common suspensions are at high concentration, and of very complex microstructure. However, to make progress and to explore the physics behind suspensions, we make some assumptions listed in Remarks 3.1–3.2. We also assume that the particles are small with $Re \ll 1$, but with $Pe \gg 1$ (non-Brownian particles), Sect. 3.2. There are many books dealing with suspensions, for instance, Kim and Karrila [1], Graham [2], Tanner [3].

© The Author(s), under exclusive license to Springer Nature Singapore Pte Ltd. 2026

D. Pan et al., *Langevin Analysis of Microstructured Fluids*,
SpringerBriefs in Applied Sciences and Technology,
https://doi.org/10.1007/978-981-95-2318-4_5

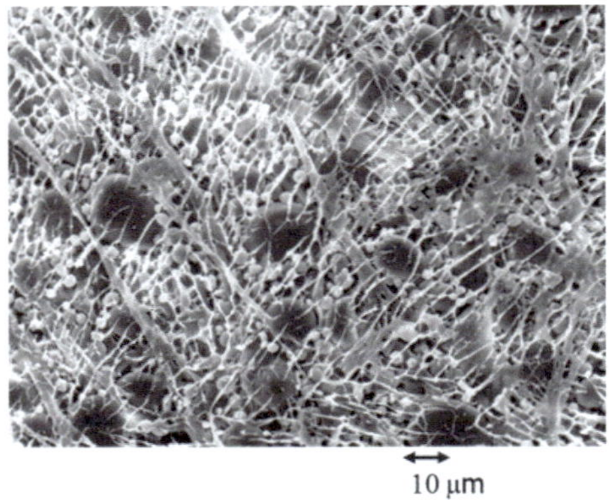

Fig. 5.1 A micrograph image of bread dough, bake break has been found as early as ~1200 BC, bread in Latin is *panis*, with *pan* as in "com*pan*ion" or in "com*pany*, presumably food eaten with companion or in company (*Source* unpublished research presentation at Rheology Group by Marcus Newberry, Sydney (2000))

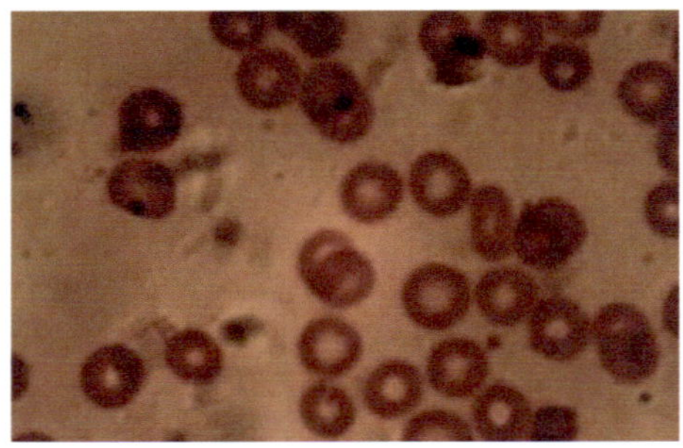

Fig. 5.2 A micrograph image of human whole blood, magnified 600X. It is rheologically a suspension of highly deformable particles (mainly red cells) in mildly viscoelastic fluid (plasma). (*Source* http://www.3dham.com/animal/bloodcompare.html, by John Alan Elson)

5.1 Viscometric Properties

The most important engineering property of a suspension is its viscosity, after all we need to pump the suspension to the point of application, and that requires at least an estimate of its viscosity. There have been many measurements of suspension viscosity, the first viscometric function, but in the early data, there was not a major effort in controlling the sample properties and flow regime, and these data may not be very helpful in our modeling effort. Thomas [4] selected data for uniform-sized rigid spherical particles in a Newtonian liquid and carefully minimized non-Newtonian, inertial, non-homogeneous, and settling effects. His data, Fig. 5.3, for 16 different sources were presented in terms of the *relative viscosity*, defined as the ratio of the suspension viscosity to the solvent viscosity,

$$\eta_r = \frac{\eta}{\eta_s}. \tag{5.1}$$

His main observations are that, 1. the suspensions behave in a Newtonian manner, i.e., provided the particles are large enough so that Brownian effects are not important;

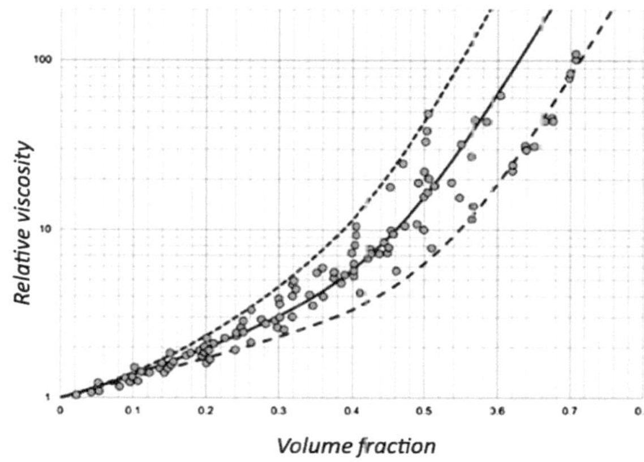

Fig. 5.3 A correlation of relative viscosity from different sources *versus* volume fraction from [4]

2. despite careful experiment techniques, the scattering in the relative viscosity data is large; 3. Krieger and Dougherty provided a good empirical fit to the data, Krieger and Dougherty [5]. There are other fits, e.g., Thomas' fit [4]. Krieger–Dougherty's fit is given as

$$\eta_r = \left(1 - \frac{\phi}{\phi_m}\right)^{-\phi_m[\eta]}, \tag{5.2}$$

where ϕ is the volume fraction of the suspended particles, ϕ_m is the maximal packing volume fraction,[1] and $[\eta] = \lim_{\phi \to 0} \Delta\eta_r / \Delta\phi$. Although the theoretical result for $[\eta]$ is 2.5 [6], it and the maximal packing volume fraction have been used as fitting parameters. Furthermore, the flow can re-arrange the microstructure, and thus measurements in a Couette rheometer yield a different viscosity to those in a parallel disk rheometer. This is an indication of flow-induced anisotropy in the suspension.

For the second and third viscometric functions, the first normal stress difference N_1 and the second normal stress difference N_2, there is a lack of data, and some recent data point to the fact that $N_1 < 0$, and $N_2 > 0$, contrary to the polymeric case, where we have $N_1 > 0$ and $N_2 < 0$. Nevertheless, we show in Fig. 5.4 some normal stress difference data from [7], for suspensions of different types of particles. It can be seen from these that both the normal stress differences and the shear stress are nearly linear with the shear rate, in contrast to polymer solutions where the normal stress differences are quadratic in the shear rate (see also the predictions of the UCM model, Problem 4.8).

Gadala-Maria and Acrivos [8] explored the memory/relaxation characteristics of suspension by a reversal shear experiment, illustrated in Fig. 5.5 for a circular Couette flow of a concentrated suspension of spheres. After the shear flow has reached a steady state, the flow was stopped; the torque (stress) reduced to zero quite instantaneously:

[1] For spheres in 3D, the maximal packing volume fraction is ~0.74, achieved by the face-center cubic structure (FCC), or the hexagonal close packed (HCP).

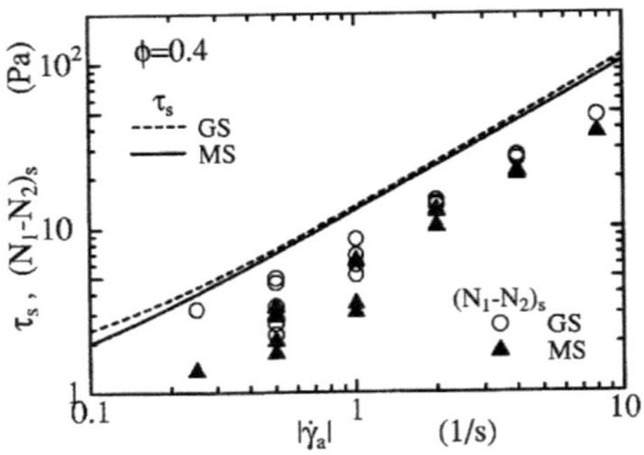

Fig. 5.4 Normal stress difference $N_1 - N_2$ and shear stress τ_s *versus* shear rate for a Newtonian suspension; measurements were done with a parallel-disk rheometer for two types of particles (labeled GS and MS); both $N_1 - N_2$ and τ_s are nearly linear with shear rate, Narumi et al. [7]

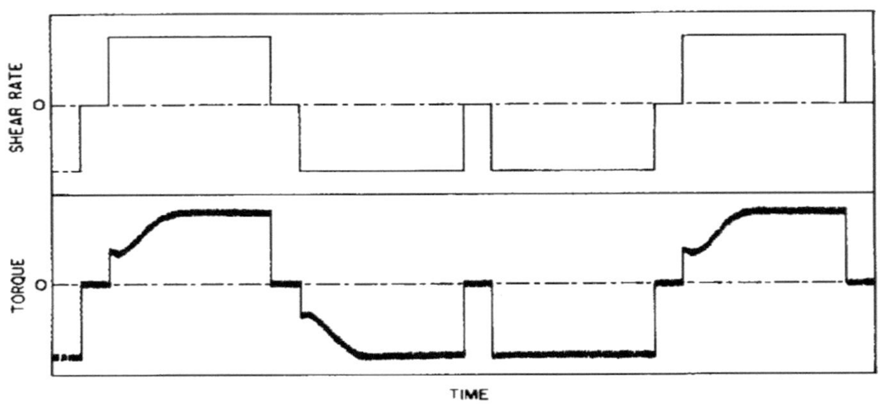

Fig. 5.5 The torque in a Couette viscometer is a measure of the shear stress [8, 9]

the fluid behaves just like a viscous fluid without memory. After a period of rest, the flow was reversed with the same but negative the previous shear rate; here the torque (stress) increased and then gradually attained the expected steady but negative previous value, thus indicating a relaxation mechanism reflecting a re-adjustment of the microstructure on shear reversal. On the other hand, if the shear flow was stopped and restarted in the same direction, the torque (stress) attained its expected steady value almost immediately.

To illustrate the transient behavior of suspension, a series of tests were done at different shear rates on a concentrated suspension, Fig. 5.6a [8, 9]. The torque (stress) increased to different steady-state level according to the shear rate imposed in a plot of the reduced torque (stress), T/T_∞ (so that all asymptote to 1), *versus* the strain $|\dot{\gamma}|t$, all the curves collapsed, indicates that the stress is a function of strain, rather than strain rate.

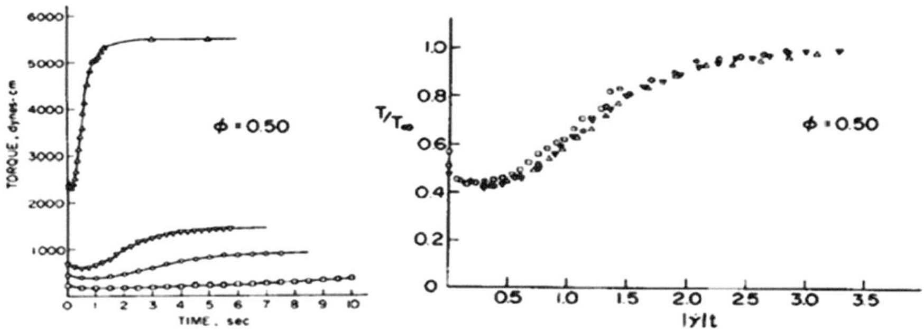

Fig. 5.6 **a** Torque as a function of time at different shear rates, from $0.15\,\mathrm{s}^{-1}$ to $2.4\,\mathrm{s}^{-1}$, different curves at different shear rates tend to a different asymptote T_∞; **b** Normalized torque T/T_∞ *versus* the strain $|\dot{\gamma}|t$, [8]

Finally, in an oscillatory flow, one expect a linear response when the strain is small. For polymer solution, this strain level is typically $\sim$0.1; however, for suspension this strain level is exceedingly small, of $\sim$0.01 or smaller.

Remark 5.1

1. Flows can re-arrange the microstructure;
2. Viscosity is sensitive function of the volume fraction, and may be correlated by the Krieger–Dougherty model;
3. Stress is a function of strain, it is a linear function of strain rate. Stopping the flow immediately reduces the stress to zero. Starting the flow in the same direction, the stress resumes immediately to its previous value; starting the flow in the opposite direction, the stress takes some time to reach its expected value;
4. The strain amplitude below which the fluid responds in a linear viscoelastic manner is typically an order of magnitude lower than that in polymer solutions.

5.2 Microhydrodynamics

With our assumptions on the Reynolds and Péclet numbers, we can safely ignore inertia and Brownian motion, and thus the equations that govern the microhydrodynamics are the Stokes equations:

$$\nabla \cdot \mathbf{u} = 0, \quad -\nabla p + \eta \nabla^2 \mathbf{u} = \mathbf{0}, \quad \mathbf{x} \in V_s \tag{5.3}$$

plus some relevant boundary conditions on particles' surfaces. Stokes equations are linear, instantaneous, and reversible in the driving data, and therefore the microhydrodynamics are also linear, instantaneous and reversible. So right away we are able to answer some points in Remark 5.1: the stress is a linear function of the strain rate (and since strain = strain rate × time, it is a function of strain). Stopping the strain rate reduces the stress to zero instantaneously. Starting the flow in the same direction, the stress also responds instateneously, starting the flow in the opposite direction, the microstructure takes sometimes to readjust leading to a relaxation of the stress.

5.2.1 Particle-Contributed Stress

To find the bulk stress in the suspension, we take the average of the stress in a representative volume V, containing enough particles to make it statistically significant. The development is parallel to that in Sect. 4.1.4. Thus, the particle-contributed stress is, *cf.* Eq. (4.23),

$$\mathbf{S}^{(p)} = \frac{1}{V}\sum_p \int_{V_p} \sigma dV = \frac{1}{V}\sum_p \int_{S_p} \mathbf{xt} dS, \tag{5.4}$$

where $\mathbf{t} = \boldsymbol{\sigma}\mathbf{n}$ is the traction on a particle's surface, with $\boldsymbol{\sigma}$ is the total stress, and the summation is taken over all particles in volume V. The contribution from particle p can be split into a symmetric part, called the *stresslet*,[2]

$$\mathcal{S}_{ij}^{(p)} = \frac{1}{2}\int_{S_p} \left(x_i t_j + x_j t_i\right) dS \tag{5.5}$$

and an antisymmetric part, call the *rotlet*,

$$\mathcal{R}_{ij}^{(p)} = \frac{1}{2}\int_{S_p} \left(x_i t_j - x_j t_i\right) dS = \frac{1}{2}\varepsilon_{ijk} T_k^{(p)} \tag{5.6}$$

where $T_k^{(p)} = \varepsilon_{kmn} \int_{S_p} x_m t_n dS$ is the torque exerted on the particle p. The particle-contributed stress is therefore given by

$$S_{ij}^{(p)} = \frac{1}{V}\sum_p \left(\mathcal{S}_{ij}^{(p)} + \frac{1}{2}\varepsilon_{ijk} T_k^{(p)}\right). \tag{5.7}$$

Very often we deal with force-free and torque-free particles, the particle-contributed stress is therefore the sum of the stresslets on all the particles in volume V.

[2] We use caligraphic S, $\mathcal{S}$, to denote stresslet, and roman S to denote the stress.

5.2.2 Dilute Suspension of Rigid Spheres

We consider now a dilute suspension of force-free and torque-free rigid spheres of equal sizes in a general homogeneous flow far from a particle. By dilute, we mean that the volume fraction satisfies

$$\phi = \nu \frac{4\pi a^3}{3} \ll 1, \tag{5.8}$$

where ν is the number density, or the number of spheres per unit volume, and a is the radius of a sphere. A representative volume V can be chosen such that $V = 1/\nu$, and in V there is only one sphere. Thus, the microhydrodynamic problem consists of a sphere in Stokes flow in an effectively unbounded fluid (note that $a/L \ll 1$, $L = V^{1/3}$ is the linear dimension of V). The superscript p on the generic particle can be omitted, and the coordinate system can be chosen at the center of the sphere. The boundary conditions for this microhydrodynamic problem are

$$\mathbf{u} = \mathbf{U} + (\mathbf{D} + \mathbf{W}) \cdot \mathbf{x} \quad \text{far from the particle, } |\mathbf{x}| \to \infty \tag{5.9}$$

where $\mathbf{L} = \mathbf{D} + \mathbf{W}$ is the constant velocity gradient for the homogeneous flow at infinity, with $\mathbf{D}$ the strain rate tensor, and $\mathbf{W}$ the vorticity tensor, with corresponding vorticity vector $\omega_i = \frac{1}{2}\varepsilon_{ijk} W_{jk}$. In addition, on the particle surface, $|\mathbf{x}| = a$,

$$\mathbf{u} = \mathbf{V} + \mathbf{w} \cdot \mathbf{x}, \tag{5.10}$$

where V is the translational velocity of the sphere, and w is the anti-symmetric tensor derived from the angular velocity $\mathbf{\Omega}$ of the sphere,

$$w_{ij} = -\varepsilon_{ijk}\Omega_k, \ \ \varepsilon_{ijk} w_{jk} = 2\Omega_i. \tag{5.11}$$

The far-field boundary condition must be interpreted as conditions far away from the particle under consideration, but not far enough so that another sphere can be expected.

We shall not pause to go into the mechanics of solving the microhydrodynamic problem (5.3), subject to boundary conditions (5.9–5.10), rather, we simply point out that this well-known solution exists in several sources, e.g. [10], and leave its verifications to Problem 5.1. In Cartesian tensor notation for clarity, this solution is, for the velocity,

$$u_i = U_i + L_{ik}x_k - \frac{a^5}{x^5} D_{ik}x_k - \frac{5D_{kl}x_k x_l}{2x^2}\left(\frac{a^3}{x^3} - \frac{a^5}{x^5}\right) x_i, \tag{5.12}$$

and for the pressure,

$$p = -5\eta_s a^3 \frac{D_{jk}x_j x_k}{x^5}. \tag{5.13}$$

From (5.12) the velocity gradient can be calculated,

$$
\begin{aligned}
\frac{\partial u_i}{\partial x_j} &= L_{ij} - \frac{a^5}{x^5} D_{ij} + 5\frac{a^5}{x^7} D_{ik} x_j x_k - \frac{5D_{kl}}{2x^2}\left(\frac{a^3}{x^3} - \frac{a^5}{x^5}\right)\left(x_l \delta_{kj} + x_k \delta_{lj}\right) x_i \\
&+ \frac{5D_{kl} x_k x_l}{x^4}\left(\frac{a^3}{x^3} - \frac{a^5}{x^5}\right) x_i x_j - \frac{5D_{kl} x_k x_l}{2x^2}\left(\frac{a^3}{x^3} - \frac{a^5}{x^5}\right)\delta_{ij} \\
&+ \frac{5D_{kl} x_k x_l}{2x^2}\left(3\frac{a^3}{x^5} - 5\frac{a^5}{x^7}\right) x_i x_j. \qquad (5.14)
\end{aligned}
$$

From this, and the pressure field (5.13), the total stress can be evaluated. In particular, on the surface of the sphere, $\mathbf{n} = \mathbf{x}/a$, where $\mathbf{n}$ is the outward normal unit vector on the surface of the sphere, and the traction $\mathbf{t} = \boldsymbol{\sigma}\mathbf{n}$ can be calculated, where $\boldsymbol{\sigma}$ is the total stress. Now, on the sphere surface,

$$
\begin{aligned}
\left.\frac{\partial u_i}{\partial x_j}\right|_{x=a} &= L_{ij} - D_{ij} + \frac{5}{a^2} D_{ik} x_j x_k + \frac{5D_{kl} x_k x_l}{2a^2}\left(\frac{3}{a^2} - \frac{5}{a^2}\right) x_i x_j, \\
\left.\left(\frac{\partial u_i}{\partial x_j} + \frac{\partial u_j}{\partial x_i}\right)\right|_{x=a} &= \frac{5}{a^2}\left(D_{ik} x_j x_k + D_{jk} x_k x_i\right) - \frac{10 D_{kl} x_k x_l}{a^4} x_i x_j, \\
-Pn_i|_{x=a} &= \frac{5}{a^3}\eta_s D_{jk} x_j x_k x_i. \qquad (5.15)
\end{aligned}
$$

From these information, we find the traction on the surface,

$$
t_i|_{x=a} = \frac{5}{a}\eta_s D_{ik} x_k. \qquad (5.16)
$$

Now the stresslet can be calculated,

$$
\begin{aligned}
\mathcal{S} &= \frac{1}{2}\int_{S_p}\left(x_i t_j + x_j t_i\right) dS = \frac{5}{2}\frac{\eta_s}{a}\int_{S_p}\left(D_{jk} x_i x_k + D_{ik} x_k x_j\right) dS \\
&= \frac{5}{2}\eta_s\left(2D_{ij}\right)\frac{4\pi a^3}{3}. \qquad (5.17)
\end{aligned}
$$

For a dilute suspension of force-free and torque-free spheres, the particle-contributed stress is, *cf.* (5.7),

$$
S_{ij}^{(p)} = \frac{1}{V}\sum_p \mathcal{S} = 5\eta_s \phi D_{ij}, \qquad (5.18)
$$

where $\phi = 4\pi a^3/3V$ is the volume fraction of spheres. Thus, the average stress for the suspension, $\mathbf{S} = \langle\boldsymbol{\sigma}\rangle$, is

$$
\mathbf{S} = -P\mathbf{I} + 2\eta_s\left(1 + \frac{5}{2}\phi\right)\mathbf{D}. \qquad (5.19)
$$

Remark 5.2

1. A rigid force-free and torque-free sphere translates with the fluid velocity and spins with the vorticity vector.
2. A dilute suspension of force-free and torque-free spheres in a Newtonian fluid of viscosity η_s behaves in a Newtonian manner, with an effective viscosity of

$$\eta = (1 + \frac{5}{2}\phi)\eta_s. \tag{5.20}$$

This is the celebrated Einstein's result.

5.2.3 *Dilute Suspension of Viscous Droplets*

In a seminal paper, [12], Sir G.I. Taylor (Fig. 5.7) extended Einstein's result (5.19) to a dilute Newtonian suspension of viscous droplets of viscosity η_1. These small droplets are modeled as spheres, moving in a Stokes motion with continuity of velocities, and shear stresses across the sphere's surface. Taylor solved the Stokes flow problem, and showed that the effective viscosity of a dilute suspension of viscous droplet is

$$\eta = \left(1 + \frac{\eta_s + \frac{5}{2}\eta_1}{\eta_s + \eta_1}\phi\right)\eta_s. \tag{5.21}$$

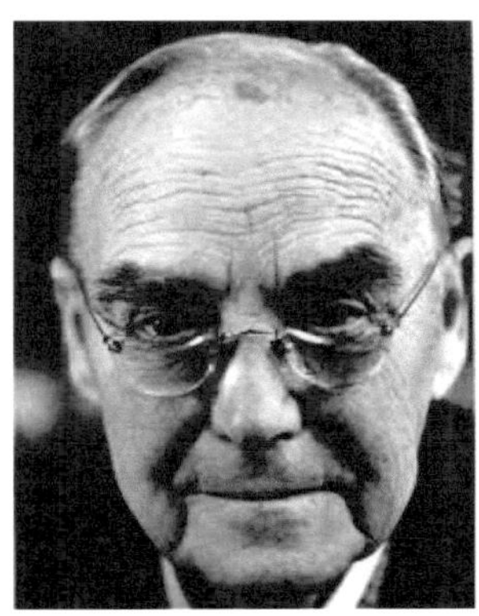

Fig. 5.7 Sir G.I. Taylor OM FRS FRSE (1886–1975) was a British physicist and mathematician who made several major contributions in Fluid and Engineering Mechanics. In a dimensional analysis on one of the Trinity tests based on a photograph, he showed that the yield of that atomic explosion scale as $E \simeq R^5\rho/t^2$. (Photograph provided in Cédric [11])

Remark 5.3 There are two interesting limits in (5.21):

1. rigid sphere limit, $\eta_1 \to \infty$. In this lime, (5.21) reduces to Einstein's result (5.20);
2. gas bubble limit, $\eta_1 = 0$. In this case, the effective viscosity of a dilute bubble suspension is

$$\eta = (1 + \phi)\eta_s. \tag{5.22}$$

5.2.4 *Passage to Higher Concentrations*

Einstein's result (5.20) is of course only valid at low volume fraction, with an error of $O(\phi^2)$. There have been efforts to find the next terms of $O(\phi^2)$ in the effective viscosity. In particular, Batchelor and Green [13] found that these depend on the probability $p(\mathbf{r})$ for the vector $\mathbf{r}$ separating the centers of the two particles. For the case of a uniform probability over accessible $\mathbf{r}$-space they found

$$\eta = \left(1 + 2.5\phi + 5.2\phi^2\right)\eta_s. \tag{5.23}$$

An important construction, known as *differential scheme*, originally due to Bruggeman [14], has been very effective in evaluating effective properties in composite materials, e.g., Taylor [15]; it has been applied to polydispersed multiphase suspensions [16], and to this scheme we turn our attention next.

5.2.4.1 Differential Scheme for a Polydispersed Suspension of Rigid Spheres

We construct the *differential scheme* by a dilute suspension of spheres of a certain initial size at a volume fraction ϕ. In this effective Newtonian fluid a dilute suspension of spheres of a much larger size is constructed; the resulting fluid is still Newtonian fluid but the solid volume fraction has been incrementally built up. This series of incremental additions of solid spheres of different sizes continues until a desired solid volume fraction is reached. One then ends up with a highly polydispersed suspension of spheres, yielding exact closed-form expressions of the effective viscosity. The construction process is illustrated in Fig. 5.8.

We begin with a dilute suspension of rigid spheres, of volume fraction $0 < \phi < 1$. The suspension is Newtonian, with the effective viscosity η given by (5.20). To a unit volume of the suspension we add an infinitesimal volume $\Delta\phi$ of (much) larger spheres. The new mixture is a suspension of spheres, at a solid volume fraction of $\Delta\phi/(1 + \Delta\phi)$. The new suspension is a Newtonian liquid, with effective viscosity given by,[3]

---

[3] Note that the current viscosity plays the role of η_s in (5.20).

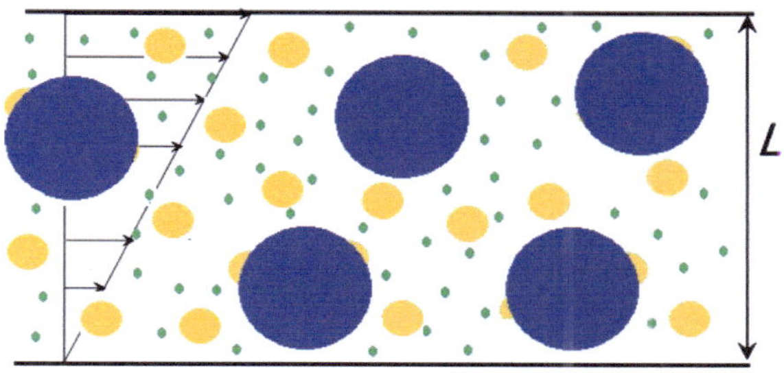

Fig. 5.8 Construction of the *differential scheme*: start with a dilute suspension of (green) spheres; then, in this effective Newtonian liquid another dilute suspension of much larger (yellow) spheres is created, raising the sphere volume fraction. This process is continued with another dilute suspension of yet much larger (blue) spheres until the desired volume fraction is reached

$$\eta + d\eta = \eta + \frac{5}{2}\frac{\Delta\phi}{1+\Delta\phi}\eta. \tag{5.24}$$

Now, as the real volume fraction increases by

$$d\phi = \frac{\phi + \Delta\phi}{1+\Delta\phi} - \phi = \frac{\Delta\phi}{1+\Delta\phi}(1-\phi), \tag{5.25}$$

we have the differential equation for the effective viscosity,[4]

$$\frac{d\eta}{d\phi} = \frac{5}{2}\frac{\eta}{1-\phi}, \qquad 0 < \phi < 1, \quad \eta(0) = \eta_s. \tag{5.26}$$

This has the solution

$$\frac{\eta}{\eta_s} = (1-\phi)^{-5/2}. \tag{5.27}$$

This has Einstein's result at the limit of low volume fraction. Relation (5.27) has been evaluated by Roscoe [17], and was found to work well at low volume fractions. At high volume fraction, he recommended replacing ϕ by 1.35ϕ, so that the maximum allowable volume fraction is $1.35^{-1} = 0.74$. The rational is that a certain amount of fluid is frozen in the gaps between the spheres at high volume fraction, causing the volume fraction to be higher that it actually is.

5.2.4.2 Differential Scheme for a Polydispersed Suspension of Droplets

We can repeat the same exercise as in Sect. 5.2.4.1 for a suspension of droplets (of viscosity η_1), with the help of (5.21), and in place of the differential equation (5.26),

[4] Hence, the name for the construction scheme.

we now have,

$$\frac{d\eta}{d\phi}=\frac{\eta+\frac{5}{2}\eta_1}{\eta+\eta_1}\frac{\eta}{1-\phi},\qquad 0<\phi<1,\quad \eta(0)=\eta_s. \tag{5.28}$$

This has the solution,

$$\left(\frac{2\eta_s+5\eta_1}{2\eta+5\eta_1}\right)^{3/5}\left(\frac{\eta_s}{\eta}\right)^{2/5}=1-\phi. \tag{5.29}$$

When the droplets are rigid, $\eta_1\to\infty$, relation (5.27) is recovered, and when the droplets are bubbles, corresponding to $\eta_1=0$,

$$\frac{\eta}{\eta_s}=\frac{1}{1-\phi}, \tag{5.30}$$

with the dilute limit (5.22), $\eta=(1+\phi)\eta_s$. The solution (5.29) allows for a maximum volume fraction of unity, when $\eta\to\infty$.[5] With limited polydispersity, the maximum volume fraction cannot approach unity, since there are interstitial spaces that cannot be filled with particles. This maximum allowable volume fraction less than unity can be incorporated into a differential model by considering a special three-component suspension, where one inclusion phase is actually made up from the solvent material (which does not contribute to the increase of the effective viscosity). Phan-Thien and Pham [16] explored this, and showed that, if the maximum allowable volume fraction is ϕ_m, then

$$\frac{\eta}{\eta_s}\sim(\phi_m-\phi)^{-5(5\phi_m-2)/6}. \tag{5.31}$$

With $\phi_m\sim 0.74$, corresponding to a FCC or HCP packing, this singular behavior is $(\phi_m-\phi)^{-1.4}$, less singular than the empirical Kieger's formula $(\phi_m-\phi)^{-1.8}$ for monodispersed suspension.

5.2.5 *Dilute Suspension of Spheroids*

We now turn our attention to a dilute suspension of rigid spheroids, orientable particles whose surfaces are described as in cylindrical coordinates $\{R,z\}$

$$\frac{r^2}{R_m^2}+\frac{z^2}{R_M^2}=1, \tag{5.32}$$

[5] This happens only when the sizes of included spheres vary from zero to infinity, which is not physically possible.

where R_m and R_M are the minor and major radii of a particle. The aspect ratio of the particle is denoted by a_R,

$$a_R = \frac{R_M}{R_m}. \tag{5.33}$$

The orientation of the particle is identified with a unit vector field $\mathbf{p}$ parallel to the major axis of the particle. The averages of this vector and its moments will provide information on the micromechanics of the particles and their contributions to the total stress.

To find the particle-contributed stress, we need the solution to the micromechanics Stokes flow problem past a spheroid. This solution has been provided by Jeffery [18] from which we learn that the orientation of the spheroid evolves according to

$$\dot{\mathbf{p}} = \mathbf{W} \cdot \mathbf{p} + \frac{a_R^2 - 1}{a_R^2 + 1} \left(\mathbf{D} \cdot \mathbf{p} - \mathbf{D} : \mathbf{ppp} \right). \tag{5.34}$$

This is known as *Jeffery's solution*. Now, if we define an *effective* velocity gradient as

$$\mathcal{L} = \mathbf{L} - \xi \mathbf{D}, \quad \xi = 1 - \frac{a_R^2 - 1}{a_R^2 + 1} = \frac{2}{a_R^2 + 1}, \tag{5.35}$$

then Jeffery's solution can be recast as

$$\dot{\mathbf{p}} = \mathcal{L}\mathbf{p} - \mathcal{L} : \mathbf{ppp}. \tag{5.36}$$

Subject to initial conditions, the solution of the non-linear problem (5.36) is also the solution to the linear problem:

$$\dot{\mathbf{Q}} = \mathcal{L}\mathbf{Q}, \qquad \mathbf{p} = \mathbf{Q}/Q. \tag{5.37}$$

5.2.5.1 Jeffery's Orbits

The components of $\mathbf{Q}$ in a simple shear flow, with shear rate in the 12-direction, are provided in Problem 5.4. With the magnitude of $\mathbf{Q}$ given by

$$Q^2 = \left(1 + a_R^2\right)\left(Q_{10}^2 + Q_{20}^2\right) + Q_{30}^2, \tag{5.38}$$

the vector $\mathbf{p}$,

$$\mathbf{p} = \left(Q_1, Q_2, Q_3\right)/Q, \tag{5.39}$$

traces out periodic paths, called *Jeffery's orbits* [18] (Fig. 5.9), with frequency,

$$\omega = \frac{1}{2}\sqrt{\xi\left(2 - \xi\right)\dot{\gamma}^2} = \frac{\dot{\gamma} a_R}{a_R^2 + 1}. \tag{5.40}$$

From Problem 5.4 we also learn that in $Q_1 Q_2$-plane, Jeffery's orbits trace out elliptical paths,

$$\frac{Q_1^2}{Q_{10}^2 + a_R^2 Q_{20}^2} + \frac{Q_2^2}{a_R^{-2} Q_{10}^2 + Q_{20}^2} = 1, \tag{5.41}$$

in which the ratio of the major to minor radii is

$$\frac{Q_{10}^2 + a_R^2 Q_{20}^2}{a_R^{-2} Q_{10}^2 + Q_{20}^2} = a_R^2. \tag{5.42}$$

Different orbits reflect different initial conditions—this is captured in the *orbital constant*,

$$C = \frac{\sqrt{a_R^2 p_2^2 + p_1^2}}{a_R p_3} = \frac{\sqrt{a_R^2 Q_2^2 + Q_1^2}}{a_R Q_3} = \frac{\sqrt{Q_{10}^2 + a_R^2 Q_{20}^2}}{a_R Q_{30}}. \tag{5.43}$$

5.2.5.2 Particle-Contributed Stress

Leal and Hinch [20] have calculated the particle-contributed stress for a dilute suspension of spheroids, *cf.* (5.4), from Jeffery solution, including the effects of Brownian forces, and we quote their results here,

$$\mathbf{S}^{(p)} = 2\eta_s \phi \{A\mathbf{D} : \langle \mathbf{pppp} \rangle + B\left(\mathbf{D} \cdot \langle \mathbf{pp} \rangle + \langle \mathbf{pp} \rangle \cdot \mathbf{D}\right) + C\mathbf{D} + d_R F \langle \mathbf{pp} \rangle\}, \tag{5.44}$$

where the angular brackets denote an average with respect to the probability distribution of $\mathbf{p}$. Without the effects of Brownian motions, we can leave out the angular brackets, and the evolution of the orientation vector is given by (5.37). In addition, the parameters called the *shape factors* A to F are functions of the aspect ratio, and d_R is the rotational diffusivity of the spheroids.

Expressions for the shape factors are complicated, but there are asymptotic values in the rod-like limit ($a_R \to \infty$), the near-sphere limit ($a_R = 1 + \delta,\ \delta \ll 1$), and the dish-like ($a_R \to 0$) limit are available, Leal and Hinch [20]; they are recorded in Table 5.1.

In a simple shear flow, the three reduced viscometric functions are recorded in Problem 5.5. In particular, the reduced viscosity is plotted in Fig. 5.10 for the limiting cases, rod-like, near-sphere, and dish-like.

The axi-symmetric elongational flow is considered in Problem 5.6, and the reduced elongational viscosity is given by

$$\frac{N_1 - 3\eta_s \dot{\gamma}}{\eta_s \dot{\gamma}} = 2\left(A + 2B + C\right)\phi \approx \frac{\phi a_R^2}{\ln 2a_R - 1.5}. \tag{5.45}$$

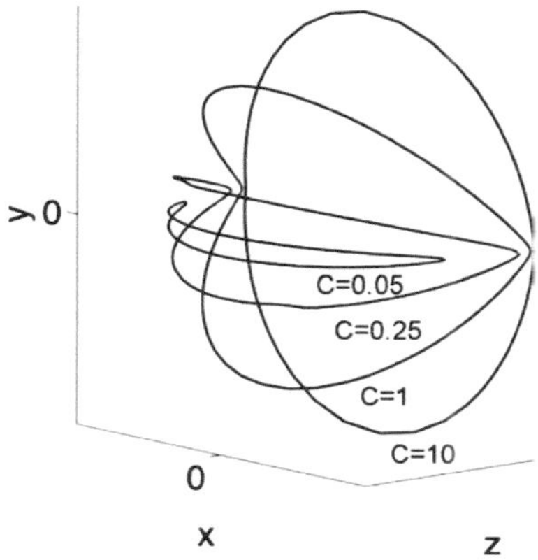

Fig. 5.9 Jeffery's orbits at different orbital constants. These orbits are traced out by vector **p**, or vector **Q**, with frequency given by (5.40). The label C on the curves denotes the orbital constant reflecting the initial conditions, *cf.* (5.43); smaller values of C indicate motions closer to the vorticity z-axis [19]

Table 5.1 Asymptotic values of the shape factors [20]

Asymptotic limit	$a_R \to \infty$ (rod-like)	$a_R = 1 + \delta,\ \delta \ll 1$ (near-sphere)	$a_R \to 0$ (disk-like)
A	$\dfrac{a_R^2}{2(\ln 2a_R - 1.5)}$	$\dfrac{395}{147}\delta^2$	$\dfrac{10}{3\pi a_R} + \dfrac{208}{9\pi^2} - 2$
B	$\dfrac{6\ln 2a_R - 11}{a_R^2}$	$\dfrac{15}{14}\delta - \dfrac{395}{588}\delta^2$	$-\dfrac{8}{3\pi a_R} + 1 - \dfrac{128}{9\pi^2}$
C	2	$\dfrac{5}{2}\left(1 - \dfrac{2}{7}\delta + \dfrac{1}{3}\delta^2\right)$	$\dfrac{8}{3\pi a_R}$
F	$\dfrac{3a_R^2}{\ln 2a_R - 1/2}$	9δ	$-\dfrac{12}{\pi a_R}$

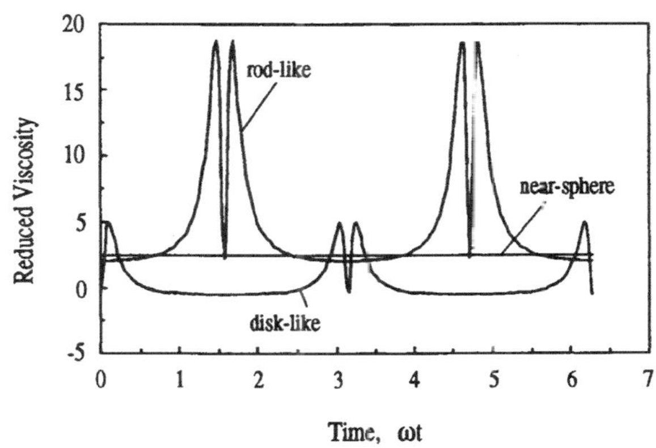

Fig. 5.10 The reduced viscosity (Problem 5.5) as a function of time. Here ω is the frequency of Jeffery's orbit, Eq. (5.40) for the three cases: rod-like ($a_R = 10$), near-sphere ($a_R = 1.1$) and dish-like ($a_R = 0.1$)

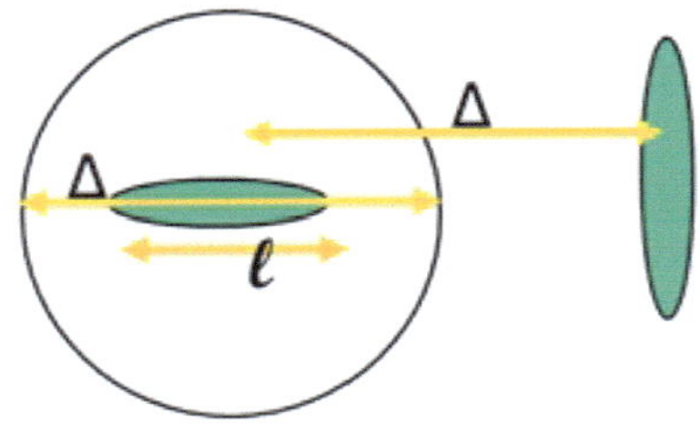

Fig. 5.11 I the semi-concentrated and concentrated volume fractions, a motion of any fiber necessarily involves a cooperative motion of neighboring fibers

Strictly speaking, the dilute assumption means that any particle can rotate freely without any hindrance from its nearby neighbors, see Fig. 5.11. The distance Δ between any two particles must therefore satisfy $l < \Delta$, so that a volume of l^3 contains only one particle, where l is the length of the particle and d is its diameter. The volume fraction therefore satisfies

$$\phi \sim \frac{d^2 l}{\Delta^3} = \frac{d^2}{l^2}\left(\frac{l}{\Delta}\right)^3 = \frac{1}{R^2}\left(\frac{l}{\Delta}\right)^3, \quad \phi R^2 < 1. \tag{5.46}$$

Thus, the reduced elongational viscosity is only $O(1)$ in the dilute limit, not $O(R^2)$ as suggested by the formula (5.45). As the concentration increases, we get subsequently into the semi-dilute regime, where $1 < \phi R^2 < R$, the isotropic concentrated solution, and the liquid crystalline solution. The reader is referred to Doi and Edwards [21] for more details. The suspension with $\phi R > 1$ is called concentrated, where the average distance between fibers is less than a fiber diameter, and therefore fibers cannot rotate independently except around their symmetry axes. Any motion of any fiber must necessarily involve a cooperative motion of surrounding fibers, see Doi and Edwards [21].

Problems

Problem 5.1 Show that the solution (5.12–5.13) is indeed the solution to the Stokes flow (5.3) for a sphere with boundary conditions (5.9–5.10).

Thus show that the force $\mathbf{F}$ and the torque $\mathbf{T}$ on the sphere are given by

$$\mathbf{F} = \int_S \mathbf{t} dS = -6\pi\eta_s a(\mathbf{V} - \mathbf{U}) \tag{5.47}$$

$$T_i = \varepsilon_{ijk}\int_S x_j t_k dS = -4\pi\eta_s a^3 \varepsilon_{ijk}\left(w_{kj} - W_{kj}\right). \tag{5.48}$$

Deduce that, for a force-free and torque-free sphere, it translates with the fluid velocity and spins with the vorticity vector, i.e., $\mathbf{U} = \mathbf{V}$ and $\mathbf{w} = \mathbf{W}$.

Problem 5.2 Verify that (5.27) and (5.29) are indeed solutions to (5.26) and (5.28), respectively.

Problem 5.3 Explore the multiphase suspension and verify relation (5.31). The reference [16] will be helpful here.

Problem 5.4 In a simple shear flow problem, show that the solution to (5.37) is

$$\begin{aligned} Q_1 &= Q_{10}\cos(\omega t) + a_R Q_{20}\sin(\omega t) = \sqrt{Q_{10}^2 + a_R^2 Q_{20}^2}\cos(\omega t - \phi) \\ Q_2 &= Q_{20}\cos(\omega t) + a_R^{-1} Q_{10}\sin(\omega t) = -\sqrt{a_R^{-2} Q_{10}^2 + Q_{20}^2}\sin(\omega t - \phi) \\ Q_3 &= Q_{30} \end{aligned} \tag{5.49}$$

where $\mathbf{Q}(0) = \{Q_{10}, Q_{20}, Q_{30}\}$,

$$\begin{aligned} \omega &= \sqrt{\frac{\xi}{2}\left(1 - \frac{\xi}{2}\right)\dot{\gamma}^2} = \frac{1}{2}\sqrt{\xi\,(2 - \xi)\,\dot{\gamma}^2}, \\ &= \frac{\dot{\gamma} R}{R^2 + 1}, \end{aligned} \tag{5.50}$$

with shear rate $\dot{\gamma}$, and

$$\tan\phi = \frac{a_R Q_{20}}{Q_{10}}. \tag{5.51}$$

Problem 5.5 In a simple shear flow of shear rate $\dot{\gamma}$, show that the reduced viscosity, the reduced first normal stress difference and the reduced second normal stress difference are given by

$$\frac{\langle\sigma_{12}\rangle - \eta_s\dot{\gamma}}{\eta_s\dot{\gamma}\phi} = 2Ap_1^2p_2^2 + B\left(p_1^2 + p_2^2\right) + C, \tag{5.52}$$

$$\frac{N_1}{\eta_s\dot{\gamma}\phi} = 2Ap_1p_2\left(p_1^2 - p_2^2\right), \tag{5.53}$$

$$\frac{N_2}{\eta_s\dot{\gamma}\phi} = 2p_1p_2\left(Ap_2^2 + B\right). \tag{5.54}$$

Problem 5.6 In the start-up of an elongational flow with a positive elongational rate $\dot{\gamma}$, show that

$$\begin{aligned} Q_1 &= Q_{10}\exp\{(1 - \zeta)\dot{\gamma}t\}, \\ Q_2 &= Q_{20}\exp\left\{-\frac{1}{2}(1 - \zeta)\dot{\gamma}t\right\}, \\ Q_3 &= Q_{30}\exp\left\{-\frac{1}{2}(1 - \zeta)\dot{\gamma}t\right\}, \end{aligned}$$

so that the particle is quickly aligned with the flow in a time scale $O(\dot{\gamma}^{-1})$. At a steady state, show that the reduced elongational viscosity is given by

$$\frac{N_1 - 3\eta_s\dot{\gamma}}{\eta_s\dot{\gamma}\phi} = 2A + 4B + 3C \approx \frac{a_R^2}{\ln 2a_R - 1.5}. \tag{5.55}$$

References

1. S. Kim, S.J. Karrila, *Microhydrodynamics: Principles and Selected Applications* (Dover, Unabridged Edition, New York, 2005)
2. M.D. Graham, *Microhydrodynamics, Brownian Motion, and Complex Fluids* (Cambridge University Press, Cambridge, 2018)
3. R.I. Tanner, *Engineering Rheology*, revised edition edn. (Oxford University Press, Oxford, 1992)
4. D.G. Thomas, Transport characteristics of suspension: VIII. A note on the viscosity of Newtonian suspensions of uniform spherical particles. J. Coll. Sci. **20**, 267–277 (1965)
5. I. Krieger, T. Dougherty, A mechanism for non-Newtonian flow in suspensions of rigid spheres. Trans. Soc. Rheol. **3**, 137–152 (1959)
6. A. Einstein, *Investigations on the Theory of the Brownian Movement*, ed. by R. Fürth, Trans. A.D. Cowper (Dover, New York, 1988)
7. T. Narumi, H. See, Y. Honma, T. Hasagawa, T. Takahashi, N. Phan-Thien, Transient response of concentrated suspensions after shear reversal. J. Rheol. **46**, 295–305 (2002)
8. F. Gadala-Maria, A. Acrivos, Shear-induced structure in a concentrated suspension of solid spheres. J. Rheol. **24**, 799–814 (1980)
9. F. Gadala-Maria, The rheology of concentrated suspensions. PhD thesis, Chemical Engineering, Stanford University (1979)
10. J. Happel, H. Brenner, *Low Reynolds Number Hydrodynamics* (Noordhoff International Publishing, Leyden, 1973)
11. Cédric, Geoffrey ingram Taylor: The visionary behind Taylor dispersion (2023). https://nanoscale-metrix.com/geoffrey-ingram-taylor-the-visionary/
12. G.I. Taylor, The viscosity of a fluid containing small drops of another fluid. Proc. Roy. Soc. A **138**, 41–48 (1932)
13. G.K. Batchelor, J.T. Green, The determination of the bulk stress in a suspension of spherical particles to order c^2. J. Fluid Mech. **56**, 401–427 (1972)
14. D.A.G. Bruggeman, Berechnung verschiedener physkilisher konstante von heterogene substazen. i. dielektrizitatskonstanten und leitfahigkeiten der mischkorper aus isotropen substanzen. Ann. Phys. **24**, 636–664 (1935)
15. G.I. Taylor, A differential scheme for the effective moduli of composites. Mech. Mat. **4**, 1–16 (1985)
16. N. Phan-Thien, D.C. Pham, Differential multiphase models for polydispersed suspensions and particulate solids. J. non-Newt. Fluid Mech. **72**, 305–318 (1997)
17. R. Roscoe, The viscosity of suspensions of rigid spheres. Br. J. Appl. Phys. **3**, 267–269 (1952)
18. G.B. Jeffery, The motion of ellipsoidal particles immersed in a viscous fluid. Proc. Roy. Soc. A **102**, 161–179 (1922)
19. A. Carlsson, F. Lundell, L.D. Söderberg, Fiber orientation control related to papermaking. J. Fluids Eng. **129**(4), 457–465 (2006)
20. L.G. Leal, E.J. Hinch, Theoretical studies of a suspension of rigid particles affected by Brownian couples. Rheol. Acta **12**, 127–132 (1973)
21. M. Doi, S.F. Edwards, *The Theory of Polymer Dynamics* (Oxford University Press, Oxford, 1988)

Chapter 6
Epilog

"A Journey of a Thousand Li Begins with a Single Step", Lao Tzu

Microstructured suspensions come in many forms of different complexity, often at high concentrations where the motion of one component involves the cooperative motions of near-by (and possibly far-field) particles. Their modeling is truly a challenge. We end this short course with an epilog, repeating the steps that we have used in Chaps. 4–5, and cite some examples (Fig. 6.1).

1. The first step is to single out the common "element" in the suspension—it may be a sphere, or a pair of spheres, or a strand, or a fiber—and model its motion (kinematics). In this modeling, try to incorporate simple kinematics only capturing the essential physics of the situation. The detailed kinematic information may not be necessary at this point.
2. Calculate the stress tensor as seen from the macroscale. This is invariably a volume average, or, if Brownian motion involved, an ensemble average.
3. Attempt to derive the constitutive equation. Closure assumptions may be needed for a close-form constitutive equation.
4. Apply the constitutive equation to some basic flows, and validate the constitutive equation. If necessary, go back to step 1, with more refined assumptions in the kinematics, but remember, simplicity often is the best.

We now cite a couple of examples, network theory for a concentrated polymer solution and a concentrated monodispersed rigid-sphere suspension.

6.1 Network Theory

This section is patterned after Lodge [2], Phan-Thien and Tanner [3]. Here, a concentrated polymer solution is modeled by entangled polymer strands (Fig. 6.2), each strand, consisting several monomer units, is a Gaussian chain, Sect. 4.1.3, with entropic force $\mathbf{F}^{(c)}$ between the two temporary junctions Eq. (4.15).

© The Author(s), under exclusive license to Springer Nature Singapore Pte Ltd. 2026
D. Pan et al., *Langevin Analysis of Microstructured Fluids*,
SpringerBriefs in Applied Sciences and Technology,
https://doi.org/10.1007/978-981-95-2318-4_6

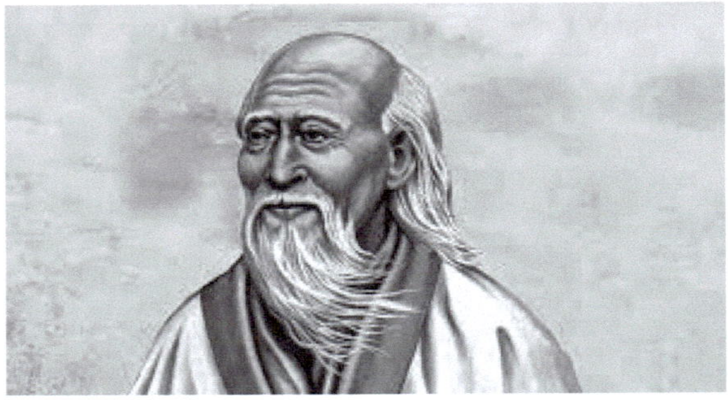

Fig. 6.1 Lao Tzu (*ci.* 571 BC), a semi-legendary Chinese Philosopher, one of his famous saying is "a journey of a thousand li begins with a single step". Another quote attributed to him, very relevant to this course is "knowledge is a treasure, but practice is the key to it". (Photograph provided in [1])

In this case, the polymer stress is, *cf.* (4.27),

$$\mathbf{S}^{(p)} = \int \mathbf{F}^{(c)}\mathbf{R}\phi(\mathbf{R}, t)\, d\mathbf{R} = \frac{3kT}{Na^2}\int \mathbf{R}\mathbf{R}\phi(\mathbf{R}, t)\, d\mathbf{R}$$
$$= \frac{3kT}{Nb^2}\langle \mathbf{R}\mathbf{R}\rangle = H\langle \mathbf{R}\mathbf{R}\rangle, \tag{6.1}$$

where $H = 3kT/Nb^2$ is the entropic spring stiffness, with (uniform) N units and Kuhn length b in the strand, and $\phi(\mathbf{R}, t)$ is the probability density function for the process $\mathbf{R}$.

Now to solve for the motion of $\mathbf{R}$ may be physically challenging, since its motion is cooperative, de Gennes [4], Doi and Edwards [5]. A useful engineering assumption that leads to the *Phan–Thien–Tanner* model is

$$\dot{\mathbf{R}} = \mathbf{L}\mathbf{R} - \xi\mathbf{D}\mathbf{R} = \boldsymbol{L}\mathbf{R}, \quad \boldsymbol{L} = \mathbf{L} - \xi\mathbf{D}, \tag{6.2}$$

where ξ is a parameter reflecting the inefficiency of stretching in a straining motion of the strand. This motion for $\mathbf{R}$ is called *non-affine* motion assumption.

The stochastic process in $\mathbf{R}$ is assumed to be a birth-death process, with the rate of creation of network strands to be isotropic $g(\mathbf{R})$, and the rate of destruction of strands to be proportional to the network density, $-h\phi$, where h is a coefficient. Thus

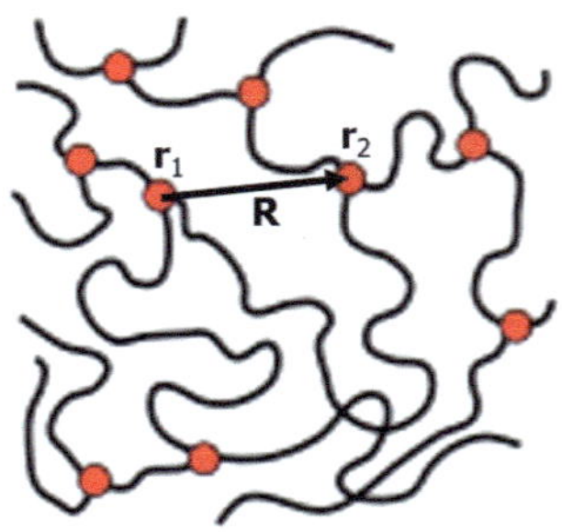

Fig. 6.2 In the network model for concentrated polymer melts and solutions, a polymer strand between two temporary entangled points $\mathbf{r}_1$ and $\mathbf{r}_2$ is denoted by $\mathbf{R}$

$$\frac{d\phi}{dt} = \frac{\partial\phi}{\partial t} + \mathbf{u}\cdot\frac{\partial\phi}{\partial\mathbf{x}} + \dot{\mathbf{R}}\cdot\frac{\partial\phi}{\partial\mathbf{R}} = g - h\phi. \tag{6.3}$$

Next, from the stress (6.1) and the assumed non-affine motion (6.2),

$$\begin{aligned}\frac{d}{dt}\mathbf{S}^{(p)} &= H\int_{\mathbf{R}_0}\left[\left(\dot{\mathbf{R}}\mathbf{R} + \mathbf{R}\dot{\mathbf{R}}\right)\phi\left(\mathbf{R}, t\right)J + \mathbf{R}\mathbf{R}\frac{d\phi}{dt}J + \mathbf{R}\mathbf{R}\phi\frac{dJ}{dt}\right]d\mathbf{R}_0\\ &= \mathcal{L}\mathbf{S}^{(p)} + \mathbf{S}^{(p)}\mathcal{L}^T + H\int_{\mathbf{R}}\mathbf{R}\mathbf{R}\left(g - h\phi\right)d\mathbf{R},\end{aligned} \tag{6.4}$$

where we have converted the integral into that on a reference configuration, with the use of the Jacobian of transformation,

$$J = \det\left(\frac{\partial\mathbf{R}}{\partial\mathbf{R}_0}\right), \qquad \frac{dJ}{dt} = J\mathrm{tr}\left(\frac{\partial\dot{\mathbf{R}}}{\partial\mathbf{R}}\right) = 0. \tag{6.5}$$

Note that the derivative of J can be found from Sect. 1.8.1 of [6]. Finally, the configuration integral of $\mathbf{RR}$ over g returns an isotropic tensor,

$$H\int_{\mathbf{R}}\mathbf{R}\mathbf{R}g\,d\mathbf{R} = G\mathbf{I}, \tag{6.6}$$

and the following constitutive equation results,

$$\frac{d}{dt}\mathbf{S}^{(p)} - \mathcal{L}\mathbf{S}^{(p)} - \mathbf{S}^{(p)}\mathcal{L}^T + h\mathbf{S}^{(p)} = G\mathbf{I} \tag{6.7}$$

This constitutive equation, known as *Phan-Thien-Tanner* model has been extensively used in software, and still is very popular in polymer engineering community, see Huilgol and Phan-Thien [7]. There are variants of the model [8], including a more recent *generalized Phan-Thien-Tanner* model by Ferrás et al. [9]. There are other kinematics for the motion of $\mathbf{R}$ as well, for example, reptation concepts due to de Gennes [4], tube and chain model of Doi and Edwards [5] to which the readers are referred.

6.2 Concentrated Suspensions

There are models that can explore the high volume fraction regimes; the most rigorous and complete studies are for periodic arrays of spheres in Stokes flows, Sangani and Acrivos [10], Zick and Homsy [11]. There are other models making use of the transfer of forces between two near-touching generic spheres, Goddard [12], Phan-Thien [13], Phan-Thien et al. [14], and we briefly describe the latter here.

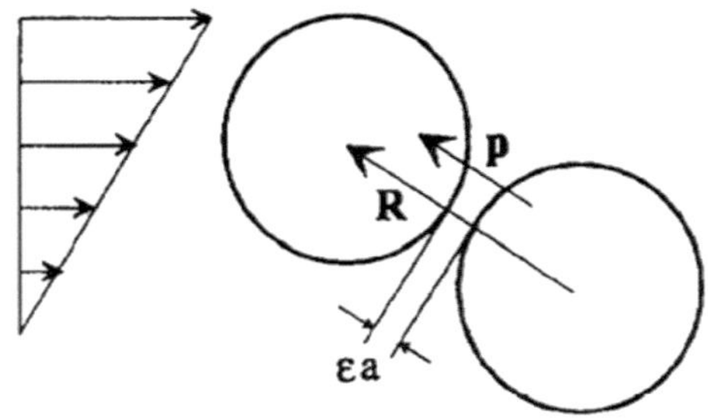

Fig. 6.3 A generic sphere and its near-touching neighbor in an average motion

Figure 6.3 depicts a generic sphere with its near-touching neighbor, both of radius a and the gap between the two is ϵa, where ϵ is a small parameter. The stresslet on the generic sphere is, *cf.* (5.5),

$$\mathcal{S}^{(p)} = \frac{1}{2}\int_{S_p} (\mathbf{xt} + \mathbf{tx}) dS = \frac{1}{2} a \langle \mathbf{pF} + \mathbf{Fp} \rangle, \tag{6.8}$$

where the load transfer between the two spheres occurs mainly at the near contact region where $\mathbf{x} = a\mathbf{p}$, with $\mathbf{p}$ is the unit vector along the line of centers. The remaining integral over the sphere surface S_p of the traction can be approximated by the lubrication force between the two spheres; it consists of a shearing force,

$$\mathbf{F}_{sh} \approx \pi \eta_s a \mathbf{U}_{sh} \ln \epsilon^{-1} = f_{sh} \mathbf{U}_{sh}, \tag{6.9}$$

a squeezing force,

$$\mathbf{F}_{sq} \approx \frac{3}{2} \pi \eta_s a \mathbf{U}_{sh} \epsilon^{-1} = f_{sh} \mathbf{U}_{sh}, \tag{6.10}$$

and a force due to spheres' rotation, of the same order of magnitude as the shearing force—see Kim and Karrila [15] for the asymptotic results on shearing, squeezing and rotation forces.

The particle-contributed stress is, keeping only the leading terms in ϵ (the squeezing force)

$$\mathbf{S}^{(p)} = a n f_{sq} \langle \mathbf{p} \mathbf{U}_{sq} \rangle. \tag{6.11}$$

The front factor on the right side of (6.11) is a function of the volume fraction ϕ, by treating ϵ as a function of ϕ; in fact it may be regarded as a fitting function of the volume fraction. We shall omit the angular brackets, since there is no fluctuation in $\mathbf{p}$.

Next, the relative motion of the two spheres has been shown to be [15],

$$\begin{aligned} \dot{\mathbf{R}} &= \boldsymbol{L} \cdot \mathbf{R} - (\xi - \zeta) \mathbf{D} : \mathbf{ppR}, \\ &= \boldsymbol{L} \cdot \mathbf{R} - \boldsymbol{L} : \mathbf{ppR}, \end{aligned} \tag{6.12}$$

where $\mathbf{R}$ is the center-to-center vector ($R/a \sim 2$), $\boldsymbol{L} = \mathbf{L} - \zeta\mathbf{D}$ is the effective velocity gradient, $\mathbf{D}$ is the strain rate tensor, and

$$\zeta = \frac{16}{3}\left(\frac{a}{R}\right)^5 - \frac{25}{3}\left(\frac{a}{R}\right)^8 + O\left(\frac{a}{R}\right)^{10}, \tag{6.13}$$

$$\xi = 5\left(\frac{a}{R}\right)^3 - 8\left(\frac{a}{R}\right)^5 + 25\left(\frac{a}{R}\right)^6 - 35\left(\frac{a}{R}\right)^8 + O\left(\frac{a}{R}\right). \tag{6.14}$$

From the $\mathbf{R}$ motion (6.12), we find

$$\dot{R} = R(1-\xi)\mathbf{D} : \mathbf{pp}, \tag{6.15}$$

The squeezing velocity is $\mathbf{U}_{sq} = \dot{R}\mathbf{p}$, and thus the squeezing force is

$$\mathbf{F}_{sq} = f_{sq}R(1-\xi)\mathbf{D} : \mathbf{ppp}, \tag{6.16}$$

leading to the particle-contributed stress

$$\mathbf{S}^{(p)} = \mu(\phi)\mathbf{D} : \mathbf{pppp}. \tag{6.17}$$

This, combined with (6.12) is our constitutive relation. To take into account fluctuations due to spheres interactions in the $\mathbf{R}$-motion, we may consider injecting random noise into Eq. (6.12); this is treated as an exercise, refer to Phan-Thien et al. [14] for guidance and predictions in simple flow problems (closure assumptions are required to obtain a close-form constitutive equation).

In this short course, we have gone a long way toward understanding and appreciation of Langevin techniques in the analysis and modeling of microstructured suspensions. We sincerely hope that the techniques will be useful for your research career and that you enjoyed the course, and re-emphasize the need of doing problems by a quotation from Lao Tzu "knowledge is a treasure, but practice is the key to it".

References

1. T. Dean, Big thinkers: Laozi and zhuangzi (2019). https://ethics.org.au/big-thinkers-laozi-and-zhuangzi/
2. A.S. Lodge, *Elastic Liquids* (Academic Press, New York, 1964)
3. N. Phan-Thien, R.I. Tanner, A new constitutive equation derived from network theory. J. Non-Newt. Fluid Mech. **2**, 353–365 (1977)
4. P.G. de Gennes, *Scaling Concepts in Polymer Physics* (Springer International Publishing AG, New York, 1979)
5. M. Doi, S.F. Edwards, *The Theory of Polymer Dynamics* (Oxford University Press, Oxford, 1988)
6. N. Phan-Thien, N. Mai-Duy, *Understanding Viscoelasticity: An Introduction to Rheology*, 3rd edn. (Springer International Publishing AG, Berlin, 2017)

7. R. Huilgol, N. Phan-Thien, *Fluid Mechanics of Viscoelasticity: General Principles, Constitutive Modelling, Analytical and Numerical Techniques* (Elsevier, Amsterdam, 1997)
8. N. Phan-Thien, A nonlinear network viscoelastic model. J. Rheol. **22**, 259–283 (1978)
9. L.L. Ferrás, M.L. Morgado, M. Rebelo, G.H. McKinley, A.M. Afonso, A generalised Phan–Thien-Tanner model. J. Non-Newt. Fluid Mech. **269**, 88–99 (2019)
10. A.S. Sangani, A. Acrivos, Slow flow through a periodic array of spheres. Int. J. Multiphase Flows **8**, 343–360 (1982)
11. A.A. Zick, G.M. Homsy, Stokes flow through periodic arrays of spheres. J. Fluid Mech. **115**, 13–26 (1982)
12. J.D. Goddard, An elastohydrodynamic theory for the rheology of concentrated suspensions of deformable particles. J. Non-Newt. Fluid Mech. **2**, 169–189 (1977)
13. N. Phan-Thien, Constitutive equation for concentrated suspensions in Newtonian fluids. J. Rheol. **39**, 679–695 (1995)
14. N. Phan-Thien, X.J. Fan, B.C. Khoo, A new constitutive model for monodispersed suspensions of spheres at high concentrations. Rheol. Acta **38**, 297–304 (1999)
15. S. Kim, S.J. Karrila, *Microhydrodynamics: Principles and Selected Applications* (Dover, Unabridged Edition, New York, 2005)

Index

© The Editor(s) (if applicable) and The Author(s), under exclusive license to Springer Nature Singapore Pte Ltd. 2026

D. Pan et al., *Langevin Analysis of Microstructured Fluids*,
SpringerBriefs in Applied Sciences and Technology,
https://doi.org/10.1007/978-981-95-2318-4

MIX
Papier aus verantwortungsvollen Quellen
Paper from responsible sources
FSC® C105338

If you have any concerns about our products,
you can contact us on
ProductSafety@springernature.com

In case Publisher is established outside the EU,
the EU authorized representative is:
Springer Nature Customer Service Center GmbH
Europaplatz 3, 69115 Heidelberg, Germany

Printed by Libri Plureos GmbH
in Hamburg, Germany